Joseph James Kinyoun

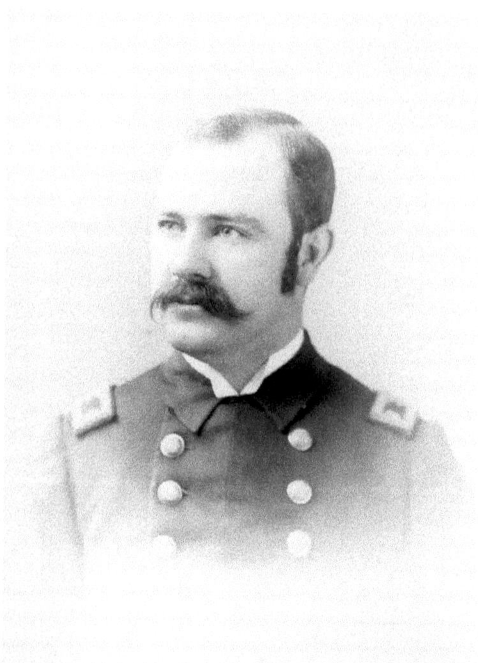

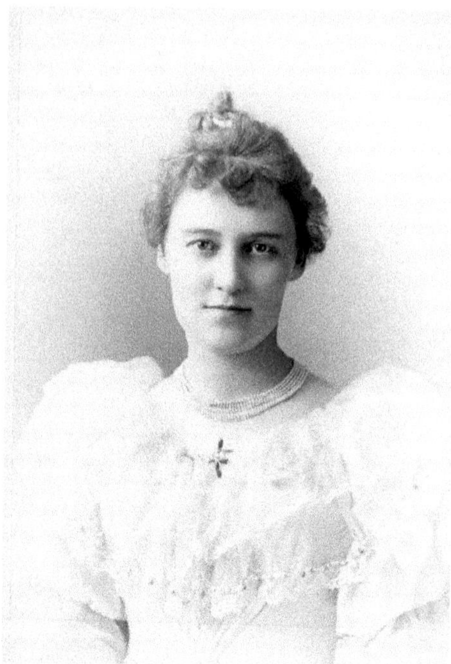

Dr. Joseph J. Kinyoun, assistant surgeon, U.S. Marine Hospital Service, Staten Island, 1887, and Elizabeth Perry Kinyoun, his wife, in presidential reception dress, Washington, D.C., 1887.

Joseph James Kinyoun

Discoverer of Bubonic Plague in America and Father of the National Institutes of Health

JOSEPH K. HOUTS, JR.

Foreword by David M. Morens, M.D.

McFarland & Company, Inc., Publishers
Jefferson, North Carolina

ISBN (print) 978-1-4766-8290-7
ISBN (ebook) 978-1-4766-4373-1

Library of Congress and British Library
cataloguing data are available

Library of Congress Control Number 2021044597

Front cover image: *inset* Dr. Joseph J. Kinyoun, assistant surgeon, U.S. Marine Hospital Service, Staten Island, 1887; UMHS Quarantine scuttle *Gen Stenberg*, bearing quarantine flag on bow and United States flag on stern, San Francisco Bay, 1890 (author collection)

Printed in the United States of America

McFarland & Company, Inc., Publishers
Box 611, Jefferson, North Carolina 28640
www.mcfarlandpub.com

To my loving family:
wife Noreen, son Joe III, daughter-in-law Kristin,
daughter Katie, son-in-law Brandon
and my four wonderful grandchildren,
Charles Kinyoun Houts, Mara Collins, Mary Cate
and Marin Claire Lorenz.

They are truly the greatest thing
to have ever happened in my life.

Love,
Dad

Acknowledgments

First and foremost, I want to acknowledge and thank my family for all their patience and support during the process of writing this book. Second, I thank the following people at the National Institutes of Health: Dr. David M. Morens, Senior Advisor, National Institute of Allergy and Infectious Disease; Barbara Faye Harkins, retired Chief Historian; Victoria Harden; Dr. Paul Theerman, former Head of Images and Archives, History of Medicine Division, National Library of Medicine; Intern Eva Ahrens; and, lastly, Dr. Anthony Fauci, Director, National Institute of Allergy and Infectious Diseases. These individuals from the National Institutes of Health, especially Dr. Morens, have been invaluable to my completion of this book.

And as always, I owe gratitude to my longtime mentor, Dr. William E. Parrish, retired from Westminster College and Mississippi State University. He has been of paramount help not only in his editing, but his ongoing encouragement to complete this manuscript and my other historical publications.

As a final note, I want to thank my great-grandmother Lizzie Kinyoun and my grandmother Alice (Allie) Eccles Kinyoun Houts. Between these ladies, they preserved and documented the family's rich history and provided safekeeping to those papers documenting its past. Without this archive, all my publications would have been lost to the ages. I am eternally indebted to them for their foresight in conserving and passing these papers on to me. My grandmother Allie was the family historian, and she alone instilled in me the love of not only history, but also our family's role in the making of America.

Table of Contents

Foreword

BY DAVID M. MORENS, MD

His life spanned the Civil War, the Spanish-American War, and the First World War. The young son of a North Carolinian soldier in the first of these, he served in uniform in the second. An unabashed patriot, as an old man dying of cancer he pulled strings to serve yet again in the last, the hoped-for War to End All Wars. He lived just long enough to see the 1918 armistice, dying on Valentine's Day 1919. By then, he had been almost completely forgotten. Carved on a marble memorial to the District of Columbia's war dead, his name has remained unnoticed for more than a century, as millions of citizens passed unaware through the city's grand Municipal Center, a stone's throw from the White House.

Yet Joseph James Kinyoun (1860–1919) was among the most important Americans of any century, his legacy touching the lives of every American today: he founded the Hygienic Laboratory, which became the U.S. National Institutes of Health; founded the biologics program that became the Food and Drug Administration; brought life-saving drugs, serums and vaccines to America from the European laboratories of Robert Koch and Louis Pasteur, and then taught the nation's doctors how to use them. When necessary, he did so at his own personal expense. He co-founded major medical professional societies, and led his country into a new era of medicine that has prolonged American life expectancy by almost 40 years.

That Kinyoun was forgotten is not a historical accident, but the tragic outcome of high-stakes political backstabbing. Investigating the infamous 1900 San Francisco "Chinatown" bubonic plague epidemic, Kinyoun was the first in the United States to diagnose the deadly disease, precipitating a bitter "states' rights" fight between the federal government, which wanted to step in and control the epidemic, and California's governor, who wanted to keep the feds out. The political face-off descended into madness when the governor accused Kinyoun of being a bioterrorist who had started the epidemic by inoculating the bacterium into dead bodies. Kinyoun and his colleagues eventually ended the epidemic. But Kinyoun had become a pawn on a vicious political chessboard. A federal-state compromise, brokered in the White House, exonerated Kinyoun of bioterrorism but pushed him into disgrace and retirement. Mourned as a hero by scientists of an earlier era, Kinyoun's 1919 death went unnoticed by the war-weary public, and has remained so.

Now, more than a century later, the remarkable story of the life of Joe Kinyoun is finally told by great-grandson Joseph Kinyoun Houts, Jr. After Kinyoun's 1919 death, all of his papers, documents, and many artifacts, memorabilia, and other objects had been carefully boxed up by Kinyoun's eldest daughter; many of these are now unearthed by Mr. Houts and assembled into this important biography. The result is a remarkable chronicle that reads like a Hollywood tale of "triumph and tragedy." (In fact, the Kinyoun family had, in the early days of cinema, actually refused to authorize a proposed film biography.) Houts' book is the story not only of a forgotten hero, but of the growth and development of American biomedical science through the Gilded Age, into the age of progressive optimism, and beyond. Kinyoun's achievements and struggles, his powerful love of country, his grounding in religion and family, his modesty, his lasting optimism, and his sorrowful exile from the scientific establishments he had helped build will surely resonate with modern readers who seek to find and restore a better America. This unexpected biography of a completely forgotten American hero opens a window on an important period in our history, and on the personal and intimate life of one who helped to shape it. It is rare, but immensely rewarding, to discover unknown heroes who have changed our world.

David M. Morens, MD, is an infectious disease scientist at the National Institute of Allergy and Infectious Diseases, National Institutes of Health (NIH), in Bethesda, Maryland. The NIH, the world's foremost medical research organization, was founded in 1887 by Dr. Joseph J. Kinyoun.

Introduction

The purpose of this introduction is to provide the reader with a general understanding of bubonic plague and an overview of its history. The story yet to unfold tells the saga of how it came to the United States and, more importantly, its reception on arriving in this part of the New World. At the time of its arrival, modern medicine had started its evolution. However, old ways and habits have always been hard to change, especially when it comes to science. Nothing could be truer than when these Old World discoveries came to America.

As part of this new thinking, the country had sent some of its brightest doctors to study under the best and brightest of their counterparts in Europe. Within this new breed of American physicians was Dr. Joseph J. Kinyoun, an assistant surgeon with the Marine Hospital Service. While abroad, he studied under Pasteur and Koch.[1] Because of this experience, he brought back new medical perspectives and treatments for the country. Nonetheless, in 1899, after Kinyoun assumed the role of federal quarantine officer for the port of San Francisco,[2] his credentials were severally called into question. These queries stemmed from the potent and unwavering self-interests of the political, commercial, social, economic and media giants of not only the city, but California as well. And unfortunately for all the parties concerned, bubonic plague made the United States its permanent new home.

American medicine at the turn of the 20th century could be described as a profession in transition. The old ways were being replaced with newer techniques and theories from Europe, but the process proceeded slowly. As a side note, in 1898, the United States had just defeated Spain in the Spanish-American War and now stood before the world as a military and to some degree an imperial power.

The country had pretty much been settled, which led it to look outward, not only militarily, but, more importantly, commercially. Its industrial base had grown significantly, leading it to engage and trade in the world's vast expanding markets. With its new acquisitions in the Pacific, a new commercialism developed, especially for the West Coast's three major harbors: Los Angeles; Seattle; and San Francisco, the largest port.

The only way for the country to reach these markets was the sea, by either sailing to or accepting ships from other nations into its ports and harbors. As merchant ships came and went, so did the plague microorganism imbedded in the bellies of fleas riding upon the fur and skin of rats. This can be seen in the Third Pandemic, which started in China, moving from Canton to Hong Kong and then to India before moving onward to other lands.[3]

The terror and horror of the plague had not gripped the world to such a degree since the Great Plague of London. Yes, periodic episodes of the disease did reoccur, and it slowly traveled around the world. However, not until the Third Pandemic did its presence reappear with the same onslaught of suffering, despair and death as in the early great epidemics. Only a matter of time remained, though, before it would disembark upon some American shore.

More importantly, the world could be said to be shrinking in the late 19th century because of expanded trade and new commercial ties, even though transportation could still be considered rudimentary. The steamship, the railroad, and the intercontinental oceanic telegraph and telephone lines were drawing nations closer together—for better or for worse. This opened up a whole new age of discovery and exploration on an entirely different level with resulting new perspectives for the world.

The problem with the Third Pandemic lay in its duration. Originating in 1855, the disease continued to wreak havoc across the planet, especially in the Far East, and by 1899 it had reached Honolulu in the Hawaiian Islands. Symbolically, the plague had now landed on an American shoreline, waiting to take the next step to the country's mainland.[4]

As a final note, Paul-Louis Simond's discovery had illuminated the transmission of the disease, how the organism spread and infected humans. In relation to the premise of this book, only one year separated his finding and the first suspected case of plague entering the harbor in San Francisco aboard the ship *Nippon Maru* from Hong Kong on June 27, 1899. Within days of its arrival Dr. Kinyoun quarantined the vessel and the first rumblings of a subsequent uproar started surfacing.[5]

Because of the scant time—one year—between these two events, it may be little wonder why the doctor encountered opposition to his detection of plague. It was unlikely that Simond's rat-flea connection had yet become widely known, or accepted, by the scientific community. News still traveled rather slowly in the late 19th and early 20th century. Furthermore, even though one scientist may have determined the rat-flea link, it still meant others in the profession would conduct their own investigations. Such a process, and a parallel outcome, could take years to substantiate. As a result, Kinyoun stood alone for the most part in trying to convince not only the public but also his peers of the medical truth in his discovering the plague in San Francisco.

Understanding Plague

Before one can understand the true meaning and impact of this story concerning the career of Dr. Joseph James Kinyoun, the reader must have some knowledge about *plague*. Probably, few other words in all the world's dialects have instilled more fear and anguish than this one. The term has gone by many names with each evoking equal shudders of horror, hopelessness and impending doom. Other common references include *pestilence*, *epidemic*, *wrath of God*, *pandemic* and the ever-ominous

Black Death: words and phrases uttered since time began, by ancient civilizations to the present, all meaning most certain death.

As notorious as the term has become, it also bears a certain degree of ambiguity. Throughout history, it has often been used to describe a whole host of other horrible and deadly diseases, lethal contagions not in fact the plague. Common examples of mistaken identity have included smallpox, measles, diphtheria, cholera and typhus. The reason for these possible misidentifications stemmed from a lack of medical understanding and classification as to a particular disease's appearance, symptoms and effect on the victim. The ancients in many cases believed all such mass, deadly infestations to be a plague of some unknown type.

Besides these early misconceptions, it must be understood that the disease has at least eight variants, if not more, meaning that the term encompasses more than one manifestation. In truth, probably only one genre actually exists, per se, but because of the types, degrees, or distinctions in the infection, it almost possesses chameleon-like characteristics, as so noted by the leading medical scientists. Other diseases have the ability to advance in severity. And although plague contains this same component, the changes in its demeanor might better be classified as stages, as opposed to a separate disease.

Yersinia pestis

From a scientific standpoint, the plague bacterium first became isolated in 1894, almost simultaneously, by two bacteriologists, while studying it in Hong Kong during the Third Pandemic. These men were Alexandre Yersin from Switzerland and Shibasaburō Kitasato from Japan. Yersin would be credited with its discovery, as opposed to Kitasato, because the latter's findings had fallen into some dispute. In honor of the leading 19th-century bacteriologist Louis Pasteur and his institute, Yersin named the organism *Pasteurella pestis*. He, like other scientists and doctors of the time, had studied with Pasteur.[6] However, in 1967, the scientific community reclassified the organism and changed its name to *Yersinia pestis*, or *Y. pestis*, as commonly abbreviated, in honor of its discoverer.[7]

Many may wonder what the terms *bacterium* and *pestis* mean in simple English. Bacterium is singular for *bacteria* coming from the New Latin derivative of the Greek word *bakterion* and diminutive of the noun *baktron* meaning a staff. In English, it means "a large, widely distributed group of typically one-celled microorganisms … chiefly, parasitic or saprophytic … disease-producing."[8] The actual plague bacterium is rod-shaped, like a staff in appearance, which may explain its link to this definition. *Pestis*, on the other hand, derives from the Latin word of the same spelling and is defined as an infectious disease, plague, pest, pestilence, or death.[9] When the words are combined a new connotation comes forth: a singular microorganism capable of transmitting and inflicting great bodily harm, or even death, upon its infected victim. Accordingly, plague represents a living microorganism, which can spread to other living organisms with resultant sickness and death.

Carrying the definition further, one must understand the composure, or intrinsic nature, of a microorganism. The word means smallness in size, whereby it cannot be seen with the naked eye.[10] Only through the use of a special lens, or microscope, can the living cell be clearly seen and identified. Furthermore, a bacterium microorganism can have several dispositions, notably either parasitic or saprophytic.[11] The former describes an organism that lives and feeds internally, externally, or at the sacrifice of the host, while the latter describes an organism living on a dead or decayed host.[12] Here the host is the other organism the bacterium has chosen to invade or prey upon.[13]

Fleas and Rats

Plague needs a host in order to survive and replicate itself. The disease can be spread by numerous methods and transports. In 1898, Paul-Louis Simond, a French scientist who had also been working in Hong Kong at the same time as Yersin and Kitasato, discovered the connection between rats and fleas as being the spreading agents. He documented through experimentation how a healthy rat would die after being bitten by a flea from a dead plague-infected rat. With rats having a common presence with humans throughout the ages, his findings were eventually accepted by others because of this interrelationship.[14] By this breakthrough, a connecting path arose establishing plague as being "transmitted from animal to animal and from animal to human by bites from infected fleas."[15]

The transmission factor operates when the rod-shaped bacterium lodges in the flea's intestines and gorges on its blood. With the flea already infected, it in turn infects the rat. Other fleas partaking of the same rat will then become infected, and, while still alive, move to other rats, repeating the cycle. Even with this scenario, there has been further speculation that the rat carries the bacterium and infects the flea. In either case, the flea is the transferring agent because it migrates from animal to animal. After it becomes infected, the rat, too, can operate as a moving agent by ferrying the infected flea to other hosts. Once a rat is infected, its bite can also become the means by which the disease is spread to other rodents and animals, including humans.[16]

Concerning the rat, one particular species, known as the black rat, stands out as the primary culprit in the disease's spread. This creature originally came from India and has also been referred to as a "weed species," meaning it can survive in a feral environment. Of special note, the black rat lives around humans. This rodent has been credited with being the chief flea agent carrying the bubonic plague. Its migration to the rest of world probably started in the 5th century AD as it snuck aboard ships or other modes of transportation during this period. The animal's passage can be attributed to its agile physical abilities; it could climb the ropes at ship moorings or hide in containers, thereby gaining passage to other lands. On disembarking, it intermixes with other rats and rodents, which become infected with the bacterium creating a focus, or starting point for the disease and its eventual proliferation.[17]

Besides the flea and rat connection, subsequent research has also determined that periodic plague outbreaks occur among rodent populations, which gives the disease additional origins. Once it gains a new frontier, it is said to become endemic, meaning the bacterium will permanently remain in an area and subsequent outbreaks will crop up going forward.[18] As previously stated, when this happens, infected fleas leave the dead host and seek a living one, infecting a new victim. If the outbreak becomes severe, then the likelihood of it infecting humans increases because the fleas must expand their feeding territory in order to survive. This cycle can continue unabated, until such time as both the carrier and host die, thereby ending the process.[19]

If the cycle becomes accelerated, then an epidemic can occur, decimating thousands, or worse, a pandemic. An epidemic involves a rapidly spreading disease[20]; a pandemic is an epidemic affecting a large group of individuals over a sizable geographical area.[21] In the Middle Ages, plague epidemics would evolve into pandemics within a relatively short period of time. Today, the likelihood of a plague epidemic and pandemic is low, except possibly in third-world countries where technology and sanitation may lag behind present-day knowledge. With the advent of modern medicine and the development of proven plague antibiotics in 1943, victims receiving an early diagnosis and treatment will most likely survive, thereby limiting its further transmission.[22]

In ancient times, effective medication to treat plague victims did not exist. In addition, public hygiene and sanitation were primitive, leading to fertile breeding grounds for rats as disease carrying hosts. Not until the rat population decreased through modern sanitation and extermination techniques, along with the discovery of curative drugs, would plague epidemics become a less frequent occurrence.[23]

Besides rats, other mammals have been known to be carriers. In all, more than 200 animals have been identified as hosts. Most common are prairie dogs, chipmunks, ground squirrels, mice and even domestic cats, rabbits and dogs.[24]

The Disease

How does one know they have the plague, and what can they expect? The disease bears several common traits, which a trained physician should be able to detect early and successfully treat. The first sign of the bacterium is usually extremely painful and swollen lymph nodes. As the nodes swell a bubble called a *bubo* forms, protruding from the skin. Bubonic plague derived its name from this condition. Other symptoms include swelling in the armpits and groin, high fever, confusion, restlessness, physical exhaustion, shock and coma.[25]

Within two to six days of contracting the disease, the victim will begin to experience symptoms. If left untreated, the bacterium advances in severity and will commence a transformation into other elements of the disease. One such variant occurs as the bacteria spread through the bloodstream and bleed into the skin leaving black blotches. The discoloration may explain the reason for the plague being called the Black Death in the Middle Ages. This phase also goes by the name of septicemia and, besides affecting the skin, will also enter the organs. Additional clinical features include chills, abdominal pain, and prostration.[26]

After entering the bloodstream, it can advance into the lungs, where in one to three days it will become pneumonic. At this stage, the plague enters into its most virulent and fatal stage. No longer does its spread occur from fleas to rodents and then to humans, or animal to human. Now it spreads from human to human by the simple act of an individual coughing and the resulting spray of infected droplets being released into the surrounding air. At this juncture, hundreds of people can come into contact with it within a small radius. Of additional concern, the mortality rate of victims becomes accelerated and in some cases death can occur within a day of exposure.[27]

Bubonic plague, septicemia and pneumonic plague probably represent the disease in its worst and most dangerous forms. These variants are extensions of the other, if left untreated and allowed to multiply. The end result will most likely be death. Other types exist and are referred to as cellulocutaneous, meningeal, hemorrhagic, pharyngeal and asymptomatic. All of these variations have similarities and in some cases affect different areas of the host.[28]

Treatment of plague has become almost routine; outcomes are good if the disease is diagnosed and treated early. Several antibiotics can be used: streptomycin, tetracycline, gentamicin, chloramphenicol and sulfonamides. Within this group, streptomycin has proven to be the most effective and has become the preferred medication.[29]

As with any deadly illness, the sooner antibiotics can be administered to the patient, the greater the prospects of survival. This is especially true with plague. Although mass epidemics are now rare, it will always be part of the organic life stream. In the United States, one in seven victims dies each year.[30] Once it becomes endemic to an area, subsequent outbreaks can occur periodically.[31] So it stands to reason that early detection and treatment are paramount for not only the patient's well-being but also the prevention of its further propagation.

Origins

Many scientists and scholars have attempted to decipher the origin of plague. In all honesty, civilization may never be able to answer this question. The best explanation of where and when bubonic plague first emerged can be found in William H. McNeill's book *Plagues and Peoples*. He offers a very critical and thorough rationale as to the disease's evolution, setting forth a convincing timeline of its first and subsequent appearances.[32]

McNeill puts forth the conclusion that plague can be traced to three originating points, or foci.[33] He places these centers in the Himalayan foothills bordering China and India, followed by the area of what he calls the Great Lakes of Africa, with the other center being along the Eurasian steppes running from the Ukraine to Manchuria. In his opinion, the bacterium planted itself not only in the black rat, but also in other burrowing rodents, where the disease could survive underground during seasonal changes. The first of these origins arose in the Himalayan foothills, followed by its progression to the burrowing rodents in Africa and lastly to the Eurasian steppes.[34] In other words, the flea and black rat partnership initiated its spread from a starting point in the Himalayas by infecting other rodents, then to Africa and the Mediterranean, followed by its eventual sweep through Europe.[35]

Many arguments can be put forth claiming the plague has existed since early time. However, those records documenting accounts of ancient epidemics may in fact not be plague, when examined by modern-day authorities. McNeill asserts bubonic plague most likely did not leave its early environs of the Himalayas until the 6th century AD and from this area slowly expanded its reign to the other continents. Other significant occurrences were in the 14th, 16th and 19th centuries, with each outbreak having devastating consequences on the populace. The plague did present itself at other times in between these periods, but the 6th, 14th, 16th and 19th centuries saw the bubonic type at its greatest height of mass infection and mortality and in turn established the disease's reputation as probably the most lethal shadow of death yet to afflict humanity.[36]

Early Plague Epidemics

As far back as the Bible's Old Testament, several of its passages have recorded the existence of vast plagues. However, these scourges have never been truly identified as being the bubonic plague, or the Black Death of medieval times. Historians, scientists and other experts have differed in their opinion as to the true nature of these epidemics, with some believing them to be plague and others suggesting smallpox, measles, cholera, diphtheria or typhus.[37]

One of the earliest biblical reports may very well be seen in one of the 10 pestilences visited upon Ramses, the pharaoh of Egypt, as foretold by Moses in the early chapters of Exodus. Moses had beseeched Ramses to free the Israelis and warned the king of subsequent wraths if he did not. However, each time the pharaoh denied their freedom the fury of God came upon his kingdom in hopes of persuading his reconsideration. The fifth and sixth of these pestilences to befall the Egyptians are called plagues. The fifth fell upon animals and the sixth upon animals and people with boils, or sores erupting upon their flesh.[38] The animal to human connection bears a remarkable resemblance to the proven transmission factor of flea to rat, followed by rodent to human. This may only be coincidental, but it has probably led biblical scholars to draw a strong correlation between the two.

The 10th pestilence also bears some relation. After Pharaoh rebuffed God and Moses for the ninth time, the Lord sent a mysterious cloud across the land claiming the lives of Egypt's first born, including Ramses' son. Finally, after so much loss and devastation had been visited upon his kingdom, the king allowed Moses and his people to leave Egypt. The question arises, though, of whether this ominous cloud could have been the pneumonic form due to its swiftness and lethality.[39] One will never know for sure, but again a convincing parallel to these pestilences can be drawn from these passages in Exodus.

Another famous biblical account of the disease can possibly be found in the book of Samuel. Within this Old Testament scripture, the story relates how the Philistines conquered the Israelis and as part of the day's bounty they carried off the sacred Ark of the Covenant. They placed the Ark in the temple of their god, Dagon, in the city of Ashdod. However, within two days, their idol of Dagon lay in ruins on the temple's floor. From this site, the Philistines moved it to Gath, where tumors broke out on the people. Fearing its continued presence, they moved the Ark to another city, Ekron, where once again tumors broke out among the inhabitants. Finally, after possessing it for seven months, the Philistines returned the Ark to the Israelis.[40]

Of great interest, though, is the actual biblical account of this story. In Chapter 6, the priests tell the people to return it to Israel, but to make a guilt offering before doing so, in hopes of appeasing their God. The offering is to consist of "five golden tumors and five golden mice, according to the number of the lords of the Philistines; for the same plague was upon you and upon your lords."[41] The words tumors and mice in this passage may bear special meaning due to the interconnection between them and the appearance of plague. First, the tumors could be the buboes forming in the lymph nodes evidencing the onslaught of the bubonic variant. Second, the mention of mice draws special recognition in that rats, a biological cousin of mice, are the initial carriers of the bacterium. Accordingly, the usage of mice in this passage might suggest the related animals are one and the same creatures. These stories may again be only coincidental, but, on the other hand, they may represent some of the earliest references to the disease.

Early biblical scholars have viewed the accounts in Exodus and Samuel as some of the first evidence of the disease. In truth, these ancient tales do contain some intriguing parallels to several elements in today's modern diagnosis of the illness. But in actuality, are these accounts truly the first signs of the disease, or a description of divine intervention in the progression of the Jewish and Christian faiths? At best, this is an extremely complicated question to answer with any certainty. Modern scholars have been more reserved and skeptical on this matter, especially since accurate records remain unavailable as to the identity of the disease.[42] For the true believer, these ancient accounts will represent the disease's presence in the world, as a result of God's wrath, whereas those in the scientific and historical professions, although believers themselves, will most likely require further proof as to the accuracy of these descriptions, as opposed to faith.

Lastly, as mentioned before, many epidemics occurring during ancient times were probably not plague, but some other highly infectious and deadly disease, with smallpox and measles being the most likely culprits.[43] Probably, the superficial appearance of these diseases upon the victim's skin may explain their association with plague. Most apparent are the red sores erupting to the skin's surface as the infection advances, which to an untrained eye could mimic the disease.[44] As bubonic plague intensifies, dark blotches form under the skin, partially explaining it being confused with these other illnesses.

It could be argued that the words *plague* and *epidemic* became synonymous with each other. With science being in an embryonic state, an accurate distinction between various ailments could not be made conclusively. Moreover, records of ancient plagues either did not provide enough information in order to make a modern diagnosis or the data has become lost through the ages. The two words appear to have been used as a "catch-all" for those diseases infecting major portions of civilization during these early times.

The Great Plagues

Most historians acknowledge the first major bubonic plague outbreak as occurring in AD 542–543, during the reign of Emperor Justinian. It became known as the Plague of Justinian and originated in Lower Egypt, spreading in AD 540 to the port city of Pelusium. Next, it entered Alexandria on the Mediterranean Sea, where it advanced northward to the empire's capital of Constantinople. Justinian ruled the eastern Roman Empire and had embarked on a campaign to reunite the western and eastern divisions in an attempt to reestablish Rome's former glory.[45] One account claimed it lasted off and on until AD 590, by which time it may have killed more than 100,000,000 individuals by some estimates.[46]

The Western Empire had fallen into a state of shambles after its fall in AD 476, but the Eastern Empire had flourished, especially under Justinian. Trade with all lands had become an important staple of its economy, bringing many ships and overland caravans into its borders. The black rat from India may have been the primary agent in bringing the bacterium as a stowaway on trading ships, along with overland carriers from the east, eventually arriving in the capital.[47]

A secretary to Justinian, named Procopius, wrote an account of the plague. His description has led present-day researchers to acknowledge the disease not only as plague, but as its most severe variant, pneumonic.[48] Two factors point to its presence. First, the illness reportedly spread from person to person and had a high fatality rate. Second, it lasted only two years. The pneumonic form moves very swiftly in its transmission and burns itself out in a short period of time from the simple fact it has consumed all available hosts.[49] These elements—human-to-human contamination and its relatively short but rapid reign—strongly suggest the epidemic was plague. In support of this conclusion, Procopius reported that upwards of 10,000 people a day were dying in the capital during its height.[50]

The next great epidemic started in 1346 north of the Black Sea, proceeded to travel throughout the far reaches of Europe, and lasted until 1361. It became known as the Black Death because of the dark blotches appearing underneath the victims' skin as the infection advanced through the bloodstream. Within a few years it reached pandemic proportions, lingering for several centuries by periodically resurfacing and invading new areas as it marched farther westward and northward across Europe.[51] Estimates vary on the death count, but, conservatively, the Black Death may have claimed upwards of 25,000,000 lives.[52]

The origins of the Black Death can be traced to the Crimea, where it broke out during the Mongol siege of Caffa. The city had become a trading center, and the disease probably arrived from the Eurasian steppes, carried by the Mongols. From this location, it traveled along the trading and shipping routes connecting the east and west, in short order absorbing Europe. Once again, the black rat and its infected fleas journeyed to new civilizations as countries expanded their outreach militarily and commercially, as evidenced by the Mongol's military operation against Caffa.[53]

The disease, being endemic, would also resurface in previous areas, again with devastating results. After breaking its eastern confines, it proceeded to move around the world. One thing was becoming apparent, though, in its transmission, and this factor could be seen in the bacterium showing up in ports. As world trade expanded, the black rat and its deadly companion, the flea, were steadily making their way around the globe. Absent a seafaring vessel to carry both, the plague might have remained somewhat contained on the continent of Europe.[54] However, the Great Plague of London showed how the pestilence could navigate the high seas and land in new lands virgin to the disease's wrath. The London plague lasted from 1665 to 1666, and claimed an estimated 100,000 lives.[55] Historians have concluded that the plague ended with the Great Fire of London in 1666, but in fact the plague more likely had run its course after becoming pneumonic, which would explain the rapid rise in deaths towards its end.[56]

The last of the great plagues started in China around 1855, and in many respects it represents not only the basis but also the beginning of this book.[57] The outbreak became known as the third pandemic and claimed an estimated 12,000,000 victims in China and India alone before stretching out to other places around the world.[58]

The plague began as bubonic but in time transitioned to pneumonic.[59] Apparently, it surfaced when a revolt started in the province of Yunnan. After putting down the rebellion, the returning Chinese soldiers carried the disease back with them. To the southwest, the province borders Tibet, India and Myanmar, all in close proximity to the Himalayan mountains, where the disease had lain in wait for centuries before its transport into China proper. Upon its entry, it broke out with intermittent frequency until 1894, when it spread to Canton and the nearby port of Hong Kong, a British protectorate at the time. By 1896, it had reached Bombay, India, and after further advancing into the country's interior, it killed all told an estimated 6,000,000 people.[60]

The plague moved to other countries, mainly through their ports, where at this point it gained the attention or the alarm of those individuals in the medical community who were knowledgeable of microorganisms and the spread of infectious diseases.[61] The medicinal titans in the 19th century were without question Louis Pasteur and Dr. Robert Koch. These men, along with several others, led the way in advancing modern medicine into today's world.

Fortunately, many other gifted individuals had studied under and with these men. One such individual who had studied with Dr. Pasteur was bacteriologist Alexandre Yersin, the man credited with discovering the bacterium and who subsequently named it after Pasteur and his institute.[62] Other former students and associates grasped the seriousness of the disease and started applying their knowledge to its cure and containment. As McNeill set forth in his book, the horror of the plague in Europe still remained a vivid memory and likely spurred these individuals to immediate action.[63]

I

The War Was Now Over

Returning Home

At the start of the American Civil War, Dr. John Hendricks Kinyoun had eagerly joined the 28th North Carolina Infantry Regiment, serving as captain of Company F.[1] As the war progressed, he would be assigned to Winder Hospital in Richmond, Virginia, at the same time as Union General George B. McClellan commenced his Peninsula Campaign in the spring of 1862.[2]

By the fall of 1863, with the South having suffered staggering losses at Gettysburg and Vicksburg, it desperately needed field surgeons. As a result, he had been reassigned to the newly formed 66th North Carolina Infantry Regiment as its surgeon.[3] But two years later, on April 26, 1865, the remnants of his regiment stood in shattered disrepair as their army surrendered to Union General John M. Schofield officiating on behalf of General William Tecumseh Sherman at Durham Station, North Carolina.[4] When mustered into service the regiment had roughly 1,100 men. But at Durham Station only 64 were present to turn in their arms. Within a week, he had returned home to Yadkin County.[5] For him and many others, the war was now over.

When he had enlisted as a volunteer on June 18, 1861, he was a young father. His and Mrs. Kinyoun's firstborn, Mary Elizabeth, had arrived on May 20, 1858. Sadly though, she had died before his joining the service. Her death would soon be followed by the birth of their first son, Joseph James, on November 25, 1860.[6]

A Changed Land

On returning home, things were much different. Money did not exist because all anyone now had was worthless Confederate money. People could only pay for goods or services through barter and with what the few greenbacks that came into circulation. Across the South, and in Yadkin County, the economy lay in shambles.[7]

Within the year, the doctor, along with his wife, realized that staying in Yadkin County and trying to find sufficient means to support their family would be an ongoing challenge. Eventually, they decided to move to Missouri. It too had been the center of a great deal of civil unrest, conflict and misery during the war. The state in many ways could be thought of as an extension of the Old South, in light of it having been a slave state.[8] Their journey brought them to Centerview, located on the western side of Missouri, roughly nine miles west of Warrensburg, the county seat of Johnson County.[9]

Prosperity and Sorrow

The town consisted of a mere scattering of houses and exemplified a small rural community. John was a physician and also a former lawyer, but the general area had little need of these services. After some searching, he landed a job splitting rails—a remarkable contrast to his educational background, but an endeavor dictated out of need, not pride.[10]

Before the war, he had spent a year at Wake Forest College in North Carolina followed by his enrollment at Columbia College in Washington, D.C., eventually graduating from Union College in Schenectady, New York. This was followed by entering law school at Columbia University, but after a short period of practicing law, he decided it was not an honorable profession. He then entered Bellevue Medical School in New York, graduating in 1859.[11]

In time, his medical services would be utilized by his neighbors and the surrounding area. He even became active in local politics as a Democrat. He served as president of the board of regents of the State Normal School in Warrensburg for six years, where his son Joe received his primary education. Later, he won election as the mayor of Centerview and served one term.[12] Of special note, in January 1893, several of his friends petitioned President Grover Cleveland in hopes of securing his appointment as the consul general of the Hawaiian Islands. Senator Francis Cockrell, a former Confederate general, supported the appointment, as did several other prominent Missourians. Consideration had also been given for his appointment as the consul general of Nassau in the Bahamas.[13]

Besides politics, he joined the Masonic Corinthian Lodge No. 262, A.F.A.M. and became a member of the Baptist Church. He also belonged to the Home Library Association of Chicago, Illinois. Membership in professional associations included the John Hoden Medical Society, the Missouri State Medical Association and the American Public Health Association. At his death, he would be the only doctor within a 40-mile radius.[14]

The family prospered, and other children joined Joe and his sister Lula Alice. They were followed by Flora Ridings, Estelle Keziah, Nellie and John Conrad. Nellie died in 1870 and John Conrad in 1871.[15] Mrs. Kinyoun herself died unexpectedly on March 27, 1872, of pneumonia.[16] Devastation probably best summarized the family's emotional state in 1871. He now had a household of children to raise by himself. Joe, age 12, and his siblings were without a mother.

The doctor would remarry in 1879, to Mrs. Martha E. (Carmichael) Hammond. Her husband had been killed during the war.[17] The job must have appeared daunting to the new wife and stepmother of four children. However, the family soon gelled, and the household took on a sense of normalcy. The couple would not have any children.[18]

Death and hardship were commonplace for most frontier families in the 19th

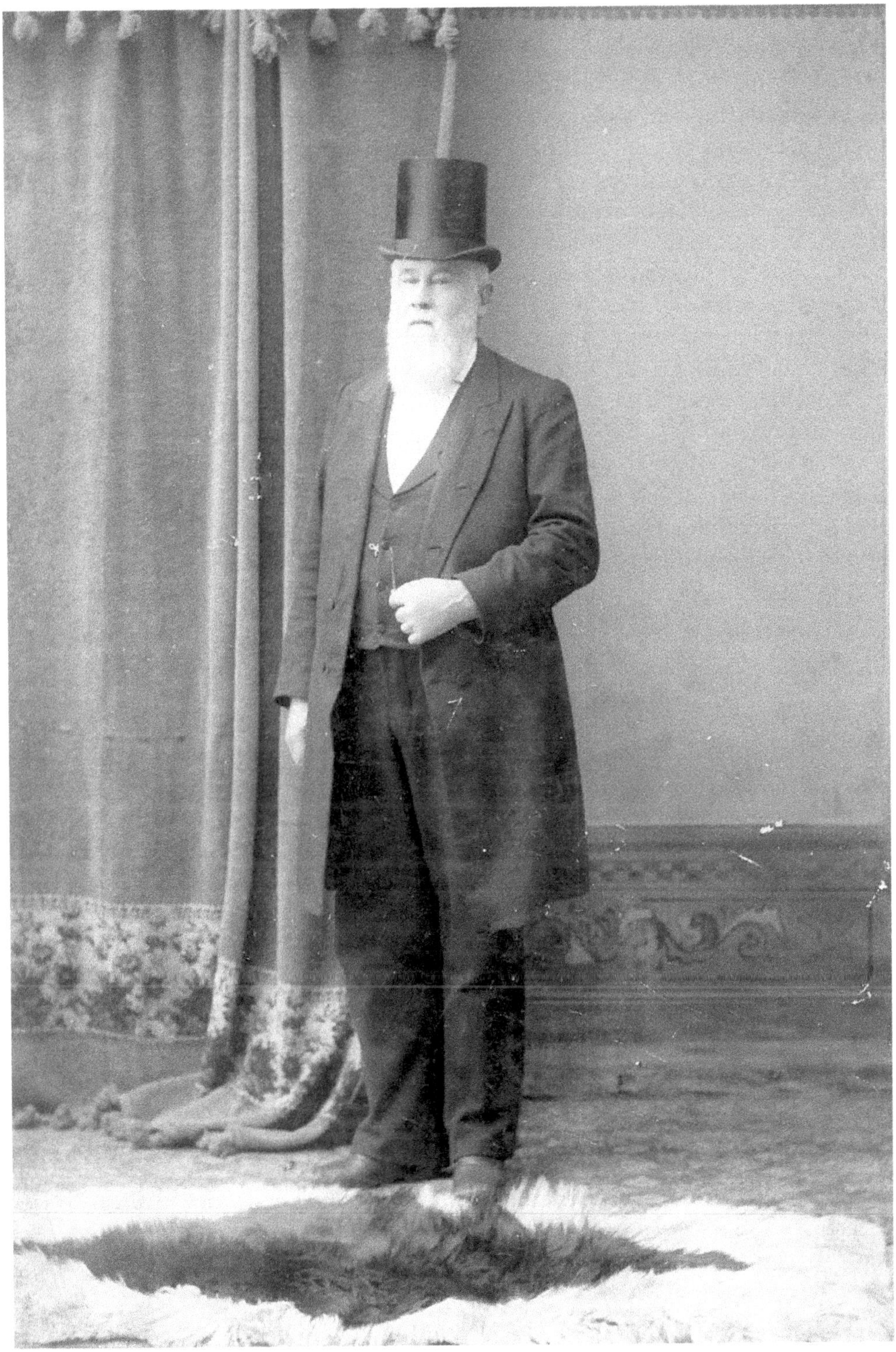

John Hendricks Kinyoun, father of Joseph Kinyoun.

century. Infant mortality ran high, which explained in part why many people had large families. Life consisted of many challenges. For the most part, the people earned their livelihood from the land. Western expansion had been a driving force in the settlement of the country long before the war. Afterwards, it experienced continued growth as the nation strung its railroads across the continent, opening up vast new territories for hungry settlers to stake a claim to and call home. Regardless, wherever they went, disease, drought, famine, outlaws and hostile Indians confronted them. America was taming the West and in the end would win the struggle, but as with all things in life the costs were high and at the expense of the indigenous Native Americans.

After many years of what could be considered a period of upheaval, a sense of stability and prosperity returned to the household. Joe had probably been affected the most by all these disruptions. During his first five years, he rarely saw—or had the opportunity to get to know—his father because of the war. On his return, this strange man moved the family to what must have appeared to be a foreign land. To further complicate his life, other children arrived in the family who obviously competed for attention. Two siblings died early after birth, followed by the death of the only person he had consistently known and loved, his mother.

Bellevue

In the span of a few years, Joe had grown up and decided upon a career in medicine, following in his father's footsteps as he entered Bellevue Medical College. Up unto this time, medicine in the United States lagged behind its European counterparts.

During the Civil War this became apparent as thousands of Union and Confederate troops perished not from battle, but from the effects of infectious disease. This occurred because of their exposure within the armies and the treatment of wounds.[19]

By the conflict's end, the application of several basic elements of medical care had become standard. These essentials included sanitation, general hygiene, proper ventilation, nutritious food and the urgency of patient treatment. After the war, a new understanding and study of medicine began to take place.[20]

Medical education in America could at best be described as rudimentary, lacking in the fundamental principles of applied scientific instruction and analysis. Eventually, medicine would be viewed more as a science, as opposed to a process of trial and error. Prior to the war, formal medical education remained somewhat archaic. Many members of the profession had only attended a few medical classes or lectures. Others merely read a book and, after a few years of mentoring by a seasoned doctor, would venture out on their own claiming to be knowledgeable in the trade.[21]

By 1882, American medical knowledge and the training of new physicians had become much more learned in its approach, though the country still remained behind Europe and its ongoing medical advancements. Of special note, the French have been credited with having the greatest influence on American medical advancement during the first half of the 19th century.[22] This influence would continue into the second half through the influence of men like Louis Pasteur, Dr. Robert Koch in Germany and Dr. Joseph Lister in England.[23]

Bellevue Hospital Medical College stood out in America as one of the foremost medical centers in the nation in 1882. It started in 1736 as a New York City hospital and has been acknowledged as the country's first. The college's origin could be described as humble, consisting of only a six-bed infirmary and located in City Hall Park as part a workhouse and correction house constructed on the grounds of the city commons.[24]

Bellevue would grow in stature, eventually becoming a school of firsts: the first municipal hospital, the first association between a hospital and a medical school, the first municipal sanitation code, the first school of nursing, the first laboratory in pathology and bacteriology, and many more. Other notable schools existed in the United States, but for the most part Bellevue distinguished itself far above the others. A new era in medicine had begun, and the graduates of Bellevue and other similar medical schools entered the mainstream entrusted with a new way of application.

The New Physician

In the spring of 1882, Kinyoun received his medical degree from Bellevue.[25] He also received three certifications from the school. The first acknowledged his completion of Private Instruction in Operative Surgery and Surgical Dressing.[26] The second confirmed that he completed the course of Medical and Toxicology Chemistry by the Chemical Laboratory of the Bellevue Hospital Medical College.[27] The third recognized his completion of studies in gynecology.[28]

With his degree and certifications, it could be said his education exceeded the known boundaries of American understanding of infectious diseases and their consequences. His studies had included anatomy, physiology, surgical anatomy, matriculation, obstetrics, analytical chemistry, a heavy dose of sanitation, public hygiene, and pathology, combined with the use of the microscope and other meaningful courses.[29] The school had made him a medical pioneer, but the country did not totally understand or accept new medical enlightenments.

Kinyoun also attended St. Louis Medical College, completing courses in medical jurisprudence, diseases of women and children, therapeutics and *materia medica*.[30] In addition, he practiced medicine as an intern at the Hospital of the City of St. Louis[31] and the Hospital of the Sisters of Charity in St. Louis between 1880 and 1881.[32] This provided him with general knowledge.

After his schooling, he returned to Centerview and began practicing medicine with his father. One thing remained, though: he had to learn the practical application of his studies, what many refer to as "experience in the field." He no longer sat in the classroom or stood in a laboratory bent over a microscope. Now he had to learn how best to use this newfound knowledge for the betterment of others.

Romance

Not everything in his life revolved around academics. Courtship and eventual marriage would enter his world. While in medical school, he started writing to a young lady also from the Centerview area by the name of Susan Elizabeth Perry, who went by Lizzie.[33] Her family had been early settlers in Johnson County, arriving in 1848.[34] Probably, the two of them had likely known each other beforehand. In a letter dated May 9, 1881, he wrote, "Miss Lizzie, Can I have the pleasure of calling to see you next Friday evening, May 12th? Very respectfully submitted J.J. Kinyoun."[35] The courtship bloomed into love.

Lizzie's parents were Nathan Washington Perry and Catherine Elizabeth (Houx) Perry. They were married on May 3, 1859. Catherine's sister, Susan Dorothy Houx, married Nathan's brother Amos Mueron in 1858. Unfortunately, as a result of giving birth to Lizzie on February 17, 1860, Catherine died on March 3, 1860. Her sister Mahala Margaret breastfed Lizzie while at the same time nursing her own daughter. Sadly, Susan died of consumption and asthma in 1859.[36] Nathan remarried on January 7, 1862, and his new wife, Betty Rice Moore, raised Lizzie.[37]

Catherine's maiden name had been Houx.[38] The Houxs had settled in Missouri prior to it being a state, sometime between 1813 and 1816. They have been credited with being one of the first settlers to bring slaves into the territory.[39] A brother, Robert Washington Kavanaugh Houx, rode with the guerrilla chieftain William Clarke Quantrill during the Civil War, as did his uncles Matthias Houx and Robert Morningstar Houx.[40] Accounts vary, but it is believed that all three rode with Quantrill when his gang of raiders burned Lawrence, Kansas, to the ground on August 21, 1863.[41]

On August 14, 1877, Lizzie received acceptance into W.E. Ward's Seminary for Young Ladies located on 15 Spruce Street in Nashville, Tennessee.[42] The school's 1880–1881 announcement stated in its forward that the seminary was for girls only.[43] Further, "co-education of the sexes has been tried in many places, but it is on the decline. We do not believe it best.... But what parent wishes his daughter to be put to such a use refining boys.... And in every school of boys there are coarse and vulgar ones."[44] Her report card for the April 1878 term showed marks of 95 or 100 in all her classes.[45]

In 1882, she graduated and returned to Johnson County.[46] Like the Kinyouns, her parents were of means and could afford to send their daughter away to what those in this period called a "finishing school" for young ladies. She and Joe appeared to have a lot in common, especially in regards to receiving a higher education. In 1880 America, going to college remained somewhat of a rarity in comparison to the overall population.

In his last semester at Bellevue, Joe wrote a long letter, dated February 19, 1882, to her concerning a variety of topics. He mostly complained about everything. The winter was too harsh, and he states he was tired of the snow, cold and New York as a whole. He did point out, though, that the city handled the snow removal all right and dumped it in the river. Graduation was nearing, and he told her that only two more weeks remained in the session followed by a week of exams. Of some interest, he explained he would not be returning home after commencement, but would be staying to take an extra course called Hospital Physicians, which had not been available during the regular semester.[47] The reason he wanted to take the course stemmed from his personal motto of "Excelsior."[48] Finally, he stated how much he wanted to see her and his yearning to finish school because of its rigors.[49]

After several months of practicing medicine with his father, he experienced what all new physicians eventually encounter, the death of a patient. In a letter to Lizzie dated December 21, 1882, Joe reported that Frank Engle's child had membranous croup and died after 36 hours. After the child's death, the doctor sought advice from another physician by the name of Dr. Hunt on his handling of the patient. The doctor told him that nothing more could have done to save the child.[50] However, this did not seem to satisfy him because he further wrote, "Almost feel like quitting medicine sometimes."[51] Lizzie's uncle, the Reverend James Houx, officiated at the funeral.[52] Regrettably, part of any doctor's practical education has been the handling of life and death situations. Medicine has always provided joy when people recover from an illness. Unfortunately, death remained a large part of the practice and how one avoided and handled its consequences truly defined the success of a physician.

His letter continued, but in a happier tone, when he talked about their approaching wedding in June 1883. He told her that all the arrangements from his side had been made, except getting married.[53] Joe concluded by saying the next year would be better, implying their marriage, and ended by wishing her well for Christmas and the new year. He finished by writing, "Good by [*sic*] love-for this time, ever devotedly, Joe."[54] On June 27, 1883, the two were married in Centerview.[55]

Pursuing Other Dreams

The newlyweds settled down in Centerview. Joe would go to work for his father as a country physician. The couple had a baby girl on June 14, 1884. They named her Bettie Kinyoun.[56] In October 1885, they purchased some land from her uncle, Bob Houx.[57] Apparently, they were expanding their real estate holdings, which had been a common trait among various family members.

So after four years of working with his father, Joe ventured into another avenue of medicine. He had acquired a special interest in clinical microscopy and bacteriology and wanted to learn more about the nature of microorganisms, or germs. In furtherance of this interest, he returned to New York in 1885 and entered the Carnegie Laboratory, enrolling in the courses of pathology and bacteriology in order to expand his knowledge in these areas.

Kinyoun became the laboratory's first student, and the facility in its own right had become the first laboratory in the country. As time would further demonstrate, he and this laboratory would represent a strange irony for both in the next two years. After his graduation in 1882, Bellevue had started offering a course on microorganisms. He undoubtedly wanted to broaden his recent studies by taking these courses at Carnegie.[58]

II

The Marine Hospital Service

The New Path

After completing his course work at the Carnegie Laboratory, Kinyoun set his sights on becoming a surgeon with the Marine Hospital Service (MHS). He probably knew the organization's admittance standards would be strict. Apparently, he had had an interest in the Service prior to his graduation from Bellevue, as evidenced by literature in his possession concerning its structure dated 1881.[1]

He sent a letter dated February 15, 1886, inquiring about the qualifications for admittance.[2] Supervising Surgeon-General John B. Hamilton (hereinafter Surgeon General) responded on February 18 setting forth the requirements. His correspondence elaborated: "Candidates, in presenting their applications for examination, should state their age, the medical school or college of which they are graduates, and furnish testimonials from at least two persons as to their professional and moral character."[3] The document stated he would be notified as to the time and place when the examining board would meet with him.[4]

Kinyoun proceeded in securing testimonials. He contacted an old family friend, Senator Francis Marion Cockrell. The senator had been a Warrensburg native, and after receiving his degree from Chapel Hill College, he became a member of the Missouri Bar in 1855. When the Civil War commenced, he joined the Confederacy, eventually achieving the rank of brigadier general after the battle of Vicksburg in 1863. In 1874, he ran for the U.S. Senate in Missouri, winning the seat and serving for 30 years. Being from the Warrensburg area, like the Kinyouns, the two families had become close friends.[5]

Senator Cockrell replied to him on February 23, 1886, stating he would send an endorsement as to his "professional and moral character and render you any other services I can, in securing for you the appointment you desire."[6] On his United States Senate stationery, dated March 22, 1886, to Surgeon General Hamilton, he expressed his profound endorsement of Kinyoun, and also praised his father. In the second paragraph, he wrote:

> Dr. Joseph J. Kinyoun is a most promising young physician and surgeon, has had fine opportunities, is intelligent, honest, sober, moral, upright, industrious, attentive, reliable, ambitious, and deserving, and has proven himself a skillful and successful physician and surgeon. I feel a personal interest in his success. I desire that he shall be invited and given an opportunity to be examined at the very first examination, please do so and advise me and oblige. Yours truly, F.M. Cockrell[7]

Copy.

Dr. John B. Hamilton,

Sup Surgeon Gen'l,

Sir,

Having known Dr. Joseph J. Kinyoun of Centerview, Johnson Co., Missouri, for quite a number of years I bear testimony to his excellent moral and professional character. He is a young man of energy, industry, honesty and promise in his profession.

Yours truly,

(signed) Thos. T. Crittenden

Ex. Gov. of Mo.

Letter of recommendation from Thomas T. Crittenden, former governor of Missouri, to Dr. John B. Hamilton, supervisory surgeon-general.

Another noteworthy endorsement came from former Missouri Governor Thomas T. Crittenden, also from Warrensburg. In a handwritten letter,[8] he asked the governor for a recommendation and explained his reasons for wanting to join the Service:

> I wish to change my field of work to one that offers the most facilities to pursue systematic investigations on medicine, something almost impossible to the Country Practitioner. The Marine Hospital Service I think offers the best inducements of any of the Government Departments-and at the same time the remuneration is sufficient to enable me to live comfortably.[9]

In response, the governor also sent a letter to the Surgeon-General highly recommending the doctor for admission into the Service.[10]

The aspiring applicant had secured the two required testimonials from probably the most powerful and influential men in his home state. Of special note, Cockrell and Crittenden practiced law together in Warrensburg, so he did not have to search far for the recommendations. The Kinyouns had been close to the Crittendens, as well as the Cockrells, as evidenced by an invitation to the marriage of one of the governor's children.[11]

He did not stop at securing just the two required letters for his application. He obtained four others, probably as added precaution. These endorsements were from Dr. Herman M. Biggs and Dr. Frederic S. Dennis of the Carnegie Laboratory at Bellevue Hospital Medical College; Dr. A. Flint, Jr., also from Bellevue Hospital Medical College; and Dr. Frank L. James, editor of *The St. Louis Medical and Surgical Journal* and president of the St. Louis Society of Microscopy.[12]

In late March 1886, Dr. Kinyoun received a letter from Hamilton inviting him to

Washington, D.C., for the purpose of presenting himself for examination before the Board of Examiners to be conducted on April 5, 1886. The surgeon general instructed him to report to the chairman, Surgeon P.H. Bailhache.[13]

Of further interest, Senator Cockrell sent a second letter to the surgeon general in April. The content was similar to that of his previous letter.[14] However, the letter had an added tone of sincerity in the last two sentences, when he stated, "He will prove a most valuable addition to your corps. I am anxious for hin [sic] success and trust his record will show him to be the best man appointed."[15] The senator went so far as to say that Dr. Kinyoun lived seven miles from his home.[16] With the doctor having completed his examination before the board, the senator likely was using his influence to accentuate his desire that he receive appointment.

Within a week after his examination, Hamilton reported he had received a score of 73.6 out of a possible 100, with 70 being the passing level.[17] He further informed him that he ranked "No. 5, on the list of successful candidates."[18] The same day, Hamilton wrote Senator Cockrell and informed him Kinyoun had passed the examination and within a year would receive appointment to the Service. He pointed out that the doctor ranked No. 5 and would have to wait his turn. He further stated his pleasure in him after having had several conversations.[19] Senator Cockrell forwarded the surgeon general's letter to the doctor[20] with the comment, "With my sincerest best wishes. F.M. Cockrell."[21]

Political connections have always been important for individuals aspiring to careers in government. Other correspondence would show that Kinyoun admired the senator and on occasion would seek his advice, especially years later when he became embroiled in the plague crisis in San Francisco. It could be said the senator had become his mentor. Cockrell had gained great respect as a leader and politician over the years in Washington. This became evident in Hamilton's timely response to him concerning Kinyoun's passing the necessary admission requirements.[22]

Years later in 1917, future surgeon general Thomas Parran worked for Kinyoun, while completing his studies at Georgetown University Medical School. The doctor served as the head of the District of Columbia Health Services. Parran worked in the laboratories and stated that his going into public health, as opposed to private practice, resulted from his association with him. He described him as an old man at the age of 56 at the time of their association.[23]

He related an interesting story about him. A year after graduating from medical school, Parran advised the doctor he intended to sit for the entrance examination for the Public Health Service, the successor to the Marine Hospital Service. Kinyoun told him to come see him before taking the examination. He entrusted him with an old rabbit's foot and imparted how he had the item with him when he took the examination in 1886. It seemed a patient had given the doctor the rabbit's foot. Parran stated that he, too, had the rabbit's foot with him when he took the exam. He passed and received the highest score out of eight other candidates. Kinyoun would not let him keep the item, however, and Parran returned it to him.[24]

Copy.

United States Senate,

Personal. Washington, D. C.

April 10, 1886

Gen'l John B. Hamilton,

Supervising Surgeon General U. S. M. H. Service

My dear Gen'l,

If I am not able to present this in person please consider it a personal call. I have known Dr. Joseph J. Kinyoun of Centerview Mo., for many years. He resides in my native county and only seven miles from my home.

He is a thorough gentlemen, honest, reliable, truthful, energetic persevering, intelligent, lauoably ambitious in his profession, sober, moral, agreeable and pleasant. I regard him as one of the most promising physicians of his age in our state.

No mistake will be made in his appointment

He will prove a most valuable addition to your corps. I am anxious for hin success and trust his record will show him to be the man to be appointed,

Yours truly,

(signed) F. M. Cockrell

Second letter of recommendation: from Senator Francis M. Cockrell to Supervisory Surgeon-General John B. Hamilton, April 10, 1886.

By year's end in 1886, Kinyoun would become an assistant surgeon with the Marine Hospital Service. His first assignment would be to the port of New York.[25] In a few months, not only his career, but also the future path of American medicine and research would be changed forever. Before this change can be fully appreciated, the history of the country's medical progression must first be understood. As with all great institutions, his new employer had evolved over many decades.

Origins and Creation of the MHS

The Marine Hospital Service traces its origins to the British Empire and America's colonial times. Britain, being an island nation and the superpower of the time, maintained its vast holdings primarily because of its large navy. Through this form of transportation, it ferried troops to keep and expand its realm along with establishing a network of commerce stretching around the world. Because of the empire's seafaring requirements, its sailors were constantly exposed to new lands, dangers and diseases. Soon, it became evident a medical system needed to be set in place that could cope with the large caseload of its sick and injured mariners.[26]

Shortly after the defeat of the Spanish Armada in 1588, a hospital for seamen was founded in Greenwich, England for members of the Royal Navy. The hospital originated out of a public response to aid those seamen injured during the battle. To pay for the service, sailors were charged a sixpence per month. In 1696, Parliament under the reign of King William III further expanded the service by enacting a law allowing for the permanent well-being of sick, injured, or incapacitated mariners at the now Royal Hospital at Greenwich. As before, a charge of sixpence was deducted per month from every sailor's wage. Other measures would follow, continually expanding health care for seamen. In essence, this measure became one of the first prepaid medical plans.[27]

Colonial America and its seamen also became subject to the tax starting around 1729. The fee went for the support of the Royal Hospital in Greenwich, a fair distance for colonial sailors to reach in time of need. Consequently, various colonies assessed a similar tax on mariners, with Pennsylvania being the first.[28] Other colonies— Massachusetts, New York, Virginia, Delaware and North Carolina—would follow with some type of sailor relief measures. Much like Britain, the colonies were dependent in large part on oceanic commerce for their survival.[29]

After the Revolutionary War, the young nation struggled with many issues confronting its newfound existence. The care and support of the country's sailors became an early concern. In the First, Second and Fourth Congresses the issue had been raised, but with no definitive action taken.[30] Finally, after several efforts to enact a measure, the Fifth Congress passed a bill on July 16, 1798, titled "An Act for the relief of sick and disabled seamen."[31] President John Adams signed the legislation into law.[32]

With the act's passage, the Marine Hospital Service came into existence. The legislation placed the Service under the jurisdiction of the Treasury Department. Similar to the British acts, 20 cents per month would be deducted from every sailor's wages in order to finance the law. Each ship was to provide an accounting of all its crew and pay the tax upon entering port. Those not complying, or falsifying the accounting report, would be subject to a $100 fine.[33]

The measure contained five comprehensive sections. Besides collecting a fee from seamen, the measure stated that the funds would be used to care for sick and disabled mariners arriving in the country's different ports. Further, the president could call for the construction of hospitals. Lastly, it called for the president to appoint directors for the marine hospitals established in various harbors. The directors would be in charge of collecting the sailor's assessment (later transferred to the collectors of customs at ports) and administering the hospital in their respective seaports.[34]

As time passed, the law would be revised, broadening the scope of the original measure. On March 2, 1799, Congress amended the legislation, broadening its coverage to include men and officers of the navy as well as members of the merchant marine. By these amendments, nearly all United States seamen would be covered and could seek assistance in a marine hospital.[35]

More important, the original statute and its subsequent revisions represented two milestones. First, the 20-cent monthly charge amounted to probably the first tax to be enacted in the young nation. Second, it became the country's first prepaid medical system.[36]

After its passage, events unfolded rapidly. In the early summer of 1799, President Adams appointed Dr. Thomas Welch as the agency's first medical officer assigned to Boston. A temporary hospital was established on Castle Island in the harbor, and by March 1800, he had drafted regulations for its administration. In 1802, Congress allocated $15,000 for the establishment of a permanent hospital in Massachusetts, with Boston becoming the selection site. In January 1804, the new hospital opened, whereupon Dr. Welch retired from his position.[37]

Other hospitals were established in Charlestown, South Carolina and New Orleans, Louisiana; eventually other cities, including some in the interior of the country—St. Louis, Missouri, Napoleon, Arkansas, and Paducah, Kentucky—got hospitals too. On September 30, 1850, Congress approved funding in the amount of $50,000 for the construction of a hospital in San Francisco. The network of hospitals now crossed the land.[38]

By 1870, the Service had expanded so much that Congress decided to reorganize it. The legislation made it a bureau under the Treasury Department. As a result of the Service's ongoing expansion combined with the commercial growth of the nation, it became necessary to centralize its control over all the hospitals. The statute similarly increased seamen's wage tax to 40 cents per month. However, by 1884, Congress rescinded the tax in its entirety and replaced it with a tonnage fee on shipping, in effect until 1906. At this time, the financial support of the Service became the direct responsibility of the government.[39]

In April 1871, Dr. John Maynard Woodworth became the supervising surgeon of the Marine Hospital Service. Later in 1875, his title became supervising surgeon general in recognition of his reorganizing the organization. In effect, he became the first surgeon general of the United States.[40] During the Civil War, he had been put in charge of an ambulance unit attached to General William T. Sherman in his march to the sea through Georgia in the autumn of 1864, after the fall of Atlanta. Woodworth later wrote about the experience in a pamphlet, telling how more than 100 men under his care made it to Savannah, Georgia, without any loss of life. The publication gained him notoriety, which probably aided in his appointment.[41]

Quarantine Measures

Along with establishing a network of port hospitals around the country, the Service and several appendage organizations imposed other protective measures for the purpose of limiting the entry of infectious disease. These actions can be seen in the evolution of the nation's quarantine and immigration policy. Having a consortium of hospitals provided more of a treatment than a solution. Without a stopgap procedure to limit the introduction of foreign maladies, the problem would never be corrected, which meant limiting the sources, or carriers. Ever since the three great plagues, governments started imposing quarantines on incoming ships, commerce and individuals in hopes of stopping this pestilence at the ports.

Venice created a procedure in 1348 to assess suspected vessels, cargo and passengers. By 1403, the city had set up a quarantine post outside its boundaries in hopes of barring the plague. Over time, multiple quarantine stations sprang up around the Mediterranean Sea. Ships suspected of carrying a communicable disease, or coming from a land containing one, were frequently quarantined for 30 days. After a while, the 30-day period proved unreliable, so it became 40 days. Quarantine means 40.[42]

Besides the plague, ships spread other terrible diseases, most notably yellow fever, smallpox and cholera. The people in the United States had little immunity to these infections, as evidenced by a deadly yellow fever outbreak in the nation's capital of Philadelphia in 1793 that claimed more than 4,000 lives. This epidemic became so severe the government had serious concerns as to whether it could function. The epidemic lasted through 1794, and reoccurred from 1796 to 1798. The government decided it had to enact some measure that could prevent future outbreaks.[43]

During the spring of 1796, Congress received a bill proposing the imposition of a national quarantine system. Already, six states had enacted similar measures. Nevertheless, when the matter came up for debate, the issue of "states' rights" dominated the discussion and led to a watered down version of the bill. Even so, on May 27, 1796, Congress passed the National Quarantine Act. But, contrary to setting up a federal system, the legislation only allowed the government to assist those states asking for enforcement of their respective quarantine statutes.[44]

Unfortunately, the legislation remained wholly wanting in protecting the young nation. In 1798, during President John Adams' annual address, he once again appealed to Congress for a more comprehensive law. To his credit, the Quarantine Act became law in 1799, repealing the former statute. Much like its predecessor, the new statute limited the government's reach. The act did require all federal port employees to comply with local and state health ordinances. Further, in time of epidemics, the president could move the seat of government to a non-infected location. Lastly, the president could acquire warehouses for the storage of merchandise confiscated off vessels suspected of having been exposed to contagions arriving from other ports.[45]

Roughly 75 years later, new measures were undertaken to reinforce and strengthen the country's system. Surgeon General John M. Woodworth reorganized the Service due to the previous law not adequately protecting the nation. In 1875, he issued instructions to all the Service's medical officers outlining their responsibilities and new expanded quarantine procedures. He advocated for a more comprehensive law, which would place it under the jurisdiction of the federal government, as opposed to the individual states. To his credit, on April 29, 1878, Congress enacted another quarantine act that placed control with the United States government.[46]

Woodworth went on to further enhance the effectiveness of the Service by centralizing the control and operation of all marine hospitals into the government, as opposed to being a patchwork administration on the state level. He also established strict admittance standards for candidates into the Service. Prior to this change, many doctors employed by the agency had been chosen on the local level to serve at a particular station. Through legislation, he had this practice abolished, whereby future officers did not receive appointments to specific locations.[47]

The surgeon general died on March 14, 1879,[48] at the age of 41. One of his remaining goals had been to establish a national quarantine service, but with his death this concept remained unfulfilled. Woolworth had revolutionized the direction of the organization. He placed it on a new footing to better serve and protect not only the country's mariners, but at last the nation as a whole in the prevention of the importation of deadly maladies.[49]

On April 3, 1879, Dr. John B. Hamilton replaced Dr. Woodworth as the country's second surgeon general.[50] A month before his appointment, the National Board of Health came into being, with instructions "to report directly to the President."[51] Congress empowered the Board to set up quarantine sites at various ports and to focus primarily on the intervention of yellow fever, cholera and smallpox. The obvious problem with this new Board lay in its overlap with the Marine Hospital Service. In effect, there were now two government agencies entrusted with much of the same power and purpose. Still, one saving grace for the Service rested in the Board's enabling legislation, which limited its life to four years, so on March 2, 1883, it lapsed into history, as ratified by a new Quarantine Act on February 15, 1883.[52]

Under this act, administration of those quarantine stations established by the National Board of Health was merged into the Marine Hospital Service. In addition, the Service would take charge of all public health matters as previously set forth in the 1878 Quarantine Act. Other laws would follow that further expanded the scope and outreach of the agency. Measures were enacted in 1888, 1890 and 1893.[53]

The Quarantine Act of 1893 solidified the Service's control over quarantine matters and ordered the placement of quarantine officers in foreign ports. The officers would be responsible for observing local health conditions and securing for each ship bound for the United States a bill of health from the departing port issued by the American consul. Of notable interest, from 1899 to 1900, bubonic plague appeared in Naples, Marseille and Genoa. Acting in response to this concern, the Service placed officers in 14 European ports until its abatement. All of these laws continued to reorganize and enhance the efficiency of the agency. Most importantly, though, they placed matters of quarantine, previously controlled in large part by the states, under the jurisdiction of the federal government.[54]

In 1876, Hamilton left the army and became an assistant surgeon with the Marine Hospital Service. Similar to Dr. Woodworth, he envisioned how the Service should grow, especially in the enactment of further quarantine measures. Although he and Woodworth removed a considerable amount of public health control from the states, they still fostered cooperative efforts between the two levels of government. By his retirement in 1891, Hamilton had achieved much of the necessary protections to guard the nation not only from pestilence outside the country's borders, but also from those already within.[55]

Immigration Controls and a New Identity

In tandem with the passage of quarantine laws was the enactment of various public health immigration statutes. Ironically, the United Sates had been a nation of immigrants except for the Native Americans. However, things changed, and a land of once open doors soon found the need to limit its accessibility. Early immigration laws primarily sought to limit the different mix of immigrants—different from the individuals of Northern European origin who came during colonial times—arriving in the mid-19th century.[56]

This became evident with the Chinese Exclusion Act curtailing immigration from China. During the building of the transcontinental railroad, the Chinese migrated to America in vast numbers with many helping in the construction of the railroad. However, the exodus became too large, so restrictive laws were passed barring them and denying their ability to become naturalized citizens.[57] Those Chinese already present ended up in the larger cities and lived apart from the general population in what became known as Chinatowns, mostly notably in San Francisco.

In time, immigration controls dealt more with public health issues. There occurred an increase of migrants who were sick or mentally disabled and who had criminal backgrounds. The country did not have the social service system to care for these individuals. Furthermore, health officials did not want diseased entrants carrying highly infectious and deadly diseases into the United States. In response, Congress passed a succession of immigration statutes between 1882 and 1885 aimed at denying entry to select types of people infected with various afflictions. These measures also established deportation guidelines for violators. With the passage of an expanded act in 1891, the Marine Hospital Service became the administrator of those measures relating to issues of public health.[58]

The Service did not have the capacity to handle the ever-swelling arrivals from 1881 to 1920. To correct this matter, it established entry stations where foreigners could be examined and screened for health problems. Ellis Island outside New York became the nation's largest facility. These facilities also served as hospitals. On a person's recovery, they would be examined and, if found unsuitable, would be deported.[59] This system worked well, and helped in containing the spread of disease.

The Service greatly served the public health needs of the young republic. And as the nation grew, so did the importance and authority of the agency. Three obstacles confronted it, which in time would be overcome. These impediments involved the issue of "states' rights," an effective quarantine system, and, lastly, a public health immigration policy. The agency overcame other challenges, especially the transition from archaic medical practices to the germ theory. However, from an administrative standpoint, these barriers ultimately dissolved in favor of the organization.

On July 2, 1902, Congress changed the Service's name to the Public Health and Marine Hospital Service to better reflect and represent its purpose. Lastly, on August 14, 1912, President William H. Taft signed another reorganization act again changing its name. After 114 years, the name Marine Hospital Service had been deleted with the stroke of a pen. Henceforth, the agency would be called the United States Public Health Service.[60]

III

The European Influence

The Birth of Modern American Medicine and a Small One-Room Lab

At the age of 26, Kinyoun returned to New York. On entering the Service, he joined the ranks of an organization in its 88th year. In 1886, there remained one final scientific frontier for the Service to cross and conquer: the germ theory of medicine.[1]

At some point in his education, he had learned about the germ theory. This concept set forth the idea that microscopic organisms, invisible to the naked eye, caused disease and its spread amongst people. Before this theory, the causation factor of diseases had remained in many respects a mystery. The microscope added much to proving this theory.[2] In effect, medicine and science became one with each greatly complementing the other.

Fortunately for him, the European approach as to how germs operated within and upon the human body had come to light at the same time as his generation entered medical school.[3] Proof of this statement can be seen in the courses offered and taken by him and his father at Bellevue and their later application of this knowledge.[4] During John Kinyoun's tenure, hygiene had become an important area of study and even more so after the Civil War with the establishment of the Council of Hygiene and Public Health in 1865.[5] Kinyoun's studies included sanitation, public hygiene, pathology, chemistry and use of the all-seeing microscope.[6] Even at the Centre View Academy, founded by both men, he listed his position as Professor of Chemistry and Microscopy.[7]

Within a year of his appointment to New York, he created the one-room Laboratory of Hygiene for the purpose of researching infectious diseases, the predecessor to today's National Institutes of Health (NIH). Through his many studies, and using the microscope, he had come to embrace the germ theory as fact. This new wave of thinking had been greatly advanced by this instrument, which allowed doctors and scientists to see—through magnification—previously invisible organisms called bacteria. It showed them how microorganisms caused disruption and death in the human body.[8]

He increased his learning after graduating from medical school by taking courses in pathology and bacteriology at the Carnegie Laboratory.[9] The laboratory originated on the top floor of the Service's hospital on Staten Island.[10] Surgeon Walter Wyman headed the New York station, where Kinyoun had been assigned as his first appointment. Wyman would eventually become the country's third supervising surgeon general upon John Hamilton's retirement in 1891. The two men would have a long association going forward.[11]

One of the key pieces of equipment in the laboratory was a Zeiss microscope Kinyoun had purchased, similar to the one used by Koch. The facility was modest, and he performed the simplest of tasks himself, including stoking the coals in the stove to keep warm. Within the first year, he had isolated the cholera bacillus, showing fellow doctors this deadly organism for the first time.[12] As time advanced, he became a strong advocate for research and received the support of both Wyman and Surgeon General Hamilton. Within a short period, Wyman named him the laboratory's director.[13] The doctor became so impassioned about research that, even before establishing the lab, "he personally drafted the legislation enabling creation of the Hygienic Laboratory."[14]

At the same time, the Service was again in jeopardy of losing its identity and being replaced by another health agency. In early 1888, a bill entered Congress after being favorably passed by the Committee on Commerce. The proposed legislation called for the creation of a Bureau of Health under the jurisdiction of the Interior Department.[15]

This new organization would administer all public health matters going forward, except quarantines, which would be the only duties left to the Service. The measure had been proposed by members of the former National Board of Health.[16] It had lasted from 1879 to 1883. It, too, had infringed on the Service and its supervision of public health. Fortunately, it had a sunset clause of four years.[17] Its former members, led in part by Dr. Billings, still wanted to usurp control of those matters governing the nation's health from the Service.[18]

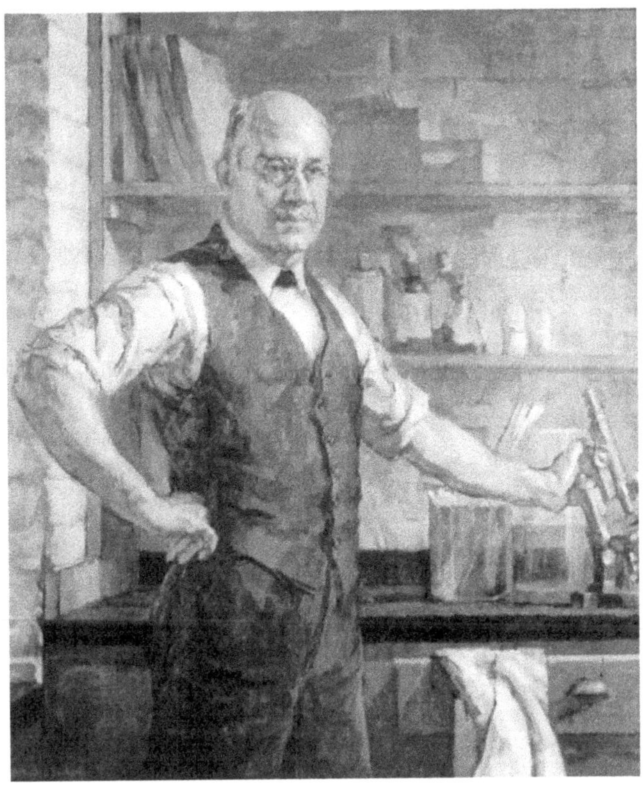

Dr. Kinyoun and his Zeiss microscope, National Institutes of Health.

Hamilton opposed the bill and asked to appear before the Committee. Billings had previously testified in support, claiming the legislation would provide medical research. As part of his testimony, he requested it not be published, which was agreed to by the Committee, meaning it could not be made public.[19]

In February, Hamilton addressed the group with a surprise announcement. He stated that the Service had a laboratory headed by Kinyoun. As proof, he directed the assembly's attention to the recent publication of the *Weekly Abstract*, wherein it set forth the lab had uncovered the presence of cholera in New York. He elaborated, stating that the findings had been verified by Drs. Armstrong and Kinyoun and confirmed by Dr. Biggs of the Carnegie Laboratory. The surgeon general replied that the doctor had studied bacteriology for five years,[20] the implication being that he had become a qualified expert in the field.

In response, a committee member told Hamilton that the bill called for ongoing research. He replied that Dr. Guiteras, formerly with the National Board of Health and attached to Havana, Cuba, had worked at the lab. He emphasized that Kinyoun worked full-time. His statement implied there was no need for another laboratory, especially one staffed by a former associate of the bill's proponents.[21] Hamilton had cleverly demonstrated his political finesse by this testimony.

He reported the employ of Dr. Stenberg, who had also been with the National Board of Health, stating his skills were being used in the study of yellow fever.[22] In essence, the surgeon general's testimony killed the bill. He countered its proponents not only with the creation of the Service's laboratory, but also with the employ of former National Board of Health physicians as researchers attached to it.

The agency once again had been saved, but at the same time Kinyoun had been thrust into the political limelight. As events would further unfold, he and his laboratory became the scientific heartbeat of medical research in the United States. In time, the facility would evolve into the National Institutes of Health, today the world's largest health research center and complex.[23]

The Titans

The creation of the Hygienic Laboratory can be attributed to three reasons. The first and foremost resulted from the medical revolution occurring in Europe closely preceding the time Kinyoun and others had entered medical school. Second, after graduation, he continued his studies focusing on microbiology and pathology. After he joined the Marine Hospital Service, he journeyed to Europe and studied under the new titans of medicine. And lastly, he brought this newfound knowledge back to the United States, turning it into practical applications for the Service.[24]

Without this new wave of thinking, combined with its scientific research, there probably would not have been this laboratory. For the most part, the epicenter of this learning took place in France, Germany and England.[25] But, who were these individuals that Kinyoun had studied with and what had they discovered that would change medical thinking forever?

As documented in the family's records, Kinyoun studied with Drs. Robert Koch, Paul Ehrlich, Friedrich Loeffler, Emil Behring, Émile Roux, Rudolf Virchow, Élie Metchnikoff and Louis Pasteur.[26] Further evidence suggested he may have met

Dr. Alexandre Yersin, who had recently been credited with identifying the bubonic plague organism, while at the Pasteur Institute.[27] He also met Shibasaburō Kitasato, who had also been credited with discovering the plague bacterium, during his travels.[28]

The most prominent individuals within this genre of scientists and physicians were Louis Pasteur of Paris, France, and Dr. Robert Koch of Berlin, Germany. Ironically, Pasteur did not have a medical degree, nor did he consider himself a doctor. Instead, he was a chemist and scientist who later pursued biology, which eventually led to his pursuit of medical research as a bacteriologist.[29] He followed a path similar to that of 18th-century Italian researcher Lazzaro Spallanzani, a priest. Spallanzani had debunked the theory of spontaneous generation, which held that microorganisms self-generated themselves into tiny particles of being. Through successive experiments, and with the use of a microscope, he proved organisms could reproduce independently and spread by air.[30]

Pasteur's research expanded on these findings and not only reaffirmed air as the carrier, but also showed that bacteria traveled by attaching to dust particles. Next, he studied anthrax in cows and established it could be eradicated through vaccinations. The same proved true in his research on hydrophobia, or rabies. Pasteur produced a cure for the disease by injecting a victim for 14 days with a serum. But more importantly, he proved the germ theory by showing the world how the invisible can invade and wreak havoc within the human body. And finally, he created the Pasteur Institute, an ongoing scientific research center.[31]

Dr. Robert Koch has been called "the father of modern bacteriology."[32] His first experience with medicine occurred while serving as a country doctor. Like Pasteur, he was asked by the local farmers to explore the disease anthrax, which decimated herds of cattle and infected people. He had recently purchased a microscope, and through its lenses he could see the bacterium. A cure had been developed, but Koch wanted to understand its life cycle, especially how the microorganism could lie dormant in the ground but then reemerge with the same lethality. After many tests, he developed a culture and found that the microbes could shrink and transform themselves into spores, or a state of dormancy. When the right conditions would return, the spores reverted back to an active bacillus. Koch's findings were published in 1876, and immediately he became world renowned. The results of this discovery further reaffirmed Pasteur's earlier conclusion of bacteria being carried through the air on dust particles.[33] In other words, the transmission concept had been proven again.

He further refined his methodology through experiments with potatoes and as a result developed a gelatin substance called agar that allowed scientists to grow bacteria in a pure form, as opposed to retrieving samples from infected animals and individuals. This new breakthrough allowed researchers the ability to place a specific disease with a specific germ. As a result, an exact measurement of identification and proof had been created, removing many of the age-old mysteries and superstitions from medicine.[34]

Next, he tackled tuberculosis, but had difficulty seeing the microbe and establishing its cause. While on this quest, Paul Ehrlich was at his laboratory conducting research. Ehrlich, who later uncovered syphilis along with a cure, had done extensive work on identifying various diseases through dyes and stains. He assisted Koch with this problem and, in 1882, allowed him to see the contagion. Kinyoun also studied under Ehrlich, which probably explained where he learned about the use of dyes and stains in his identifying bacteria.[35]

Koch studied other diseases and traveled to various regions of the world to visit and take samples of other deadly microorganisms. He first worked on cholera in Egypt, where he isolated the microorganism and concluded that it originated through infected waters. He then turned his attention to bubonic plague and concluded that the flea on infected rats was its transmitting agent. Other maladies examined by him included sleeping sickness and malaria. Although Koch never developed a cure for the many diseases he researched, he did bring the science of bacteriology forward into the modern era. Now doctors, scientists and researchers could literally put a name and face together with a disease and the corresponding germ causing the sickness. His postulates on how to isolate, produce and identify a germ have survived to this day.[36]

Besides Pasteur and Koch, other medical titans were emerging upon the scientific and medical forefront. Élie Metchnikoff studied the bloodstream and through his research uncovered secrets as to the mechanics of the body's immune system. Originally from Russia, he had settled in Sicily and set up a laboratory studying the digestive process of fish. He observed the functions of leucocytes, or white blood cells. In time, he theorized these cells would attack invading bacteria, as evidenced by seeing these cells congregate around an open wound and sores. He called these cells phagocytes, from the Greek word for cell eaters.[37]

Pasteur heard of his theory and offered Metchnikoff laboratory space at his institute so he could advance the concept of phagocytes through further study. He eventually proved his theory by repeated experimentation with various groups of animals and the use of the microscope. Phagocytes respond to any invasion of the body by moving to the injured area and consuming the bacteria. His findings demonstrated how these cells could literally move through the walls of blood vessels in order to reach the infected site. However, he mistakenly believed phagocytes represented the body's only immune system. Although partially right, he overlooked antitoxins acting as chemical agents in the bloodstream, which helped prevent bacteria from spreading. He wrote a book titled *Immunity in Infectious Diseases* and for his work won the Nobel Prize in Medicine.[38]

While in Germany, Kinyoun also worked under Dr. Rudolf Virchow,[39] who has been called "the father of modern pathology."[40] It became known as the study of the origin, structure and nature of disease. The science derived from the word *pathogen*, which meant a disease-causing microorganism. Virchow believed and furthered the concept that the human body consisted entirely of cells. He claimed the cell represented life in its basic and truest form. In the end, he proved all organisms were composed of cells.[41]

His research demonstrated how cells contracted a disease, being cells too, and the body's reaction to their presence.[42] He referred to diseases as "damaged"[43] cells. If these cells, or diseases, invaded an organ, then its operation would be interrupted, or cease, possibly leading to death. If a diseased cell entered the blood, it could affect the body's normal functions. Once again, the microscope led the way for him to prove his theories and show others how diseased cells damaged normal cells. In time, cures would follow from this study with the microscope allowing physicians to see how a cure suppressed an infection.[44]

Virchow looked at diseases as a condition of society, believing poverty, overcrowding, a poor diet and even oppression contributed to their occurrence. Other achievements included his discovery of leukemia and coining the terms *thrombosis* and *embolism*. Other studies included the human spinal cord, nervous system and the origin of epidemics. But in the end, he always came back to cells as being the building blocks of all life forms, especially those in the form of bacteria, which ended life. His accomplishments went a step further, besides his concept about cells. He learned how to stop infectious maladies and find cures, allowing the afflicted to recover from various diseases. Truly, his methodology exhibited greatness and took medicine a giant step forward.[45]

In addition to these medical revolutionaries, Kinyoun studied under Emil Behring, Émile Roux and Friedrich Loeffler while in Europe.[46] Behring had been a protégé of Robert Koch in Berlin, and Roux worked at the Pasteur Institute in Paris. This triumvirate collectively studied and brought about a cure for diphtheria, a dreaded childhood disease usually resulting in death. Loeffler had studied under Koch, too, and collected samples of the infection. Through the use of a dye, he uncovered the clump-like bacillus colony causing the illness. Yet he could never trace the disease from the throat and determine its spread within the body. He theorized the malady must somehow pass from the primary area of infection to other areas, which in turn would kill the victim.[47]

Roux improved on Loeffler's discovery and, along with Alexandre Yersin, he began working on diphtheria. After reading Loeffler's report on the disease, he started conducting tests in hopes of proving the theory. Roux developed a filtering technique, allowing him to capture toxins from an infected throat. Next, he injected various animals with the substance. Following several attempts, he learned the disease had a long incubation period, but in time would spread from the throat to other parts of the body, thereby proving the theory.[48]

Behring had worked at the Pasteur Institute, in addition to being a student of Koch. He had read Roux's findings on diphtheria and embarked on a quest searching for a cure through the use of chemicals. He tested numerous formulas and in time found tri-chloride of iodine to be a successful combatant. Unfortunately, side effects occurred that did not make its usage ideal.[49]

So he started experimenting with a new approach by re-infecting guinea pigs that had survived the disease. What he discovered would change medicine forever and lead to the permanent cure of diphtheria. The guinea pigs were immune to the disease. Not being totally convinced, he repeated the test numerous times on different groups with all achieving the same successful result. Behring found that the body had developed its own agents to ward off subsequent exposures to the disease.[50]

Afterwards, he developed a serum by extracting their blood, refining it, and then injecting it into healthy guinea pigs, followed by an injection of the diphtheria bacillus. In each case, the animals were not affected by the disease.[51] Behring concluded that the serum had become what he termed an "anti-toxin,"[52] or a chemical within the blood able to survive the contagion and later protect against its reappearance.[53]

As final proof of his efforts, in 1891 he treated several children with diphtheria at the Berlin hospital using his serum. Within a short period, most of them showed signs of recovery. His research and subsequent findings uncovered the body's ability to immunize itself. The discovery became acknowledged as a major medical advancement.[54] Because of this remarkable finding, he became known as the founder of "the modern science of immunology."[55]

In 1891, Dr. Kinyoun had journeyed to Europe to research and work not only with Behring, but under all of these titans.[56] Along with his post-medical school studies, he had trained himself on the theories and approaches of these men prior to traveling overseas.[57] After he established the Hygienic Laboratory, he employed this new knowledge and started producing amazing results in biomedical research, never seen before in this country.[58]

His supervisor, Surgeon Wyman, as well as Surgeon General Hamilton, being impressed with his findings led to his being sent to Europe for further study. On his return to America, he applied the new knowledge, bringing additional proof of the germ theory by introducing different ways to detect and conquer civilization's worst maladies.[59] The evolution of his one-room lab had become an amazing success. There still remained much to be learned from his overseas studies, but with the laboratory and his persistent dedication to research, medicine in America had entered a new and promising age.

IV

The New Frontier

Kinyoun's Laboratory: The Early Years

As his first step in setting up the laboratory, Kinyoun drafted enabling legislation for its creation. The lab started in a small room at the Marine Hospital located in Stapleton on Staten Island.[1] The furnishings were modest, and the prize piece of equipment was a Zeiss microscope that he had purchased with his own money. This particular microscope had been tailored after Dr. Robert Koch's.[2] He also collected an assortment of bottles, equipment and supplies to use in his work. During the winter, he had to feed and stoke the lab's tiny stove in order to keep warm.[3]

He soon received the title of director from Surgeon Wyman. In 1887, this small room became known as the Laboratory of Hygiene, latter changed to the Hygienic Laboratory.[4] As time evolved, the enclosure would become the National Institutes of Health, today the world's largest health research center.[5] It would be reasonable to assume he had little idea that it would grow into the country's most significant and largest facility for the study of infectious diseases.

He had a passion for this new form of research. As with many passionate individuals, they prove to be successful, especially when focused on how to make the world better. With all his education and aspiration, he soon excelled at trying to understand, control and eradicate the burgeoning onslaught of germs.

Cholera

His first research centered on experimentations with cholera based on the methodologies used by Pasteur and Koch. Within the laboratory's first year, he had isolated the bacillus. The microorganism consisted of a spiral composition, which explained why it sometimes had been referred to as spirilla of Asiatic cholera. The disease originated in the small intestines and was characterized by extreme diarrhea, resulting in severe dehydration and probable death if left untreated. Throughout the ages, it had wreaked havoc on civilizations because of its highly infectious nature.[6]

In the fall of 1887, along with Dr. S.T. Armstrong, he verified the germ's presence on two steamships in New York harbor. They set forth their findings in an article written for the Service published in November 1887 in the *New York Journal of Medicine*. The article reported that the ship *Alesia* had arrived in the port on

September, carrying 600 immigrants. Eight of the passengers had died. Several passengers, suspected of having the illness, were placed in quarantine on Swinburne Island.[7]

The doctors requested that the port's health officer, Dr. William H. Smith, be allowed to conduct bacteriological tests. He agreed, and they observed the afflicted passengers and took excreta samples for experimentation. The next day they proceeded to make plate cultivations of the specimens according to Koch's procedures. On October 5, they confirmed the samples to be cholera.[8] Because of the experiment, other doctors could now see the never-before-seen organism.[9] As verification, they had Dr. Shakespeare in Philadelphia test their findings, which he also confirmed as cholera.[10]

The *Britannia*, owned by the same company as the *Alesia*, sailed into the harbor on October 13, carrying 400 passengers. It had called on similar ports in Italy as the *Alesia*, and upon entry informed authorities that three immigrants had died in route from intestinal disorders. Several days later, Dr. Smith asked the doctors to visit the ship and secure specimens from several ailing passengers. Over the course of the next 11 days, they confirmed five new cases. In each instance, they had secured samples of the victim's bowel discharge, and, through autopsying the deceased's intestines, procured specimens of watery feces for culture testing.[11]

The samples were given to Dr. Biggs, the Director of the Carnegie Laboratory, where Kinyoun had conducted postgraduate training in biology and pathology. In addition, they sent specimens to Dr. T. Mitchell Smith, the Director at the Animal Laboratory of the College of Physicians and Surgeons, for testing. All the results proved positive. By November 6, no more cases of the disease had occurred and the ship was released from quarantine.[12]

The doctors summarized their findings in three points. First, upon death, an autopsy and culture tubes should be made of infected tissue to ensure the proper diagnosis. Second, successful inoculations can be made within 24 hours postmortem. Third, although the symptoms of the victims lacked consistent definition, bacterial analysis established the cause. This article demonstrated how a scientific approach based on Dr. Koch's provided the proof, as opposed to the previous symptomatic method of diagnosis.[13]

Early in 1888, *The Weekly Abstract of Sanitary Reports*, a publication of the Service, released a report by Kinyoun concerning the water in New York Bay. Again through research, he unveiled the existence of Asiatic cholera, this time on a far greater scale than aboard steamships. In this instance, he confirmed that bacteria can sustain itself in a large body of water. His premise centered on the fact that 3,000,000 individuals lived around the area and all their sewage discharged daily into the bay. He wanted to test his theory about the water's access and the sewage's impact from a biological standpoint.[14]

After conducting numerous tests at various locations around the bay, he confirmed the disease's presence. He concluded that it likely gained a foothold, not by the dumping of sewage alone, but from the quarantine station and its release of infected waste from patients. This idea came about in part from his recent examination of the steamships *Alesia* and *Britannia* when they were placed in detention.[15] Disclosure of this discovery soon circulated across the country, as far away as the Cedar Rapids *Evening Gazette* and the San Antonio *Daily Light*.[16]

During these early days, the lab pretty much existed as an unknown to the world. Its debut came somewhat as a surprise to the American medical community. To some extent, its identity helped in preserving the Service from being disemboweled by Congress in 1888. Former associates of the National Board of Health once again attempted to persuade Congress to create a similar agency called the Bureau of Health. The Bureau would assume all public health duties, leaving only matters of quarantine to the Service.[17]

After initial hearings, the Committee on Commerce tentatively approved the measure. However, later in the year, while testifying before the Committee, Surgeon General Hamilton revealed the existence of the Laboratory of Hygiene and reported on its important findings under the stewardship of Kinyoun and several other doctors. He divulged that two doctors associated with the lab had previously been associated with the National Board of Health. Hamilton explained the laboratory had become a permanent research center for the Service. As a result of his testimony, the bill failed and the Service survived, largely due to the lab.[18]

In March 1888, the San Antonio *Daily Light* reported another accomplishment of Kinyoun.[19] In a story titled "Phosphorus Not a Disinfectant,"[20] it reported that the surgeon general had instructed him to test the effectiveness of the gas as a disinfectant for use on ships. After conducting his experiments, he concluded the substance only worked as a surface cleaner, but had no fumigation prowess because of its lack of penetration.[21]

Hamilton had made a brief mention of the laboratory in his annual report for 1888. However, in his 1889 and 1890 reports, the findings of the lab received more prominence, demonstrating how it had become an integral component of the agency. The 1889 report set forth a general overview of its operations.[22] He stated: "Its usefulness is unquestionable, but if it were transferred to this capitol much time might be saved and the work made directly a part of this bureau."[23] Yellow fever remained a menace to the country, especially in the southern regions of the nation. The surgeon general reported that the president had authorized the establishment of another hygienic laboratory at the Key West quarantine station on the Tortugas Keys because of this disease. Assistant Surgeon H.D. Geddings would be placed in charge of it.[24]

The report also summarized Kinyoun's activities. He stated that more equipment had been added to the lab, including an apparatus to cultivate anaerobic microbes in the study of the fever. Next, he related that a long series of disinfectant experiments were nearing completion for utilization in quarantines, singling out sulfur dioxide as having the greatest penetrating application. Unfortunately, the gas did not have any effect on the microorganism's spores. To the contrary, though, it proved to be effective on cholera spirillum, a non spore-bearing microorganism.[25]

The director discussed trials involving yellow fever, malaria and pneumonia. He pointed out how phosphorus pentoxide had been recommended in its treatment. Through additional testing, he proved the compound had little value. Concerning pneumonia, he conducted an examination of sputum and performed autopsies on victims, which revealed how the disease would appear localized at first, but in time would became systemic, or move throughout the body. Progress had been made, but more studies would be needed to further define its pathology and etiology. The doctor suspected there must be some other predisposed cause for the disease besides traumatism, or its transmission through a wound and other paths of entry.[26]

In concluding, he stated the lab would be working on Weigert's treatment for tuberculosis, the effect of nurses' and assistants' hands as transmitters of infectious disease in treating wounds, and the cause of anaerobic microorganisms. To finish, he complained about the small size of the laboratory, citing its lack of sufficient space to photograph experiments and other matters.[27]

At the age of 29, Kinyoun had risen to the forefront of this new frontier of medical science. A mere 10 years before, he knew little about medicine, except what he may have learned while accompanying his father visiting patients. Now, he stood as the gatekeeper to this new approach in the battle against disease. Oddly enough, he saw a possible transmission factor between a patient's illness and the lack of clean hands by those administering to the sick. But through the microscope and other new procedures it could be seen how microscopic organisms could invade the body by hand, besides by air.

Cobra Venom

In this opening remarks of the 1890 annual report, Hamilton stated with obvious pride, "The country may congratulate itself on the fact that no epidemic of yellow-fever, small-pox, or cholera has prevailed in any portion of our country."[28] Especially noteworthy was the report on the Hygienic Laboratory, given partly by him and Kinyoun. It consisted of 17 pages, as opposed to the two pages in the 1889 report. Its placement appeared more prominent, being fifth in the table of contents, compared to 16th the preceding year.[29]

His introductory comments about the lab restated the need for it to be moved to Washington, D.C., because of the confined space and touted the greater good it could offer to the Service's other hospitals. He expressed its ongoing value and need to be under the jurisdiction of the bureau, as opposed to a single port.[30]

The remainder of the report, including Kinyoun's, involved a possible new cure for the treatment of cholera and yellow fever using cobra venom from India. In a confidential letter to President Benjamin Harrison, Mr. F.A. Perroux of Calcutta advised he had a cure for Asiatic cholera. He claimed that people from several northern tribes had injected the venom into sufferers of the disease with the procedure showing curative results.[31]

Hamilton stated that Perroux had sent samples of the venom to the State Department, which he in turn gave to the Hygienic Laboratory for testing. Hamilton pointed out that Dr. Gnezda, apparently with the Service, had been studying its effects in Berlin under the direction of Koch. He did not express much support for Perroux's theory, stating that previous trials with venom on various animals had resulted in death and would probably do the same in humans. Also, he viewed any American analysis as a duplication of what Gnezda had been doing in Berlin. Nonetheless, he decided to allow the lab to conduct its own analysis, since Perroux had already supplied the samples.[32]

Perroux contacted the Unites States because he wanted verification of his claim. His theory revolved around the idea of humans having poison in their blood as part of their composition, which became depleted by cholera. He hypothesized that the cobra venom, administered properly and in the right amount, would restore the supposed human poison, allowing the afflicted to recover. Possibly he had in mind the body's antibodies, which do attempt to ward off infections upon entering the body.[33]

In subsequent correspondence, he recommended using the procedure on human patients who had "given up"[34] or were nearing death. He provided some notes on the venom, as developed by the former Indian "Snake Poison Commission."[35] Part of his synthesis centered on the coagulation of the blood. He reasoned that while blood does not coagulate in humans after death, it does in some animals.[36]

Mr. Perroux sent two packages of venom, with the first containing four samples and the second containing 14. He gave instructions on how to milk a cobra by grabbing it behind the head and pressing the fangs through a palmyra palm wrapped over a mussel shell. After extraction, the venom should be placed in a water glass and allowed to dry, until it resembles a cobweb. Next, it should be mixed with a liquid substance before administering. Finally, its application should be through an incision in the patient's arm.[37]

His instructions noted a difference between cobra and viper venom. He stated cobra venom does not poison the blood, whereas a viper's has the opposite effect. Perroux reasoned that human blood does not coagulate upon death when exposed to cobra and viper venom.[38] And he further added, "Partial coagulation of the blood is the immediate cause of choleric death."[39] Because cobra venom cannot poison the blood, it can kill cholera, since the disease does not affect the blood.[40] He postulated his theory by stating:

> The rationale is that the effects of these two conditions of functional abnormality, cobraic and choleric, on human vitality are of an opposite nature. Although each kills on entering the blood stream alone, if present together they mutually destroy the power of each other and become inert.[41]

Most venoms can be either hemotoxin or neurotoxin; the former attacks and destroys the blood, while the latter attacks the nervous system causing paralysis, and both, if left untreated, result in death. Some species of snakes carry hemotoxin and neurotoxin in their venom.[42] Perroux might not have known these modern-day facts at the time of his theory. In addition, his hypothesis may have confused antibodies in the blood with what he called poisons in the blood. Regardless, he repeatedly put forth the curative effect of cobra venom, maintaining that it would have epic positive consequences in curing cholera.[43]

In Kinyoun's report to Hamilton, he meticulously reported on whether cobra venom operated as a cure for Asiatic cholera. He substantiated his findings by stating he used the same methodology Gnezda had set forth in his paper after attending the Ninth International Medical Congress concerning cobra venom.[44]

The doctor performed a series of three tests. The first involved the effect of the venom on blood and its coagulation. The testing group consisted of a dog, mouse, cat and rabbits. All the experiments showed coagulation of the blood, which partly debunked Perroux's theory. The second round involved the germicidal effect of the venom on Asiatic cholera and several other diseases, most notably anthrax along with typhoid. Ten tests were conducted, and in each case the venom had a germicidal effect on the disease, being most effective at a three-quarters solution. The third series of tests involved seven experiments on rabbits. The tests ranged from the size of the rabbit, the method of injecting the disease and the percentage of the venom solution injected into the animal. In only one case did a rabbit respond favorably. The other cases ended in death after injection of the venom.[45]

Kinyoun finalized his report by stating that the use of cobra venom did not cure cholera, but in fact increased its severity. He did confirm that the venom can kill the disease by using a three-quarters solution. Next, he found no parallel, or antagonism, between the venom and the disease. To conclude, he affirmed it would not prevent coagulation of blood. Through careful and articulate experimentation, he had proven Perroux's theory of no value.[46]

The importance of his rather lengthy report demonstrated the application of science to medicine. This example illustrated the new process(s) of scientific research firsthand. Within three years of its establishment, the lab had become the new standard bearer for unraveling the mysteries and interactions of microorganisms and their effect on the human body. The new frontier in medicine had gained a foothold in America.

Death

Personal tragedy soon struck the Kinyoun household. In a series of six telegrams from the doctor to Lizzie's father, Nathan W. Perry, in Centerview, the tragedy unfolded with devastating news. In a cable dated February 26, 1888, he informed Mr. Perry, "Bettie is dangerously sick."[47] In another wire, he reported her to be sick with membranous croup. Later in the day, he relayed that a Dr. Janeway had apparently performed a tracheotomy as a last resort with Bettie resting comfortably.[48]

The next morning he informed Mr. Perry, "Bettie died this morning at 7 o'clock."[49] In a wire received at 7:07 p.m., he stated, "Leave New York tonight make all arrangements. Meet us at Warrensburg. Russell selected. Short service at church in Centerview. Select burial lot in Centerview Cemetery. J.J. Kinyoun."[50] On February 28, he communicated they would arrive Wednesday and would need two hotel rooms.[51]

In a strange twist of fate, Kinyoun's first fatality as a new physician occurred when a child died because of membranous croup.[52] The disease mainly afflicted young children and caused swelling in the throat and trachea making breathing difficult.[53] One has to wonder how haunted he must have felt by having the dark shadow of this disease pass through his own household to claim the life of his and Lizzie's first-born child.

Death Revisited

Later in the year, an extraordinary event transpired as reported in the *Baltimore Sun* on December 29, 1888. While visiting her parents and Bettie's grave over the holiday season, Lizzie had her mother disinterred for the purpose of seeing her for the first time.[54] Because of complications during Lizzie's birth, her mother, Catherine Elizabeth Perry, died two weeks later on March 3, 1860.[55] Consequently, she had never seen her mother's face in person. The article described the exhumation:

> The body had been placed in a metallic casket and buried in an underground vault, which was bermetically [sic] sealed. When the casket was opened Mrs. Kinyoun was utterly amazed to see that her mother's body was in just as natural and lifelike condition as it was when she was buried. Her clothing was intact, and the preservation of her body was wonderful. There was no ghastliness about the face, the complexion was as clear and delicate as to that of a living person, there was even a slight color in the cheeks, and her brow was as clearly penciled as if it had been artificially done only a few days before. Mrs. Kinyoun could see, with surprising distinctness, what she had always heard, that she strikingly resembled her mother.[56]

The reason for exhuming her mother may have stemmed from the death of Bettie. Catherine had been buried for over 24 years and by the article's description demonstrated the well-preserved condition of the body. The account ended by stating that Mrs. Kinyoun was the niece of Mrs. H.C. Eccles of Charlotte, North Carolina, and the cousin of Georgia Senator Joseph E. Brown.[57]

A New Year

As the new year arrived, so did a change of circumstances for the family. The *Baltimore Sun* reported in January 1889 that the doctor had been transferred to the Marine Hospital in Baltimore.[58] The article did not state a reason for the transfer.

On January 14, 1889, he wrote to his father about what was happening in his and Lizzie's life. While back East, the family in Missouri had been sending them eggs and butter. Kinyoun told his father that though the three-dozen eggs he had sent had arrived, most were broken, but usable to some extent.[59]

He wrote that he had entered school again, this time taking the courses of biology and pathology at the cost of $50.00.[60] He elaborated that "the two combined, are for the search for the cause of disease, and its prevention."[61] He noted,

> On the full knowledge of this depends the advancement of the science of medicine, and surgery. Some people do wish you to think that nothing is to be known in medicine except what is known and thus hedge themselves about with the wall of in flexibility [sic], and make us the shekels.[62]

These two sentences have important meaning. First, he advocated for medicine's progression and implied it moving forward as in Europe. Second, those who try to stop its advancement will make it the worse for all. For him, he would be one of the primary persons in making this transition for the country. Through his lab, steps toward this transition would advance, along with others in bringing American medicine into the mainstream.

Still, these words would in time come to haunt him, when he became the Federal Quarantine Officer on Angel Island in San Francisco Bay upon his detection of bubonic plague. It could be said by these lines, the birth of modern medicine in the United States had just arrived and, much like some newborn children, it would come into the world kicking and screaming.

He also revealed a secret to his father, stating he had been directed to study hog cholera, or swine plague as it had been technically called, under Dr. Welch, a professor from his former Bellevue days.[63] Welch wanted him to study the disease because it would "be of some benefit to the farmer as well as the sailor."[64] With some exasperation, he commented that his workload had become somewhat taxing, implying that while he remained eager to tackle these tasks, they had started to consume him.[65] He noted, "I make the morning visits—see about 50 patients, then I go over to Johns Hopkins Hospital for the afternoon,"[66] taking the biology and pathology courses.

Another important sentence appeared towards the end of the letter, where he told his father, "A bill has been reported to Congress to establish a laboratory in Washington, if it passes, I will be sent there to take charge of it."[67] The stage had now been set for the Hygienic Laboratory to be moved to the nation's capital. Within the span of two years, his tiny lab had achieved national recognition and importance. His career had started to skyrocket. In the course of the year, Congress would approve the lab's transfer, with the doctor as its first director.[68]

As previously reported in the *Baltimore Sun*, the doctor had been transferred to this port in January.[69] However, in a letter dated March 1889, the surgeon general wrote of his being relieved of duty from the hospital at Baltimore and ordered back to New York.[70] No explanation has been found for this brief interlude. It may have had something to do with his official promotion to the rank of assistant surgeon by President Cleveland, as stated in the *Sun* on January 16.[71] It more likely had to do with an expected addition to the family.

A New Child

On May 19, Betty Kinyoun wrote two letters on the same day to her husband John from New York detailing the birth of Lizzie's and Joe's second child, Alice Eccles Kinyoun. She would later be called Allie. The first letter related that Lizzie had gone into labor and had been experiencing very painful contractions. Betty expressed her deep concern for her daughter and the yet-to-be-born child.[72] Her concern led her to write, "I feel like it would break up the little family to lose her. I mean our little circle, only four of us, since dear little Bettie went to her heavenly home."[73]

Losing a child has always been a horrible and traumatic event for any couple. It will also test the strength of a relationship. Obviously, the Kinyouns had been grief-stricken, and the birth of a new child would help in overcoming the loss of Bettie. As her mother mentioned, if this new child were to die during birth, it would be catastrophic for the young couple.

The second letter was written on the same day. She reported how Lizzie's labor had lasted for two hours and the baby weighed 8¾ pounds, calling her a large baby, "fat as a large pig … she seems to resemble her father."[74] The baby's birth had taken place at the Marine Hospital on Staten Island.[75]

V

The Pursuit: 1890–1891

A Promotion and European Bound

As plans progressed for the lab's transition, Kinyoun applied for a promotion in 1890.[1] Within the organization there were three levels of rank below the supervising surgeon-general. These were surgeon, passed assistant surgeon and assistant surgeon. Upon entering the Service in 1886, he had received the rank of assistant surgeon.[2] Similar to when he initially joined the agency, he had to submit an application with letters of recommendation from physicians and pass an examination.[3]

Concerning the first part of the process, he secured three recommendations. The first came from his supervisor, Surgeon Wyman,[4] who stated, "It gives me great pleasure to bear testimony to his irreproachable conduct and habits of great industry while he served under my command at the port of New York."[5] He also received supporting letters from Surgeons John Godfrey and George Purviance, who served over him while he had been stationed in Baltimore.[6]

While Kinyoun awaited word on his promotion, Acting Secretary of the Treasury A.B. Nettleton issued a directive creating a special board. He ordered the group to study fumigation appliances for disinfecting ships in compliance with the National Quarantine Act, establish a "Supply Table" for officer use and prescribe new uniforms for the officers and employees. The board consisted of Surgeon W.W. Austin, as chairman; Surgeon Fairfax Irwin; and Assistant Surgeon J.J. Kinyoun, as recorder.[7] They were "to convene in Washington, D.C., on Monday, December 1st, 1890."[8] Surgeon General Hamilton sent a separate dispatch to Kinyoun directing the same.[9] He had now caught the attention of his superiors and, in testament to his abilities, he began receiving special assignments.

The following day, he received word of his promotion to Passed Assistant Surgeon. The order had been signed by Hamilton, Acting Secretary of the Treasury A.B. Nettleton and President Benjamin Harrison.[10] The doctor had become one of the youngest, if not the youngest, member of the Marine Hospital Service to be promoted to this position.[11]

Within weeks of his promotion, he received a directive from Hamilton relieving him of duty in New York. The order directed him to proceed to Berlin, Germany, and enter Dr. Robert Koch's laboratory to further his research training.[12] Acting Treasury Secretary Nettleton issued him an official leave of absence with the right to make application for an extension.[13]

Copy.

Treasury Department,
U. S. Marine Hospital Service,
Office of the Supervising Surgeon-General,
Oct. 7, 1890.

To the
Surgeon General,
U. S. Marine Hospital Service,
Washington, D. C.

Sir,

Assistant Surgeon J. J. Kinyoun informs me that he is about to make application foe examination for promotion and in accordance with the regulations will forward letters of commendation from the officers under whom he has served. It gives me great pleasure to bear testimony to his irreprochable conduct and habits of great industry while he served under my command at the port of New York.

Very respectfully yours,
(signed) Walter Wyman
Surgeon, M.H.S.

Letter to Supervisory Surgeon General John B. Hamilton recommending Dr. Kinyoun's promotion to passed assistant surgeon from Surgeon Walter Wyman, October 7, 1890.

On December 17, Secretary of State James G. Blaine issued him and his family diplomatic passports and a letter of introduction.[14] He also received a special letter of introduction to William Walter Phelps, Envoy Extraordinary and Minister Plenipotentiary of the United States at Berlin by Acting Secretary of State William F. Wharton, as requested by Senator Joseph E. Brown of Georgia.[15] The letter asked that the doctor and his wife be extended "Official Courtesies"[16] as representatives of the surgeon general. The Kinyouns departed for Europe in late December 1890.[17]

Coinciding with their departure, the Secretary of the Treasury, at the request of Hamilton, submitted an appropriation letter on January 23, 1891, to the Speaker of the House of Representatives, requesting $1,800 for the Service. The money would be used to rent a building for the transfer of the Hygienic Laboratory to Washington.

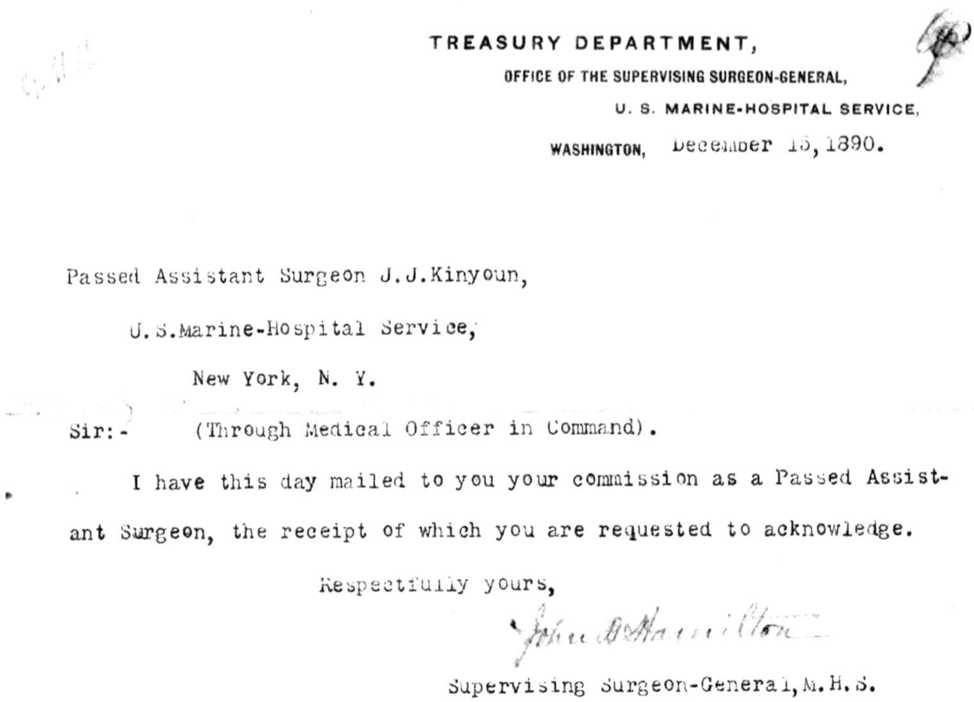
TREASURY DEPARTMENT,
OFFICE OF THE SUPERVISING SURGEON-GENERAL,
U. S. MARINE-HOSPITAL SERVICE,
WASHINGTON, December 15, 1890.

Passed Assistant Surgeon J.J.Kinyoun,
U.S.Marine-Hospital Service,
New York, N. Y.

Sir:- (Through Medical Officer in Command).

I have this day mailed to you your commission as a Passed Assistant Surgeon, the receipt of which you are requested to acknowledge.

Respectfully yours,
John B Hamilton
Supervising Surgeon-General, M.H.S.

Letter from Supervisory Surgeon-General John B. Hamilton to J. J. Kinyoun appointing him passed assistant surgeon, December 15, 1890.

The letter asked that there be two passed assistant surgeons assigned to the laboratory, as opposed to one.[18] Further, "the object of this additional detail is to station a bacteriologist permanently on duty in connection with the laboratory."[19] The laboratory would be under the direct supervision of the surgeon general.[20]

Within a few months, Congress approved the request, and, in June of 1891, the laboratory moved from New York to the fourth floor of the Butler Mansion on Capitol Hill, becoming an official entity in its own right. The Service had recently moved from F Street to the mansion. Concurrently, newly installed Surgeon General Walter Wyman, Kinyoun's former boss in New York, wanted both he and the lab under his authority[21]

Old World Medicine: Berlin and Koch's Laboratory

On January 26, Lizzie wrote her father-in-law from their residence of 101 Friedrich Strasse, III, about the many changes the family has been experiencing. She expressed excitement that, "Tomorrow will be Emperor Williams birthday and there will be great parades. There will be a procession, a troop review and the Kaiser may

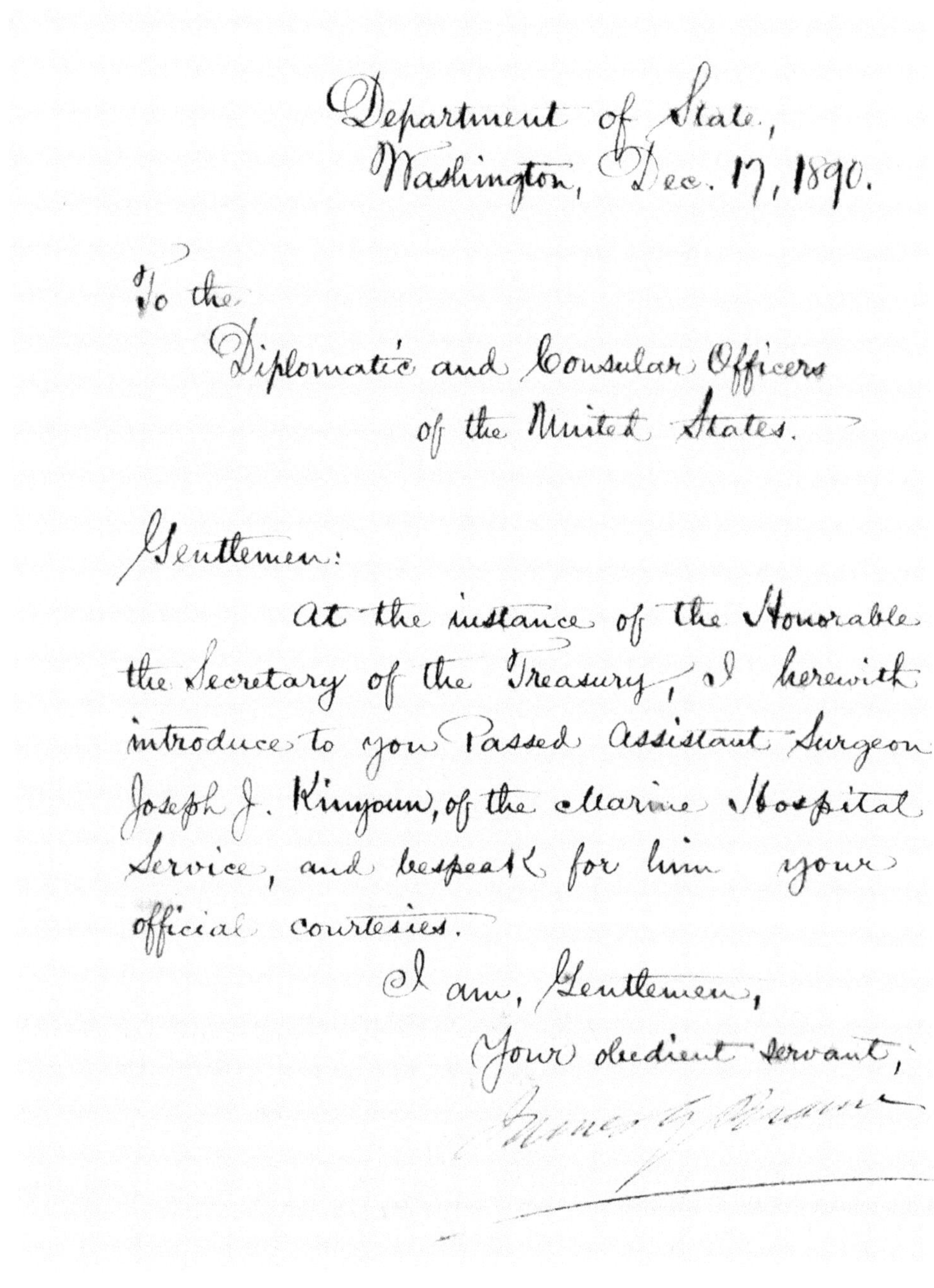

Department of State,
Washington, Dec. 17, 1890.

To the
Diplomatic and Consular Officers
of the United States.

Gentlemen:

At the instance of the Honorable the Secretary of the Treasury, I herewith introduce to you Passed Assistant Surgeon Joseph J. Kinyoun, of the Marine Hospital Service, and bespeak for him your official courtesies.

I am, Gentlemen,
Your obedient servant,

United States State Department letter of introduction for Joseph J. Kinyoun from James G. Blaine, December 17, 1890.

make an appearance, as well."[22] She wrote, "Monday night is always Royal night(,) evening dress is required."[23] Apparently, either a custom or an official event occurred every Monday evening, requiring ladies to be dressed in formal attire. This might have been when foreign dignitaries called on the crown, as part of diplomatic protocol.

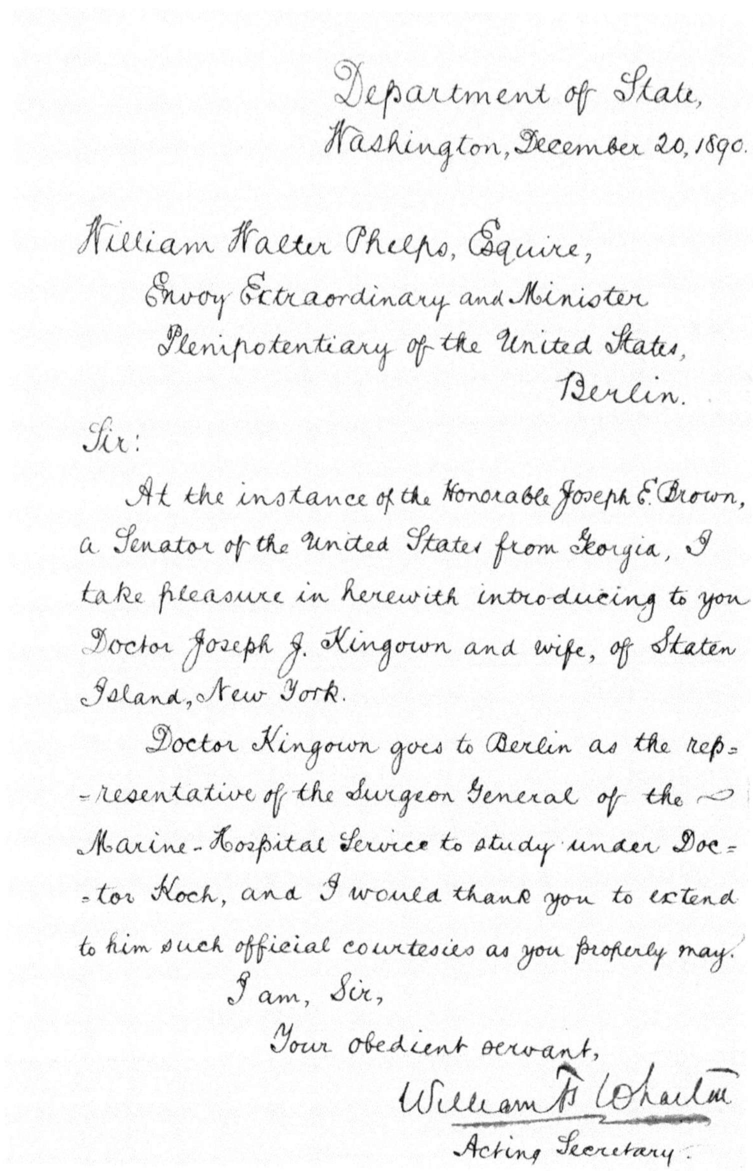
Department of State,
Washington, December 20, 1890.

William Walter Phelps, Esquire,
Envoy Extraordinary and Minister
Plenipotentiary of the United States,
Berlin.

Sir:

At the instance of the Honorable Joseph E. Brown, a Senator of the United States from Georgia, I take pleasure in herewith introducing to you Doctor Joseph J. Kingown and wife, of Staten Island, New York.

Doctor Kingown goes to Berlin as the rep-resentative of the Surgeon General of the Marine-Hospital Service to study under Doc-tor Koch, and I would thank you to extend to him such official courtesies as you properly may.

I am, Sir,
Your obedient servant,
William F. Wharton
Acting Secretary.

Letter of introduction to William Walter Phelps, Esquire, envoy extraordinary and minster plenipotentiary of the United States, Berlin, introducing Dr. Joseph J. Kinyoun and his wife from William F. Wharton, acting secretary, Department of State, December 20, 1890.

The last part of the correspondence centered on Alice, who would have been a little over a year and a half.[24] With some amusement in her pen, she explained how her daughter "writes,"[25] or more likely scribbles, every day, as if she were writing a letter to her grandfather. Lizzie concluded by saying that she takes Alice on walks, and every time she sees a dog,[26] she "barks."[27] Alice, or Allie as she would eventually be called by her grandchildren, loved dogs. By the time of her death in 1974, she claimed to have had a total of 42 during her lifetime.[28]

In a January letter to her mother-in-law, Lizzie related how the daughter of the

United States minister to Berlin, Miss Phelps, had called upon her the same day the country was celebrating the emperor's birthday.[29] She wrote what a wonderful occasion the event had been, stating, "A great gala day with the people all over Germany. Grand procession of State carriages and gorgeous uniforms and grandeur generally. The sixth prince had been christened the day before."[30] Lizzie wrote they visited the Hohenzollern Museum the following day and had seen many of the royal family's personal effects.[31]

Originally, the doctor had been assigned to Dr. Koch's institute for 30 days. Within a short period, Hamilton extended his assignment indefinitely due to the extent of the research before him.[32] As a result, he imparted this information to Missouri Senator Cockrell, stating that his stay in Berlin had been changed to an indeterminate period. He stated that a leave of absence apparently through diplomatic channel would not be necessary.[33]

Hamilton confessed that, in his opinion, the government's interests would be best served by keeping him at Koch's lab indefinitely, until he had achieved the purpose for which he had been sent to Europe. As part of his duties, Kinyoun had to send weekly progress reports.[34] He was to fully study and comprehend the inner workings of the germ theory and not only send periodic updates, but bring this knowledge back to the United States.

As a sidebar, Hamilton wrote that he wanted "to establish him [Kinyoun] here as bacteriologist."[35] He further stated that a letter had been enclosed explaining what the Bureau had planned and he would greatly appreciate the senator's support in sponsoring the bill,[36] presently before the "Appropriations Committee."[37] As can be seen from this passage, the surgeon general needed Cockrell's support. On January 23, a measure to transfer the lab from New York to Washington, D.C., had been presented to the House Appropriations Committee.[38] On clearing the Committee, it would need legislative sponsorship in the Senate, which he sought from the senator. The measure would also place Kinyoun in charge of the new facility, now being called a bureau.[39]

As previously noted, the Cockrell and Kinyoun families had been close friends for many years. Hamilton liked what he saw in him and his aptitude for research, which explained why he had been sent to Europe. It only made good political sense to have the senator spearhead the bill, especially in light of their close family relationships and the doctor being from Missouri as well. If it came to pass, it could be a possible plum for the senator, too. It never hurts to promote a potential success story— as the young doctor was becoming—from one's home state, especially when the news may turn out to have significant positive results on a national scale.

In one of his weekly reports to Hamilton, dated February 28, 1891, he wrote about his ongoing studies at the Hygiene Institute of Berlin. He stated that his work continued to progress and had actually increased because many workers had left the laboratory for some unexplained reason. Since January 3, he had been concentrating on two fields of study.[40] They involved "the production of a lymph for tuberculosis and studies in immunity to disease."[41] He also provided an account about two cases of tuberculosis he had been observing that had been receiving Koch's treatment[42] at the "…ni Chante' Heospitue."[43] Kinyoun related how the first case had recovered completely and the second had improved greatly, indicating the patient would recover.[44]

The letter, though, pointed out several issues with the treatment. First, he explained it must be administered for a lengthy period.[45] And, "at the same time I am more convinced that the remedy has but a very small range of usefulness, and is only applicable to those that are in the first stage of the disease."[46] He wrote that a gentleman named Lecnech had informed the Berlin Medical Society of "remarkable success in the treatment of tuberculosis by using Potassium Caulthardate in minute doses of 0.0002."[47] But he disputed this claim by stating that unless more was accomplished,[48] "no conclusion can be drawn."[49]

The report showed that Kinyoun had experienced, firsthand, the inner workings of microorganisms and how new experimental treatments had started making a difference. In some cases, there appeared to be progress, and in others more research needed to be conducted before a particular methodology could be considered successful. Although learning new techniques, he did not accept things at face value, as seen in his comments about Koch's treatment of tuberculosis. With his own education and experience, he looked at these European advancements with a learned eye.[50] He had to see "convincing proof of a treatment's success"[51] before he would accept its findings. As he observed about the procedure, it worked best when applied early, but more needed to be achieved before its results could be called conclusive.[52]

As part of his research, he maintained articulate logs on the cases he studied. The journal's format resembled a modern-day spreadsheet, listing the cases, or patients, on the left side of a checker-boxed sheet with top headings identifying nine procedures. The remaining boxes charted the patients' progress as each responded to the various procedures. This grid format showed how scientific application had been condensed into a written tracking system.[53] This probably had become standard by the European medical and scientific community. However, it also reverted back to the American Civil War, where the doctor's father kept a medical journal of his patients' afflictions and their progress, as had been mandated by the Confederacy's Surgeon General Samuel Preston Moore.[54]

Official Report

In the 1891 annual report, Kinyoun described in great detail his experiences at Koch's laboratory. He acknowledged that all previous arrangements had been fully complied with by Professor von Esmarch, Jr. The professor introduced him to the laboratory and set him up with those areas of interest he had requested. Esmarch had been appointed to act on behalf of Koch, who at the time was in Egypt.[55] In his absence,

Kinyoun reported, the professor would have "immediate supervision of my work."[56] The doctor stated Berlin had not only become the "military capital of Europe"[57] but also the "Mecca for physicians and tuberculous [sic] patients"[58] because of Koch's treatment. He proceeded to explain in detail the functions of the laboratory and the effects of the remedy, noting that Koch had remained quite secretive as to the elements of his discovery.[59] Much to his surprise, the medical community had developed a "mercenary spirit"[60] in attempting to learn its compounds,[61] and apparently he had found this "amusing."[62] He revealed that the city had a large hospital full of tuberculosis patients, most of whom were in the last stages of the disease and would soon perish. Adding to the influx was the worst winter Germany had experienced in 30 years.[63]

The death rate had soared, with every hospital at maximum capacity. Everyone wanted to receive Koch's lifesaving injection, and physicians hovered at the hospitals wanting to observe its effect. Because of the patient overload, arrangements had been made for Kinyoun to observe and study cases at the Charite and Moabit Hospitals. Professor Gerhardt made these accommodations for him, and he would spend the next four months studying countless cases of tuberculosis.[64]

He reported that the death rate at each hospital had become very high.[65] He wrote how Dr. Virchow, considered the father of modern pathology,[66] had given him full access to all demonstrations and examinations conducted at the Pathological Institute.[67] Virchow had become famous for proving that cells are the basic building blocks of human construction and that disease invaded cells resulting in sickness. He also espoused that disease stemmed from society's social ills and lack of sanitation.[68]

After examining numerous cases, Kinyoun concluded that Koch's vaccine had both a positive and a negative aspect. He concluded that if the treatment was administered early to the patient, then the results proved positive, resulting in recovery. To the contrary, though, if the disease had become advanced, then the treatment appeared to accelerate the illness, resulting in death. In postmortem tests conducted on a patient's sputa, the results showed no effect on the tubercle bacilli. This proved to be a surprise as to the overall value of Koch's cure.[69]

On the heels of this revelation, Virchow challenged the positive effects of Koch's tuberculin serum after conducting autopsies on victims. Contrary to its purported value, he claimed it could hasten a patient's death. He theorized that the treatment had caused a necrosis, or gangrene reaction, mirroring pneumonia of those cells harboring and emerging near the tubercle bacilli. As the necrotic cells would break away, it triggered the release of tuberculosis cells throughout other areas of the body through its transmission systems.[70] Virchow called tuberculin "a poison capable of great harms, and stated that the majority of deaths that occurred during its use were directly attributed to it."[71]

This statement sent shock waves through the medical realm with most of Koch's supporters contesting Virchow's findings. At the time of his announcement, Koch remained in Egypt. However, an apparent rebellion now ensued among the various medical camps.[72] As an outsider to this conflict, Kinyoun observed:

> It must be stated here that all observation goes to show that it is an inherent custom among the Teutonic nations, in their scholastic training, to choose a master and follow his tenets blindly, never giving nor receiving from any other, unless overwhelmed and vanquished by opposing facts and arguments.[73]

The rebellion soon died down, when countries reported similar findings, leading to Koch's followers reexamining the treatment. In time, they modified the serum and decided that a lesser dosage caused only a local reaction to the tuberculin, as opposed to accelerating the disease.[74] The approach now became "to assist nature, not as was formerly advocated."[75] The result increased cures.[76] This medical episode, or scientific upheaval, would also add to his education. It showed him how a once respected medical standard could come under question and lead to a broader scope of discussion and argument. Within nine years, he would experience the same turbulence in San Francisco over the plague.

Koch returned from Egypt and commenced modifying his tuberculin serum. He changed the substance from a liquid base to a compound crafted from precipitation. Other improvements were made to the serum that increased its effectiveness. He went so far as to acknowledge that he had not been completely convinced of its total curative prowess. In defense of the remedy, he professed its usefulness and felt it still had a positive value, if only in five percent of tuberculosis patients.[77]

Although many in the European medical community had questioned its application, he noted the Americans had abandoned its use, drawing his criticism. Even so, he encouraged his colleagues to conduct more research and improve the serum in light of its shortcomings. In response to his request, Kinyoun pointed out that at present the Hygienic Institute did not have the necessary scientific mechanical means to accommodate Koch's request.[78]

In other parts of his report, he spoke of associations with many other medical scientists of the time, including Dr. Thomas Weyl and Professor Proskauer. Weyl had conducted chemical research on tuberculosis and published an article concerning the toxic nature of tuberculin. He also spoke of work on protozoa and research conducted by Kartulius in Alexandria, Egypt, on dysentery.[79]

Before leaving, Kinyoun studied alongside three other medical giants of the period, Dr. Kitasato Shibasaburō of Japan, Dr. Emil Behring of Germany and Dr. Ernest H. Hankin of Britain, all also at the laboratory.[80] Kitasato had made the discovery of bubonic plague in 1894, along with Dr. Alexandre Yersin, with the latter receiving the credit for the finding.[81] Hankin had become a noted bacteriologist in his own right. At the same time, Kitasato and Behring performed experiments on immunizations on animals, in particular tetanus. Conversely, the treatment proved ineffective, resulting in the body's temperature rising and potentially making a patient's condition worse.[82]

Hankin shared his findings on immunizations concerning anthrax, which showed promise. He theorized that blood plasma contains bactericidal elements that he referred to as[83] "protective protein."[84] Through his trials, this element would increase, and it prevented the disease from afflicting other animals.[85] Kinyoun allowed: "If the theories of Kitasato, Behring and Hankin could be put into practical operation by immunizing persons against disease, the results would be all that could be desired."[86] It appeared a solution to the spread of disease had all but been unraveled for the world.

The Pasteur Institute

In April, Dr. Émile Roux of the Pasteur Institute, an eminent doctor in his own right, sent Kinyoun a note advising of his acceptance to study at the Institute.[87] In a dispatch from the United States legation in Paris, he received a diplomatic letter advising of his admission. It, too, acknowledged that his acceptance had been approved by Roux and directed him to arrive by May 5. The document had been signed by Bailly-Blanchard, Secretary.[88] After four months with Koch, he would now be studying at the most prominent medical research facility. Even Koch had acknowledged its greatness: he sent his architect to Paris to create a mirror image of Pasteur's facility as he started planning for a new laboratory in Berlin.[89]

Kinyoun had been sent to Paris to study

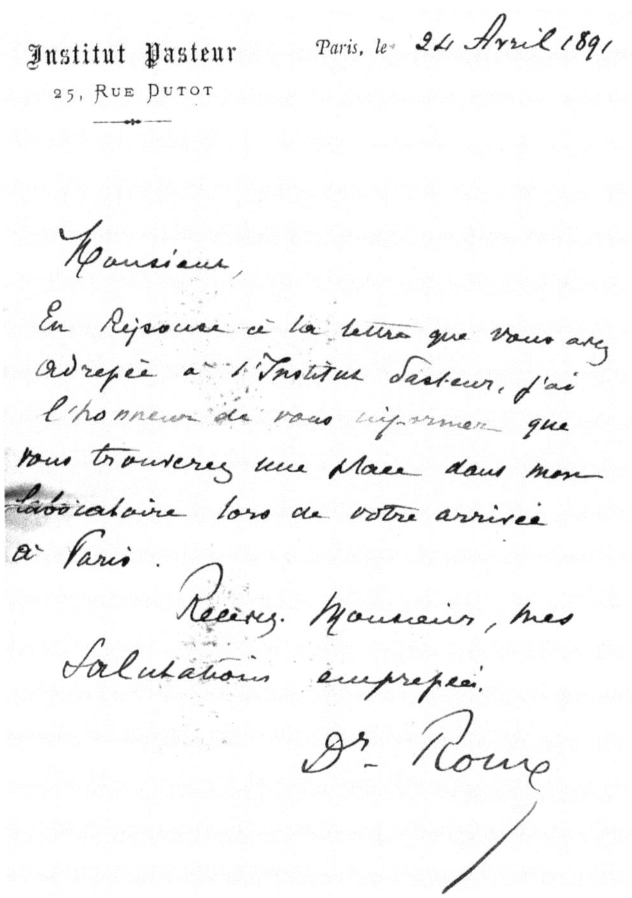

Institut Pasteur
25, Rue Dutot

Paris, le 24 Avril 1891

Monsieur,

En Réponse à la lettre que vous avez adressée à l'Institut Pasteur, j'ai l'honneur de vous informer que vous trouverez une place dans mon laboratoire lors de votre arrivée à Paris.

Recevez, Monsieur, mes salutations empressées.

Dr Roux

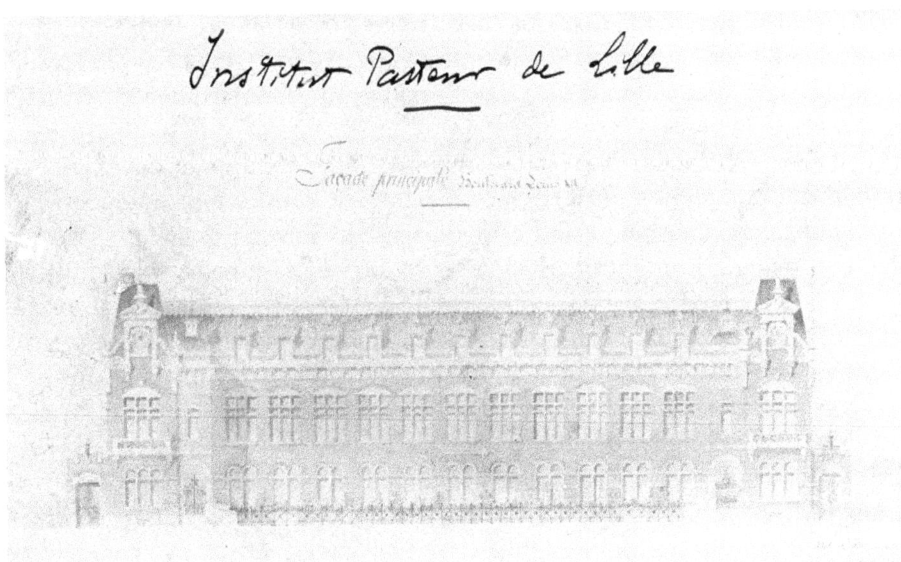

Top: **Letter from Émile Roux approving Kinyoun's admission to the Pasteur Institute, April 24, 1891.** ***Above:*** **Institut Pasteur.**

Pasteur's research and success with rabies. He even acknowledged in his report that the name Pasteur was usually used in reference to the disease. However, he pointed out such characterization to be far from the truth. In fact, he described it as the best research laboratory in existence. It not only focused on bacteriology, but biology and chemistry, in addition to rabies.[90]

In a rough draft of his weekly report to Hamilton, the doctor described the institute's floor plan,[91] commenting that

> ... the ground floor contains two laboratories—one for the preparation of the material used for inoculations against the rage [most likely in reference to rabies] and for the treatment of the cases. Another for the production and distribution of the special vaccine used for the protection against anthrax.[92]

On the second floor, he described the presence of two large laboratories for bacteriological and chemical usage with each being under the direct control of Drs. Roux and Duclaux.[93] The third floor had been set up for what he referred to as "private work special research, especially in matters pertaining to zoology, nephrology, which is under the direction of Prof. Metchnikoff."[94]

He next turned his report to rabies and its treatment. Kinyoun allowed how at first he had been skeptical about its effectiveness and the supporting statistics,[95] suspecting they may have been "padded"[96] by the French. But he later recanted his opinion, stating that further analysis had shown the disease to be very common on the continent. As an aside, he noted every effort had been taken to arrive at an accurate accounting of the afflicted and those cured. It had become required that every animal purportedly having the disease be certified by a veterinarian after examination of a piece of the animal's brain and spinal cord. Statistically, 80 percent of the cases had been verified through this process as positive for rabies.[97]

He revealed that 10,445 cases had been treated from 1886 to 1891, with an average mortality rate of 74 percent. Yet the rate had been decreasing each year, resulting in a mortality of 32 percent in 1890, a significant improvement from 1886, when it initially registered 94 percent.[98]

The reason for the change rested in a better understanding of the disease combined with the completion of the first research stage. Most important had been the decoding of the incubation period of the disease by Pasteur and Roux. They concluded that its length might be as short as 14 days or as long as six months. This discovery had resulted in the development of a better inoculation, thereby increasing the survival rate. Next, he discussed the chemical composition of the treatment and how various formulas generated different results. With this report, Kinyoun had shared this new treatment of rabies with the surgeon general in one of his weekly reports, thereby making it available to the United States.[99]

He explained how the institute provided daily inoculations to the public commencing at 11:00 a.m., noting that within 40 minutes 100 individuals can receive injections. Of additional interest, he related how the laboratory produced large amounts of the vaccine for distribution throughout France and to other countries. Kinyoun pointed out that the Institute generated considerable revenue through vaccine sales.[100]

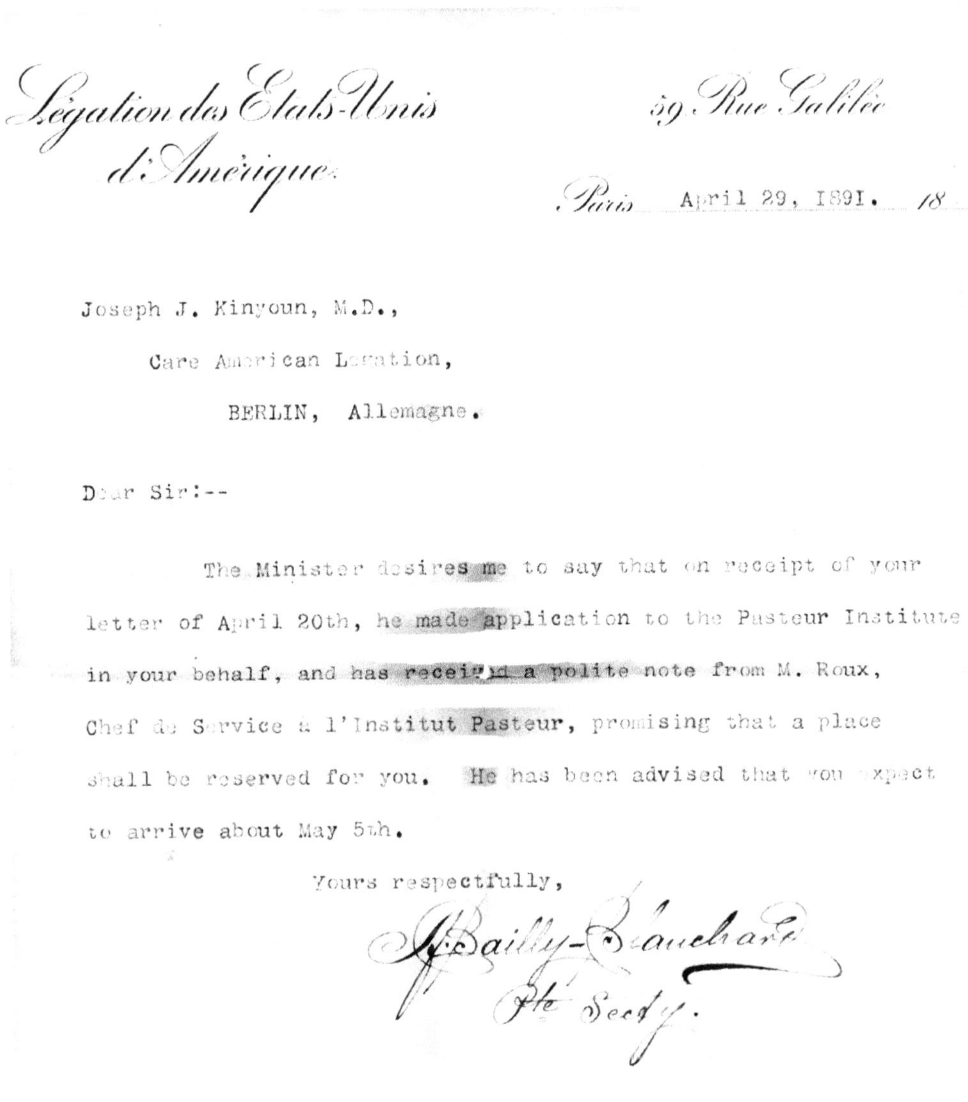

Légation des États-Unis d'Amérique. 59 Rue Galilée

Paris April 29, 1891. 18

Joseph J. Kinyoun, M.D.,

Care American Legation,

BERLIN, Allemagne.

Dear Sir:--

The Minister desires me to say that on receipt of your letter of April 20th, he made application to the Pasteur Institute in your behalf, and has received a polite note from M. Roux, Chef de Service à l'Institut Pasteur, promising that a place shall be reserved for you. He has been advised that you expect to arrive about May 5th.

Yours respectfully,

A. Bailly-Blanchard

2d Secy.

Diplomatic assignment from Bailly-Blanchard directing Kinyoun to the Pasteur Institute.

Of special note, he advised that another famous European physician had embarked on copying the Institute. In this case, Dr. Joseph Lister had replicated the Institute for Preventive Medicine, located in London, based on Pasteur's laboratory.[101] As evidenced by other research authorities constructing similar institutes modeled after Pasteur's, Kinyoun had been exposed to the world's very best medical lab.

He also wrote about studying under Élie Metchnikoff, who discovered the role of white blood cells, or the process of phagocytosis, where cells attack and devour bacteria when they enter the body. Metchnikoff showed how this process lead to the destruction of diphtheria and tetanus.[102] Kinyoun described him as "a patient, plodding, conscientious worker in everything he attempts to investigate."[103] In addition, he had written one of the most objective articles concerning the shortcomings of tuberculin. Metchnikoff brought forward the theory of antibodies in the bloodstream and immunity in organisms against disease.[104] On several occasions, he incurred the disdain of other members of the European medical community, but in the end his theory about phagocytes became the basis of a new understanding about the body's inner defenses.[105]

The Return

What had originally been billed as a month's study aboard had turned into a six-month sabbatical. While he had been overseas, changes had occurred at the Service. In particular, Surgeon General Hamilton had retired with Surgeon Walter Wyman appointed as his replacement. The doctor now returned to a new city and position, once again under the charge of his former supervisor.[106]

The first thing the doctor did was to collect his family and find a suitable home in Washington, D.C. Within a short period, they moved into a house at 210 New Jersey Avenue NW.[107] The family had been reunited and settled into a new setting full of promise and a fair amount of prestige.

After settling into his surroundings, he submitted his report to Wyman concerning developments at the Hygienic Laboratory for the preceding year, as part of the surgeon general's annual report for 1891. Since the doctor had been in Europe for half the year, most of it centered on his studies under the medical greats of Europe.[108]

At the report's end, he expressed his long-felt belief about how the Service should proceed for the betterment of the country:

> Since the laboratory has been removed from the Marine Hospital, New York, to the national capital, it has now the room and equipment requisite for proper work, and is available for general bacteriological investigations. It is hoped that appropriations commensurate with its importance will be forthcoming for its further enlargement. The subjects of hygiene and demography have not as yet received the proper amount of attention from our legislative bodies. This laboratory, situated and equipped as it is, should form the nucleus for one national in its character, and developed on the same lines as those established by Germany, France and England.[109]

With this said, he assumed command of the nation's new medical research facility nestled in the bosom of the capital.[110] As part of his report, Wyman advised the medical community that he would make sure the new laboratory would rival its European counterparts.[111] And Kinyoun stood ready to make this become a reality with his newfound knowledge.

Within a few months, Wyman increased Kinyoun's annual salary to $1,980.00, apparently to reflect his new position.[112] Now 31, he had become one of the country's leading experts and researchers on bacteriology. Although not alone, as far as the government, it was up to him to further transition the nation and its medical establishment towards the germ theory, plus provide the necessary instruction to perfect its conversion.

The next nine years could be considered a whirlwind. He would have repeated success in applying the Old World's new techniques to the New World's thought processes, establishing medicine as a science in the cure and eradication of disease. In many respects, this period could be described as not only a time of wonder, but also one of personal fulfillment.

VI

A Whirlwind of Discovery and Research: 1891–1894

A New Home

While Kinyoun was in Europe, Congress voted to move the Hygienic Laboratory to Washington, D.C.[1] The Kinyoun family moved with it. Shortly after arriving in the city, he became a professor at Georgetown University teaching bacteriology and hygiene. And from 1892 to 1899, he served as a professor of bacteriology and pathology.[2] His passion for learning became clearly evident.

Dissemination

His expertise had become became highly sought after. Before returning home, his findings had been presented in an article titled "Koch's Celebrated Lymph," printed in the *Atlanta Constitution* in the spring of 1891. He reported on an effective treatment for lupus, pointing out that while it was still expensive, the initial cost of $6,000 had decreased to $325.[3] He described how the lymph interacted with the disease, stating, "The lymph is a most deadly poison."[4] He reported that "in the first stages of a few selected cases it certainly does good,"[5] but that "in the second stage of the disease, so far as I have seen or can learn, it has in no instance been the least beneficial, but … dire results."[6]

Of major interest were his findings on rabies from the Pasteur Institute. As set forth in the Proceedings and Discussion at the Ninetieth Annual Meeting, held in Kansas City, Missouri, he read a paper on it.[7] His presentation also dealt with tuberculosis, revealing how one method of the disease's transmission was "through cow's milk."[8] He announced, "I do not think there is enough attention at present by sanitarians."[9] He related that the medical profession needed to employ a special system and apparatus to isolate the disease, as used in Germany.[10]

The same held true with diphtheria in its being passed through milk to children,[11] Kinyoun reported, noting that the best way to stop the spread of this organism was through "pasteurization,"[12] a scientific treatment whereby food in a liquid state is heated above boiling and then quickly reduced in temperature, thereby killing the bacteria, making the consumption of food products safer.[13] This new technique had been proven to greatly reduce infant mortality.[14]

The year 1892 proved to be a busy one for Kinyoun and the family. In early March, he received an assignment for special duty in New York.[15] Later in the month, he became chairman of the Board for Physical Examination of Candidates and Officers for the Service.[16] In April, Wyman appointed him as the recorder of the board.[17] His stature as a respected member of the Service had increased, significantly. It had only been six years since he had been examined by this board as a prospective candidate. Now, he served as its chair and sat in judgment of those seeking admission.

On August 13, a very special event occurred, not only for him, but for Lizzie and Alice as well. Lizzie delivered their third child, Joseph Perry Kinyoun. He had been named in honor of the doctor and Lizzie's maiden name. They would call him Perry.[18]

Following the birth, Kinyoun received several additional assignments. Within the course of a month he went to Baltimore, Philadelphia and New York. These travels involved quarantine inspections and supervision.[19]

In a September edition of *Abstract of Sanitary Reports*, he elaborated about his experience with disinfecting procedures.[20] He reported on the value of "heat as a disinfectant for clothing, bedding, textile fabrics, etc., that have been exposed to cholera infection."[21] In particular, he stated the temperature must exceed 100 degrees and be from steam heat.[22]

The report derived from his research abroad the previous year. As the article pointed out, he had experienced this process firsthand while in Berlin, London and Edinburgh witnessing the disinfecting stations and apparatuses used in the process. At the same time, he had been exposed to these techniques under the tutelage of Professors Koch, Kitasato, von Esmarch, and by Drs. Frosch and Theodore Weyl.[23]

He commented how Germany used disinfection procedures in its military branches, whereas the Russians did not[24]—an interesting observation, because as evidenced in earlier wars, the biggest killer of armies had been their exposure to infectious disease.[25] Overall, the article demonstrated the sharing of his new knowledge from Europe in hopes of educating others.

Rabies

Rabies is a fatal virus affecting the body's central nervous system. The most common transmission of the disease is from the bite of an infected animal, usually from a dog, bat, skunk, coyote, fox, or raccoon. Incubation upon being bitten can range from several weeks to a year. Victims can evidence signs of madness as the disease progresses in the brain and may exhibit a fear of water (hydrophobia). Inoculations have proven to be an effective treatment, if administered early, upon suspicion of exposure to the virus.[26]

Sometime in 1892, Kinyoun wrote an extensive paper titled "Rabies—Its Prevention and Treatment." It set forth what he had learned at the Pasteur Institute, examining the inner workings of this virus. He referred to it as a malady, transmittable from animal to animal. Further, he labeled it as a separate biological structure that should not be confused with other organisms bearing similar characteristics.[27]

He explained that the virus was mainly spread by infected canines and felines, citing dogs as the primary culprit. Russia, Spain and France had the largest number of cases ,with the southern and southeastern parts of Russia experiencing a greater toll because of wolves. He pointed out that Germany and Sweden had mostly eradicated the illness through strict enforcement procedures. Australia had remained devoid of the disease because of extensive quarantine measures. Kinyoun also dispelled the notion of rabies being a tropical illness, stating that its greatest presence occurred between December and May.[28]

Turning his focus to America, he noted laxity in addressing its prevention and treatment. He stated that skunks and dogs represented the primary carriers. After a bite by an infected animal, the disease's onslaught usually started within a minimum of six days to as long as a year, with the average being 40 days. Based on studies conducted by Dr. Roux at the Pasteur Institute, he noted that, upon entering the body, the virus gravitates to a nerve, where it proceeds through the nervous system to the brain. Roux pointed out that if the bite occurred close to the head or upper body it was more likely the incubation period would accelerate resulting in death. Furthermore, the more mentally advanced the animal, the shorter the incubation period, as noted in studies on dogs, horses and humans.[29]

Kinyoun outlined the disease's three phases, describing them as "1st, excitement of both motor and sensory systems; 2d, incoordination; 3d, paralysis."[30] Again referencing Roux, he described how the disease would become infectious within two to three days of contact. Although not initially noticeable, the body's temperature would start to rise after the third day. During its secretive period, glands begin spreading it throughout the body. Only in the third stage do the outward signs of its presence become manifest.[31]

Postmortem, the stomach shows traces of it along with the victim's spinal cord and brain. After setting forth the infectious process, he stated it had to be a microorganism. He acknowledged its elusiveness, but stressed that the disease dies a rapid death on exposure to oxygen. Air or heat also caused it to die. Lastly, he revealed that the virus does not appear in blood, possibly making its diagnosis more problematic.[32]

A considerable amount of his paper was devoted to treatment of the illness. Unfortunately for the infected person, the treatment required a series of inoculations, which could last upwards of 18 days with varying quantities per injection. Mortality transpired for two reasons: the individual waited too long to receive treatment or the bite happened in the upper portion of the body near the brain. The serum consisted of a small amount of the virus being injected daily, with each additional dose being increased slightly.[33] After describing the process, he stated that the side effects had been minimal and all lab assistants had been inoculated for their protection.[34] He praised Pasteur for developing the treatment, stating that it marked "an era in preventive medicine."[35]

Kinyoun stated that the mortality rate from rabies had continually declined in France since 1886, when the serum had been first introduced to the public. In 1886, the mortality rate had been 94 percent, but by 1890 it had decreased to 32 percent.

Another important factor in its prevention centered on the creation of other medical institutes resembling Pasteur's; 21 laboratories had recently become available in 11 countries for his treatment of rabies.[36]

As to the United States, it needed to take a more responsible role in the disease's abatement. Many towns had passed ordinances addressing the matter, he acknowledged, but enforcement appeared in many cases non-existent. He implored doctors to take the lead on educating the public and making sure laws were obeyed and enforced.[37]

He simplified the solution by offering three corrective measures in containing its further expansion and ultimate eradication. The measures were:

1. Quarantine of all imported dogs;
2. General muzzling of all dogs;
3. Preventive treatment of the disease in men.[38]

Quarantine Assignment

In September, he received orders to quarantine duty in New York to assist in supervising the disinfecting of several ships suspected of carrying cholera. He had proven his expertise after discovering the disease in the city's harbor in late 1887. This assignment would occupy him until late October. During his stay, he would inspect and disinfect the following ships: *State of Indiana*, *Herman*, *Massillia*, *Polaria*, *Nevada*, *Scandia* and *Bohemia*.[39]

On his arrival, he visited several quarantined ships on Swinburne and Hoffman Islands. The port's health officer, Dr. William T. Jenkins, placed him in charge of disinfecting those vessels harboring in the lower portion of the bay. His duties comprised no easy task because of several factors, including a shortage of manpower to assist him and crews unenthusiastic about helping. In time, he overcame these obstacles, but it still took him longer to accomplish his tasks.[40]

The one thing in his favor was his total understanding of the disinfection process. In most cases, a bichloride of mercury solution coupled with steam heat exceeding 100 degrees Celsius operated as the killing agent. All the ship's compartments had to be sealed for a minimum of two hours for the sanitization to be effective. Not only did the ship's quarters need processing, but all of its contents: bedding, clothing and even the life preservers.[41]

While treating the *Bohemia*, he ran into a unique problem involving a large group of Russians and their children. Cholera had broken out among the adults, and measles had become epidemic in their roughly 100 children.[42] Kinyoun noted their compartments were "in as filthy a condition as could be."[43] He commented how these people had little knowledge of cleanliness. Also, the mothers apparently had no idea how to use diapers because they were contaminated with feces, making conditions ripe for disease.[44]

Eventually he found the main culprit. It had spread through the food they had brought on board. In one day, 10 bushels of filth and food were removed from their compartments.[45] Yet none of the passengers or officers would lend a helping hand, pointing out their "lack of discipline and ... perfect indifference"[46] to the situation.

The doctor tried to remove the passengers from the *Bohemia* to another ship or one of the quarantine islands, but his requests received repeated denials. Unfortunately, five new outbreaks occurred on board. After two and half days, he received permission to transfer them to Hoffman Island. Immediately, he commenced cleaning the *Bohemia*. He burned most of the bedding, then disinfected the ship. He concluded that all quarantine stations should be furnished with the equipment he utilized in sanitizing the vessels.[47]

On returning to Washington, he wrote a brief memorandum about an article concerning diphtheria. Titled "Animal Immunity against Diphtheria," it discussed several of Emil Behring's experiments concerning the immunization of animals from this dreaded disease. The doctor took some exception to the author's findings, especially his claim that Behring did not have a consistent result with guinea pigs. Consequently, the author could not endorse Behring's methodology as being a reliable process in effectively immunizing animals.[48]

He remained primarily neutral in his memo, but it seemed apparent that he knew that not all methods proved initially successful and needed constant evaluation as to effectiveness. Nonetheless, another implication can be deduced from the paper. Kinyoun had witnessed how scientific research operated and therefore knew about its trials and errors.[49] Although this particular author had rejected Behring's findings, in time it might prove successful. An important aspect can be drawn from the report, and that is his ongoing research of diseases, in this case diphtheria.

Political Hankerings

Towards the end of the year, he received several letters from his father. The elder Kinyoun wanted to pursue an appointment from the Cleveland administration to be the ambassador to the Bahamas in Nassau.[50] He asked his son to submit the application, since he understood Washington's inner circles. For references, he listed Senators Vest, Cockrell, Ransom and Vance, along with references to Drs. Armen, Tarsury, and Morgan.[51]

In January, another letter arrived from his father. It contained his handwritten application addressed to the president seeking the position of Consul General of the Hawaiian Islands.[52] In his previous correspondence, he had sought the ambassadorship to the Bahamas.[53] Cleveland had become the first Democratic Party presidential candidate to win a presidential election (1884 and 1892) since before the Civil War.[54]

These were plum jobs, as today, for individuals contributing to or assisting in a candidate's election. The Democrats obviously relished the prospects of filling these positions with important and influential members of their constituency. Since the elder Kinyoun had been a longtime Democrat, he saw himself as a prospective nominee. Apparently, a list had been provided to him from which to make a selection. After looking over the other possibilities, he had decided only Hawaii would be acceptable.[55]

In a third letter, dated March 26, he reported receiving a "Letter of Endorsement" from Missouri Supreme Court Justice James Britton Gantt. However, in this case, the application had been changed from Consular of Hawaii to Cairo, Egypt.[56] It now appeared that his previous requests for assignment to the Bahamas and Hawaii had been turned down.

By August, he asked him to retrieve all the endorsements he had forwarded concerning his possible assignment to Cairo from the State Department.[57] A month later, in a letter to Lizzie, he wrote that he did not want any of the commendation letters back[58] because,

> ...as they have availed nothing, as they did in Washington as favors and appointments are made and given to their special friends regardless of merit or qualifications, and I want as little to do with this Mugruunp [sic] Administration as possible, I think it is soled [sic] out to a little Knot of Jesus in London, and what Mr. Cleveland wish or direct our Congress will do.
>
> Our Congress, both House and Senate have proved this Extraordinary Session that all have had more Mouth than Brains.[59]

Quarantine Regulations

The year 1893 proved to be another busy one for him. In a February communiqué, Wyman assigned him and five other members of the Service to a special committee.[60] They were directed to prepare "rules and regulations in accordance with the provisions of the recent Quarantine Act of Congress granting additional powers and duties for the Service."[61]

In a Senate and House Bill Memorandum issued the same week, the specific changes to the present law had been presented to committee for consideration. The memorandum stated that the Act did not change those sections of the 1878 quarantine law not annulled by the February 15, 1893, revisions. The 1889 law would remain unchanged concerning the commissioning of Marine Hospital Service officers. And the quarantine law of 1890 remained unchanged by the legislation.[62]

The act did alter and amplify three areas of importance. The first amendment changed the role of a state's and city's handling of quarantines.[63] The language was changed from "to co-operate, [sic] aid and assist State and Municipal Health Authorities in the enforcement of their rules and regulations"[64] to "to co-operate with and aid State and Municipal Health Authorities in the execution and enforcement of such needful rules and regulations as are deemed necessary."[65]

It should be pointed out that the text reading "needful rules"[66] had been highlighted in the report, stressing its importance. This change constituted a major shift, or transfer, in state and local authority in the handling of quarantines to the federal government. By this amendment, state and local laws could now be superseded by federal authority. What had once been a significant area of contention over governance had been determined in favor of not only the United States, but also its administrative agency, the Marine Hospital Service.[67]

The second amendment limited state and local quarantine powers. It specified that quarantine regulations, whether maritime, interstate, or foreign, were henceforward to be established by the commissioner of public health in conjunction with an "Advisory Board"[68] approved by the president, as opposed to the Secretary of the Treasury.[69] Once again, the phrase "Advisory Board"[70] had been underscored in the memorandum, stressing its importance. This represented another significant change to the previous statute by establishing a new governmental body. It would control all matters relating to quarantines, allowing it to direct regulations and to intervene on the state and local level.

The third amendment addressed the Hygienic Laboratory, stating: "The law establishing the Hygienic Laboratory is amplified, in the matter of regulations for its government, for details, etc., and the appointment of its Director."[71] By this amendment, the laboratory continued to be recognized and promoted as the leading scientific research body of the government.[72]

Combined with the second amendment, authority to promulgate regulations as to quarantine and health had become vested in his lab. At the age of 33, his career had in essence skyrocketed along with the importance of the laboratory in directing and dictating matters of public health. Another acknowledgment of his ability was his appointment to the advisory board that would assist the commissioner of public health in drafting quarantine regulations.

The World's Fair

In May, Wyman dispatched him to the World's Fair in Chicago to oversee the Service's exhibit, a replica of the Hygienic Laboratory.[73] Wyman wanted to tout the workings and importance of the Service at this exhibition. As part of this campaign, he addressed the 44th annual meeting of the American Medical Association (AMA) in Milwaukee, where he advocated for a uniform quarantine code. In his presentation, he spoke about an improved disinfection technique used in quarantines.[74] He gave the doctor credit for it, stating:

> A simple apparatus for carrying the gas cylinder from place to place, which at the same time can be used for weighing gas liberated, has been recently revised by Passed Assistant Surgeon Kinyoun, and may be seen in the Marine Hospital Service exhibit in the Government Building at the Columbian Exhibition.[75]

The exhibit contained three components: the first explained the purpose of the Service, the second its quarantine procedures against the entry of infectious disease, and the third the workings of the Hygienic Laboratory. As part of the display, statistics from 1871 were presented documenting all the annual medical examinations conducted by the bureau and showing how it had saved lives.[76] In order to give the exhibit a sense of realism, furniture, surgical equipment and books used in the laboratory had been reproduced so the public could visualize it firsthand.[77]

One of the more unique displays showed on a full-size, working model of a steam disinfecting machine. Another interesting section showed actual specimens of bacteria requiring disinfection.[78] The lab received special billing:

> The Laboratory of Hygiene consists of a complete Bacteriological Laboratory fully equipped with all the latest improved apparatus for investigating subjects pertaining to sanitary service.[79]

Towards the end of June, Kinyoun wrote Lizzie, complaining he had not heard anything from Washington concerning how long he would be stationed in Chicago. He expressed his boredom and said he hoped to be relieved of duty within a week. The letter, written on a Sunday, related that he had strolled through the fair and found most of the exhibits closed, including those from Japan, Great Britain, Italy and China.[80]

Of special note, he had toured the electricity building. Electricity and its illumination of buildings had recently become available, thanks to inventor Thomas Edison.[81] World fairs had always been a place of wonderment for the average person, allowing people the opportunity to see civilization's most recent discoveries and inventions. As a doctor, he was probably intrigued by this new use of electricity. Ironically, his facility stood as a scientific showcase, too, in this case the country's advancement in medical research.

Ellis Island

Not long after his return, he received an assignment to New York, mainly because of the return of cholera aboard arriving ships.[82] Of particular interest was a new immigrant processing center called Ellis Island, which had opened the year before on January 1, 1892. It had been established to augment the Service's quarantine and inspection duties.[83]

The location of Ellis Island in New York Harbor, being close to the New Jersey shoreline, made it ideal for such a task. The main building had been recently constructed, and the entire complex initially encompassed roughly 3.3 acres, but over the coming years more buildings would be erected, and through infill the island eventually would grow to 27.5 acres. Five years after its opening, the station burned to the ground. As an interesting twist to the fire's aftermath, the Treasury Department mandated henceforth all future buildings be constructed fireproof. The new inspection station opened on December 17, 1900, with 2,251 individuals passing through for inspection.[84]

The island had been established as an immigration clearing station under the control of the federal government and the Marine Hospital Service to assess the health of those individuals mainly arriving from Europe. Specifically, individuals were inspected for communicable diseases, especially the more deadly ones, like cholera and smallpox. As a rule, immigrants arriving as first- and second-class passengers did not have to go through Ellis Island, but instead received a visual on-board inspection. Because they could afford a more expensive ticket, they were thought to be people of means and therefore less likely to become wards of the government for financial or health reasons.[85]

Third-class or steerage passengers had to proceed through Ellis Island for examination. The ship quarters housing these people were usually in its bowels. More often than not the rooms were dirty and overcrowded, making the environment an incubator for disease. Another factor affecting this group stemmed from the origins of its members; they came mainly from Eastern and Southern Europe, where standards of health paled in comparison to Northern Europe. Many of them had been displaced due to persecution, famine, or war, compelling them to seek a better life in America.[86]

Although the steerage class had to go through the inspection process, most successfully passed the examination. Normally the inspections would last between three and five hours, depending on the number of daily arrivals and available staff.[87] Ellis Island processed in excess of 12,000,000 people during its tenure from 1892 to 1954.[88]

By 1954, immigration had decreased considerably because of national quota limitations. Also, the former processing of immigrants had been transferred to American embassies, or consular offices, in the country of origin, thereby eliminating the need of the island's services. In 1965, President Lyndon B. Johnson made it part of the Statue of Liberty monument, thereby insuring its preservation as a historic American icon.[89]

Cholera Again

Wyman's instructions to Kinyoun on arriving in New York were quite direct.[90] They stated:

> Your detail is that of inspector M.H.S., in the interests of medical officers of the Marine Hospital Service detailed for duty in the immigration bureau, who must certify to the safety of immigrants and baggage passed through the immigration station and in the interests of the interstate quarantine … please show these instructions to Dr. Jenkins (New York City Health Officer).[91]

This directive was precipitated by the discovery of new cases of Asiatic cholera on board the ship *Karamania*. The vessel had arrived on August 3, from Naples, Italy, and had been immediately detained. It had 21 cases that had resulted in three deaths.[92] The quarantine officer asked for the Service's assistance, so Wyman sent Kinyoun. Within the first paragraph, he cited the recently enacted Quarantine Act empowering the Service as the primary operative in containing the outbreak.[93]

He had been selected for this assignment for several reasons. Primarily, he had previously studied cholera and identified its occurrence in New York Harbor as part of his initial duties upon joining the Service. His boss at the time had been Wyman, who had confidence in his abilities. The surgeon general wanted him in charge because he had the experience. Equally important, he knew the city's public officials, the port and the quarantine facilities, and could thus proceed faster than someone else in addressing the situation.

In late August, Dr. Bailhache and Kinyoun investigated two deaths in Jersey City on the other side of the harbor.[94] The following day, he reported that one of the deaths had been from cholera. Based on this confirmation, the New York Board of Health requested a meeting with Wyman. Over the next several days, he met with public health and political officials from New York and New Jersey and reviewed with them the new Quarantine Act. He also complimented them on their early actions to abate and correct the situation.[95] By early September, no new cases had surfaced, which allowed Bailhache and Kinyoun to return to New York.[96]

Supplementing the doctors, Wyman had summoned Surgeon H.W. Sawtelle, along with Assistant Surgeon J.A. Nydeggar. Accompanying them were four private surgeons, three state board of health officers, and Dr. A. Clark Hunt, the state sanitation inspector. Dr. Bond rounded out the task force representing the board of health from New York City.[97] Wyman had assembled this group on having been requested by the New Jersey State Board of Health to intervene in the disease's containment.[98]

One may question the need for such an array of physicians. Initially, the assemblage had been formed for two very important reasons. First, the *Karamania* had docked earlier with 21 cholera cases and 3 deaths, meaning the disease continued to enter America. Second, Wyman had used the new Quarantine Act in responding to the danger and to project its expanded authority. The reason for this conclusion can be derived from two communiqués, wherein he stressed the authority of the new Congressional legislation in dealing with matters of quarantine.[99]

In October the *Russia* arrived from Hamburg, Germany containing 460 passengers with five having died, accompanied by two suspicious cases. One person had died on arrival, and postmortem tests proved the cause to be cholera. The other passengers were transferred to Hoffman Island and Swinburne Island for disinfection and observation. Later, on Swinburne Island, another passenger succumbed to the illness. Eventually, five passengers would die from the contagion.[100]

In mid–October, the doctor reported on the quarantine of the *Lyderhorn*, a Norwegian vessel. It, too, received a thorough fumigation, after which the local health officer issued a certificate of disinfection. The cost for the service was a mere $10.00.[101]

By late November, he must have been worn out from his job, because he requested a 30-day leave of absence. The leave was granted on December 4.[102] But on December 9 Wyman appointed him as the recorder of the board charged with the task of revising the quarantine regulations.[103]

As 1893 came to an end, the family received a telegram dated December 30 from Kate Houx, telling them that cousin Bob Houx had died the day before. The Houxs were relatives of Lizzie's on her mother's side.[104] Besides this sad news, the year overall had been a good one for the family. The doctor's intellect and experience continued to be relied upon by his superiors with his stature growing beyond the Service. His European education had made him not only an important asset for the agency, but also an integral part of its operations.

1894: Forward Steps

In his annual address to the Treasury Department concerning the affairs of the Service, Wyman gave a brief introductory overview of its operations.[105] He outlined its most important undertakings for fiscal year 1894:

1. Hygienic Laboratory of the Marine-Hospital Service.
2. Sanitary reports and statistics.
3. Sanitary inspection service.
4. The national quarantine stations.
5. Revision of maritime quarantine regulations.

6. Promulgation of interstate quarantine regulations.
7. Enforcement of quarantine regulations.
8. Relations of the national quarantine system to State and Local quarantines.
9. Prevalence of cholera, yellow fever, smallpox, plague, and leprosy, and special efforts of the Service to prevent the introduction or spread of the same.[106]

Kinyoun's lab ranked number one on Wyman's list. As to all these other points, he had been extensively involved with each of them. Although other surgeons in the Service assisted in these areas, in a majority of these he stood out as a leader. As the ensuing year would soon demonstrate, he continued to advance in his education and knowledge.[107] Medical research combined with its understanding and application for the nation's well-being had no boundaries for him.

The Quarantine Act of 1893 aroused suspicion from various sectors of the country. Knowing his father would take exception to it as an infringement on a state's administration of its affairs, he had tried making the distinction between supervising germs and supervising a state and its governance.[108] Kinyoun also received a letter from Dr. Richard Lewis, secretary of the North Carolina Board of Health, echoing these same sentiments. He did not like matters being centralized in the government.[109] As with any major change, the ways of old have always been hard to relinquish when confronted with the future.

Besides quarantine legislation, several important initiatives had been undertaken by him and the government. The first occurred in February, when the Honorable G.W. Shell, chairman, Committee on Ventilation and Acoustics of the United States House of Representatives, wrote to Wyman and asked him to witness a test of the Shaw Gas Tester. The apparatus would be used to examine the air quality in the House Chamber. He replied to the representative and said Kinyoun would attend the demonstration on behalf of the Service.[110]

After witnessing the experiment, he wrote a report detailing his inspection of the House of Representatives and its surroundings.[111] He cited numerous statistics in support of his findings. The analysis showed high levels of carbon dioxide, ammonia and illuminating gases. Carbon dioxide occurred mainly in the boiler room and cellar, where discarded stationery and other trash had started decomposing. Because of poor ventilation, the air did not circulate sufficiently, thereby causing much of the problem. The high increase in carbon dioxide had resulted from the exhalation of humans, as documented by the number of people in the House Chamber.[112]

Ammonia originated from respiration, followed by decomposing material found in the basement, floors and grates. Illuminating gases arose from the lighting system, where the pipes were found to be leaking. Other exceptions to the air quality had been traced to cigar smoke, spittoons and other discharges. Kinyoun recommended a whole host of corrective measures that would not be too expensive. He forwarded these recommendations to Henry Adams, the supervising architect for the House. Consequently, his findings resulted in renovations to the entire building.[113]

Concerning the second initiative, Kinyoun had written to Wyman asking him to expand the staff of the Hygienic Laboratory. He initially praised him for having supported the lab in its evolution. Yet he criticized its present state, especially its move to Washington, D.C. He stated New York offered a better setting because of its many hospitals, citing the Willard Parker and Reception Hospitals, followed by the New York Quarantine Station, the Immigration Hospital, North Brothers Island Hospital and the Marine Hospital, as examples.[114]

He argued these institutions provided all the necessary materials to detect and control disease. It seemed he had become very accustomed to these various facilities and disliked his new surroundings. He commented that, assuming the facility would not be returned to New York, the lab needed its own building, as opposed to being combined with the administrative portion of the Service.[115]

In support, he pointed out how the agency, through legislation, had greatly changed from its original purpose of attending to "sick and disabled seamen"[116]; now it supervised the health and well-being of the country.[117] He noted that the bureau now must administer all quarantines, which involved inspections and disinfections; maintain an immigration station for the medical examination of immigrants; and supervise not only maritime quarantines, but also foreign quarantine stations. The Service, he argued, should have the highest trained and experienced personnel to fulfill these responsibilities.[118]

Pressing his argument, he wrote:

> In no branch of medicine has the advance been so rapid as in that of preventive sanitation, and none more important or conducive of good.
>
> The discovery of the causes of disease, their prophylaxis and treatment, are being put to a practical test in our system of prevention, and it behooves every member of the Marine Hospital Service to be fully identified with all the advances made therein and to be in the lead.[119]

As a solution, he proposed all members of the bureau be trained in the science of bacteriology at the lab and be instructed in quarantine disinfection. He concluded by stating that his proposed solution had been discussed with several of his colleagues and they would be willing to attest to its validity. Those individuals in support included Surgeon H.R. Carter and Passed Assistant Surgeons J.H. White, P.M. Carrington and R.M. Woodward.[120]

The request must have fallen on deaf ears, because he sent a follow up letter to Wyman. Again, he implored him to take heed of his previous suggestions. It appeared Kinyoun did not like Washington because he further stressed the importance of the facilities and hospitals in New York. In this correspondence, he took a different approach. He stated that to study and combat disease the laboratory had to either move back to New York or have a separate building.[121]

One would have thought he would have been enjoyed having an entire floor for the lab on its move to the capital, especially on his return from Europe with all his newly acquired knowledge. Originally he had praised the transition. But the lab had become an integral part of the Service, as evidenced by it being placed in the same building. The political advantages of being in Washington and in the bosom of the Service would have seemed extraordinarily beneficial for him and for the laboratory. However, it appeared the quarters lacked what he previously had in New York. These letters showed his true passion in medicine, which boiled down to research alone, and having the best facilities available.

Several things had become clear in these letters. First, he foresaw the need for the agency to expand the training of its officers. Second, he appeared convinced that scientific and medical research was the mainstay of eradicating maladies. He went so far as to assert, "I feel that the solution of the yellow fever problem will be a matter of comparative ease."[122] This would be possible only if he and others were given the needed tools and accommodations. He concluded his second request stating:

> It would be my purpose to commence the investigation in the following order; viz.: the pathology and causation of small-pox, of vaccina, varicella, measles, scarlet fever, typhus and yellow fever.[123]

Most of his repeated demands would eventually come to pass, except moving the lab back to New York. Wyman knew he had a good thing in not only the Hygienic Laboratory, but Kinyoun, too, and he meant to keep both by his side. Not all would be lost, because the lab would continue to expand under his watch, although maybe not at the pace he envisioned for it and his own pursuits. One final observation based on these letters: he ran the risk of being overly persistent.

During this period, Wyman had kept Kinyoun busy with other matters. In April, he had sent him to Wilmington, Delaware, for the purpose of meeting Mr. Francis of the Kensington Engine Works.[124] The company had been working on a special disinfectant barge named the *Zamora*,[125] which operated as a sulfur furnace.[126] He instructed him to review the plans, specifications and pricing for the apparatus. On completion of its construction, the ship would be transferred to Ship Island. He also asked him to meet with Passed Assistant Surgeon Glennan regarding the price of painting the barge copper.[127]

Because of this meeting, he and Francis became partners in the invention and production of several disinfectant machines. These were the Kinyoun-Francis portable sulfur fumigator, the Kinyoun-Francis portable steam disinfector and the Kinyoun-Francis steam disinfecting chamber. By himself, he invented the Kinyoun formaldehyde gas generator. Each of these inventions had been designed and used for disinfecting ships, along with cargo suspected of harboring disease.[128] What had become a passion for research had now turned into a practical integration of knowledge into the combination of scientific discovery and mechanical application. In essence, his inventions provided the means for the Service to eradicate the invisibles killing mankind.

Wyman also sent him to attend the annual meeting of the North Carolina State Board of Health at the Board President's request. His orders directed that he explain to the gathering the recent changes in the Quarantine Act outlining the government's new position concerning interstate quarantine and maritime matters. He had, in other words, been sent as the Service's liaison concerning its expanding control over all things quarantine.[129]

Opposite, top: **Kinyoun-Francis Disinfecting Machinery, & Quarantine-Station Plan, manufactured by Kensington Engine Works, Ltd. Francis Brothers. Beach and Vienna Streets, 704 Arch Street, Philadelphia.** ***Bottom:*** **Kinyoun-Francis Disinfecting Machinery, U.S. Marine Hospital Service, Portable Chamber.**

International Congress and Diphtheria

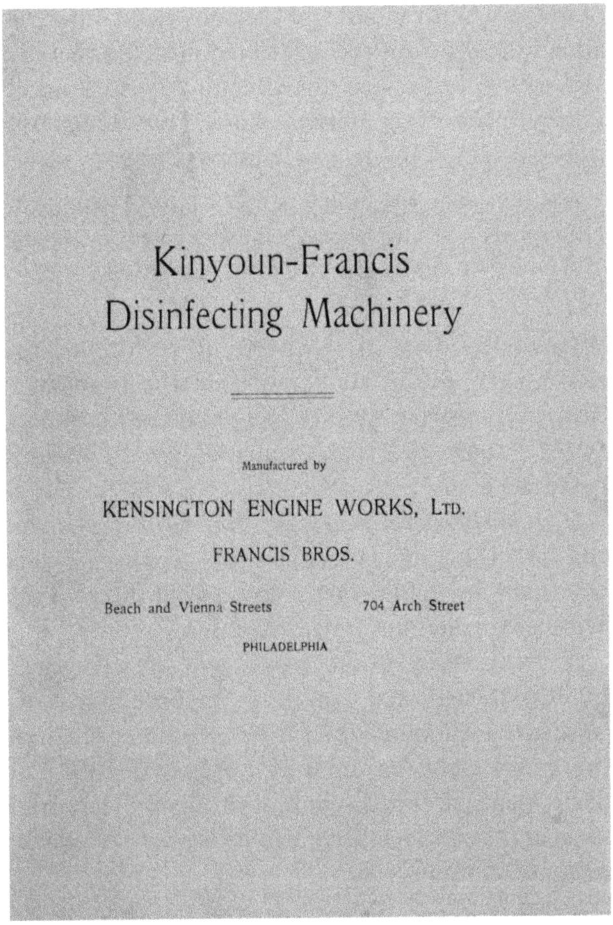
Kinyoun-Francis
Disinfecting Machinery
Manufactured by
KENSINGTON ENGINE WORKS, LTD.
FRANCIS BROS.
Beach and Vienna Streets
704 Arch Street
PHILADELPHIA

Diphtheria is a bacterium causing a high fever, weakness and the formation of a false membrane within the throat making breathing difficult. The disease is highly infectious and can be extremely fatal if left untreated.[130]

Kinyoun asked Wyman for permission to attend the upcoming Eighth International Congress of Hygiene and Demography being held in Budapest in September.[131] Before receiving a response, he went ahead and booked his passage through the Hamburg American Packet, Co. The company responded by providing free transit.[132]

He reminded Wyman

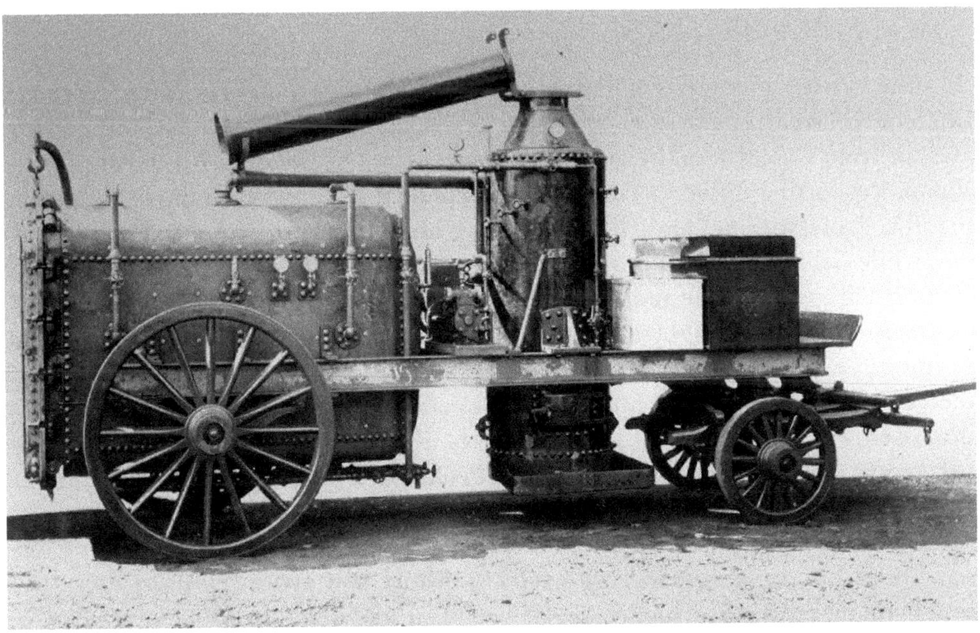

of his previous request in September 1891, after returning from Europe wanting to attend the next conference. Kinyoun stated that his attendance would be in the best interests of the Service, allowing him the opportunity to learn the newest techniques. Furthermore, the conference would be attended by most of the world's greatest medical scientists.[133] In summarizing, he wrote:

> Personally, and officially, I feel that so long as I am engaged in such investigations (scientific) it is my duty to take advantage of every opportunity afforded, to better fit myself for the discharge of my duties, especially so, when my motives are prompted by the interest which I have for the Service.[134]

Wyman approved his request and proceeded to ask the Secretary of the Treasury's permission. He stated that the Imperial and Royal Government of the Austro-Hungarian Empire had previously invited a representative from the United States,[135] suggesting that, from a diplomatic standpoint, someone should attend the conference.

He advised the secretary that sending Kinyoun would benefit the Service. In addition, the agency would pay his expenses. And since he would already be on the continent, he should spend upwards of three weeks in Bologna, Italy, studying preventive inoculations under Professor Tizzoni.[136]

On his return from Europe, he wrote a lengthy report about his experiences. The Eighth International Congress consumed most of his report, but his travels afterwards covered many other areas. He stated that the Congress focused primarily on preventive medicine and the etiology of disease. Concerning demography, few of the participants attended sessions on this subject, preferring instead those on hygiene; most of the conferees were bacteriologists.[137] Kinyoun appeared in awe of the various delegates, commenting:

> Perhaps there has never been a more brilliant assemblage of scientists at any meeting of the congress than those attending this. The delegations from the several countries of Europe were composed of men whose reputation was world-wide.[138]

The various medical scholars presented numerous papers on their research. Cholera received considerable attention as discussed by Élie Metchnikoff and Dr. Hassan from Calcutta on behalf of Dr. Ernest Hart in London. Mr. Gruber from Vienna set forth a different view on the virulence of cholera, contrary to Metchnikoff's. Professor Pagliani from Rome gave an address on quarantine methodology, while Celli, also from Rome, discussed pathogenic amoebae. Dr. Laveran spoke about malaria, but no one addressed yellow fever.[139]

One of the most important topics at the Congress was "Immunity and Immunization."[140] Those presenting papers on the subject consisted of a "Who's Who" of medicine: Metchnikoff, Buchner, Denys, Loeffler and Roux. The primary malady discussed within this context was diphtheria. Kinyoun cited Loeffler as giving the best report and commended Roux as well. Professor Welch, representing the United States and Johns Hopkins University, gave a bacterial analysis of the disease, which received favor among the delegates.[141]

Of all the presenters, he reported that Roux had given the most definitive insight on diphtheria and his serum. He had been studying the disease at the Pasteur

Institute for four years and had examined 600 cases. In initial observations of Paris hospital patients, the morality rate had been in excess of 50 percent. However, after his treatment the death rate had decreased to 26 percent.[142] Kinyoun stated that his paper clearly opened "up a broad field in the domain of preventive medicine."[143]

After the Congress, he had been ordered to visit Professor Tizzoni in Italy.[144] But the professor said he would be unable to meet with him until November.[145] In the meantime, he had been invited by Roux to visit the Pasteur Institute to learn more about the diphtheria serum.[146] During his stay at the Institute, he studied recently acquired cultures of the bubonic plague forwarded from Alexandre Yersin, who had been credited with discovering the bacterium in 1894. He likewise received a culture that he took back to the United States for further analysis.[147] By being able to witness this newfound microorganism, he became the "First American"[148] to examine it.[149]

Before heading to Paris, he went to visit laboratories in Prague, Munich and Vienna.[150] From Paris, he went to Koch's Hygienic Institute and observed his diphtheria "heilserum."[151] He rounded out his European journey by visiting the Hamburg Hygienic Institute and its work on water filtration, plus the workings of the laboratory. In addition, he met with Professor Rumpf and learned about his treatment for typhoid fever. And before heading home, he ventured to London and observed the operations of several of its labs.[152]

After returning to the States, he wrote a booklet titled *Report on the Treatment of Diphtheria by Antitoxin Serum, and Notes on the Preparation of Diphtheria.* It focused on Roux's successes and those of Koch in researching the

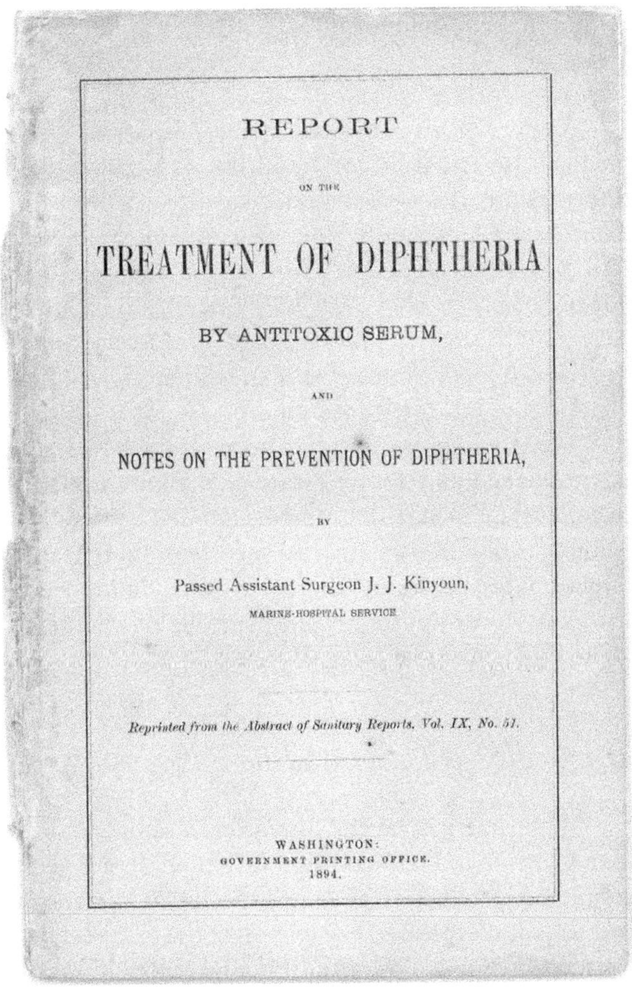
REPORT

ON THE

TREATMENT OF DIPHTHERIA

BY ANTITOXIC SERUM,

AND

NOTES ON THE PREVENTION OF DIPHTHERIA,

BY

Passed Assistant Surgeon J. J. Kinyoun,

MARINE-HOSPITAL SERVICE.

Reprinted from the Abstract of Sanitary Reports, Vol. IX, No. 51.

WASHINGTON:
GOVERNMENT PRINTING OFFICE.
1894.

"Report on the Treatment of Diphtheria by Antitoxic Serum, and Notes on the Prevention of Diphtheria" by Passed Assistant Surgeon J. J. Kinyoun, Reprinted from the Abstract of Sanitary Reports, Vol. IX, No. 51. Washington, Government Printing Office 1894.

disease. Kinyoun predicted that while the serum remained in an experimental stage, it would eventually prove successful, much as vaccinations had in treating smallpox.[153] He further elaborated:

> It appears that at last we have found a method which is not only good in one disease, but the principle [*sic*] method can be applied to many. It at last has opened a new field for work in infectious disease.[154]

It looked as if one of the European medical giants and his research had broken the yoke in finding a cure for not only this disease, but maybe others. He continued to experiment and evaluate the vaccine's inner properties.[155] After which, he reported:

> I have tried hard to find fault, to pick flaws in the statistics, but have significantly failed. The work must stand for itself.[156]

He pointed out the mortality rate from diphtheria in Europe from 1889 to 1894 had averaged around 85 percent, but at present registered under 47 percent, and appeared to be on a decline because of Roux's treatment.[157]

As part of his duties, he began imparting this information to the American medical and scientific communities. As a result, the press became electrified by the information. The news traveled fast, and within the course of roughly a month a front-page article about the new cure appeared in the *St. Louis Post-Dispatch*, *The New York Times*, *The Argus*, *Fort Wayne News*, *Daily State Press*, *The Washington Post*, *Logan Sport Reporter*, *The Daily Gazette*, *The Daily Republican*, *Weekly Wisconsin Cousin*, *The Daily Northwestern* and *The Chicago Daily Tribune*. In almost every story, he received top billing as the man who brought it to America. All the accounts were ecstatic about the new discovery.[158]

Even though the news had been received with high expectations and excitement, he cautioned it did not necessarily constitute a total cure. He acknowledged its curative powers, but stated it must be applied early on, or the patient will probably die. And regardless of its statistical successes, there would be cases where its application might not be successful. Therefore, early identification of the illness remained key to its value. More importantly, the methodology behind the serum could in all probability be used to combat other diseases.[159]

The Geddings Letter and Its Postscript

While in Paris, he had forwarded a sample of the diphtheria toxin from the Pasteur Institute to Dr. Geddings at the lab. In a five-page letter, he requested him to commence production of Roux's vaccine. He detailed the steps to be taken in its making. Kinyoun expressed excitement at the prospects of its manufacture. Horses would be needed to make the solution, and it would take over two months to create the serum.[160]

As to the right horse to use, he stated, "Any old horse will do, one which you should be able to pick up for five dollars."[161] He recommended contacting a "street car company"[162] to see if they had any used horses that they might provide free. Before injecting a horse, he prescribed a test run involving guinea pigs to determine its strength. This process would be followed by injecting the horse according to a set time period with a dosage application spanning 70 days. He advised Geddings to wait after each injection until any inflammation at the place of the inoculation had subsided before administering the next dose. He calculated the lapse between injections would vary anywhere from eight to five days, with each dosage being increased per the table set forth in his letter.[163] After the serum had reached a certain chemical level, it needed to be properly stored to keep its potency.[164]

Kinyoun reported on the different diphtheria serums being tested in different countries. Initially, he had favored Koch's, but after hearing Roux's paper on diphtheria at the Congress, he changed his position. He reported that 600 children had received the inoculation in France resulting in a considerable decrease in the mortality rate.[165] He noted that people were "flocking in [to the Pasteur Institute] from all parts of the world—some from Germany and Italy."[166] He spoke about Drs. Wasserman and Behring having developed a similar vaccine, but said that, in his opinion, it did not compare to Roux's. Of particular note: the toxin had been given to him instead of to others because of his previous associations with the Institute.[167]

Several weeks later, he sent another letter, titled "Postscript."[168] After further research and consultation with Dr. Martin, Kinyoun had decided to change his previous schedule of recommended time frames and dosage amounts. He advised that Martin had told him that the frequency and amount of the injections were excessive and needed to be scaled back.

Kinyoun stated that he had been working on a paper, "Report on the Treatment of Diphtheria by Antitoxin Serum, and Notes on the Preparation of Diphtheria," that explained everything about the serum and its manufacturing process. He hoped it would be published in the *Abstract*, a medical publication of the Service.[169] As set forth in his previous letter to Geddings, the European medical community had been "flocking"[170] to the Pasteur Institute wanting to learn more about Roux's treatment.[171] Of interest, he wrote:

> There has also been the ubiquitous American. Several have dropped in just to see how the thing worked, pumped me and then left after perhaps one or two days. As I was not as brilliant as the average American, I have not been able to master the techniques soon as they, nor did I come here for the same purpose as they. I do not care much for the passing reputation which might perchance be mine, so long as I can set the matter going properly at home, and will be doing some good to the little folks.[172]

The passage illustrated his sincerity in producing the vaccine and helping children. He was concerned more with the science than the fame others were seeking or might receive from it. He ended the postscript by stating that these passersby may achieve some "local notoriety"[173] by their casual association with the serum, which in his opinion will "do more harm to the thinking medical man and cast discredit."[174]

Once home and successful in production, he started instructing state health boards on how to replicate the vaccine.[175] He demonstrated the three steps necessary in its production that he had learned from Roux: preparation of the toxin, animal immunization, and the formulation and safeguarding of the serum.[176] In a significant first for the country, he had developed the vaccine at the Hygienic Laboratory.[177]

Public Safeguards

As the popularity of the diphtheria serum grew, Kinyoun foresaw a potential problem looming in its production and administration,[178] as mentioned in his post-script to Geddings.[179] With such a demand for its use, he and Koch warned about it being improperly made, which could lead to serious complications for a patient. He envisioned that the open market might produce otherwise dangerous and worthless versions. In order to protect the public, it should be tested and administered by trained individuals. Simply put, he wanted some type of government regulation for the manufacture of vaccines. Infectious deadly bacteria was a dangerous enough substance itself without leaving its manipulation into combative serums in the hands of laymen, untrained technicians and swindlers.[180]

At first, his recommendation received little attention. Only after 10 St. Louis children died from tainted diphtheria serum did Congress act. In 1902, it passed the Biological Control Act, leading to a separate Biological Control Division placed under the administration of the Hygienic Laboratory. This would be the beginning of many federal agencies yet to evolve and be entrusted with safeguarding the public's health and safety.[181] Some individuals have claimed that his foresight constituted the reason for creating the Food and Drug Administration (FDA) and the Center for Disease Control (CDC),[182] thereby making him the founder of these two future agencies in addition to the National Institutes of Health (NIH).

Kinyoun had become one of the country's leading medical scientists and a great visionary. At the age of 34, he had seen and achieved many breakthroughs for the advancement of medicine in America. Besides making vaccines, he had transitioned his knowledge and turned it into medical equipment allowing him to directly eradicate maladies, especially in the disinfection of ships. This allowed others the opportunity to achieve the same results with greater ease and efficiency and less loss of life. Of some irony, he had yet to reach the prime of his biological life and career. The future held great promise for him. As 1894 ended, he would continue to make more achievements that would contribute towards defending the afflicted from nature's most dreaded organisms.

VII

Widening the Realm: 1895–1896

Perfecting a Cure

Kinyoun continued to experiment with diphtheria in hopes of perfecting it. On his return, he had shared his knowledge with many others around the country. In his 1896 annual report on the lab, he commented that the medical profession had been skeptical about the serum. Through his research, he eventually demonstrated its reliability, leading many to accept its value. He noted that 76 patients had received it and only four died, resulting in a mortality rate of 5.2 percent. Just as important, the antitoxin's success correspondingly stemmed from an early detection of the illness and its immediate application.[1]

Throughout his report, he clarified several unknowns about the illness. First, he stated that its root cause derived from the bacillus diphtheria. Previously the bacillus appeared to be an inflammation of the body's upper air channels, combined with a "pseudo-membrane."[2] This meant that previous afflictions in the throat and nose were probably diphtheria, as opposed to some other disease. Second, he explained that diphtheria perhaps had been mistaken for croup, leading many to believe the latter to be the more fatal. He concluded that when croup was suspected, more often than not the disease was diphtheria.[3]

In support of his findings, he analyzed its mortality, reporting that out of 256 Eastern and Midwestern cities with a combined population of 23,209,937, there had been 50,986 diphtheria cases resulting in 11,861 deaths. Within this group, there had been 4,209 instances of croup, resulting in 2,904 fatalities. These two sections of the country accounted for the largest population centers. This indicated that the disease had not become as virulent as in the South and West, due to these regions' smaller populations. Unfortunately, children seemed to be the largest age group afflicted with it.[4]

He listed eight measures to be followed by all governing bodies. His points stressed uniform regulations, government uniformity in prevention, delegation to local health authorities, and mandatory notification of suspected cases. All cases should be assumed to be diphtheria, not croup, unless proven otherwise. Next, cases should be isolated and schools should undergo weekly inspections, including premises and books. All cases should be inoculated immediately. He also pointed out several known sources of the bacterium: milk, railway cars and steamships.[5]

The disease had been well known for being fatal. In time, the situation began to change because of early childhood vaccinations, thereby reducing the number of victims. Consequently, the country would come to view vaccinations as not only a preventive measure but also a cure.

Another Breakthrough

Smallpox is an extremely infectious, often fatal disease, brought about by the variola virus, resulting in high fever and vomiting and evidenced by rashes that can turn into blisters and may leave permanent visible scars on its survivors.[6]

Smallpox had long been a killer throughout the world and in the United States. Between November 1, 1894, and November 1, 1895, there were 3,347 reported cases, resulting in 633 deaths. The virus had spread to 30 states and to 170 counties and cities. Wisconsin had the largest number of cases with 581, followed by Illinois with 475. Most of the states affected were in the central part of the nation. The theory had evolved that it had migrated along the country's waterways, mainly from those outlets dumping into the Mississippi River system, a course estimated to run from Pittsburgh; through St. Louis; to Hot Springs, Arkansas, in the west; and to New Orleans.[7]

To abate its spread, the Service offered free vaccinations to sailors employed along these waterways. Between May and June 1895, 2,576 vaccinations were administered in New Orleans. In St. Louis, personnel inspected 52 ships and vaccinated 505 seamen. Likewise in Pittsburgh, the medical officer inspected 73 ships and 462 sailors. Within this number, 251 passed inspection, 178 agreed to be vaccinated, and 38 refused.[8] It should be recognized that vaccinations represented a preventive measure and not an antidote.

In the fall of 1893, Kinyoun had struck upon an idea on how to cure the virus. He approached the New York health commissioner, Dr. Cyrus Edson, asking his approval to visit North Brother Island and examine its smallpox patients.[9] Later, he printed his findings in an article titled "Treatment of Variola by Its Antitoxin," published by *The Atlantic Medical Weekly*.[10] Although the article did not constitute the first release of his research on smallpox, it described his development of an effective vaccine limiting its spread.[11]

After visiting the hospital, he contacted Dr. Ralph Walsh, who owned the "national vaccine farm."[12] He made arrangements to experiment with vaccinia, also known as cowpox, to test his theory about smallpox.[13] Kinyoun pointed out that Raynaud and Sternberg had proven "that the blood serum of an immune animal destroys the potency of vaccine lymph."[14] This meant that it would override the disease's poisons harboring in the lymph gland and its nodes.

Maurice Raynaud and John Miller Sternberg had become recognized medical researchers. Raynaud, a French doctor, had been a noted lecturer and writer. He had discovered an elusive vasospastic condition, where blood vessels contract in the body's limbs.[15] Sternberg on the other hand served as the surgeon general of the United States Army.[16] Noted bacteriologist Robert Koch had even referred to him as the "Father of American Bacteriology."[17] In 1892, he wrote a definitive book on the science, *Manual of Bacteriology*.[18] During his career, he conducted research on malaria, typhoid fever and yellow fever.[19] Kinyoun knew of their work and had been impressed with their findings.

At this time in America, there were two surgeon generals: the surgeon general of the United States Army and the supervisory surgeon-general of the Marine Hospital Service. Although the Service had a quasi-military structure, it served the public sector, whereas the surgeon general of the Army dealt with the well-being of the army.[20]

Concerning the lymph, it acts as a repository and transmitter of white blood cells in warding off bacteria and infections. Conversely, after an illness has become manifest, it can become a propellant of the malady, as opposed to being a repressive agent. By injecting the victim with immune cells from a previously infected party, these cells could trick the system, causing the body to reactivate its defenses and arrest the virus.[21]

Kinyoun elaborated: "It had occurred to me, as well as to others, that this fact could be utilized in the treatment of small-pox by the injection of this serum in patients suffering from the disease."[22] Based on this theory, he commenced experimentations by extracting blood from a cow that had been vaccinated earlier for cowpox. This was followed by several procedures resulting in a serum. After making a sizable amount of the compound, he forwarded it to Dr. Lewellyn Elliot, who oversaw the smallpox ward on North Brothers Island. He advised the treatment be administered to those cases showing early signs of the illness.[23]

Elliot did not have any new cases, just two where the disease had been progressing. He injected them with various levels of the antitoxin. In the first patient, the serum prolonged the victim's life by 72 hours and appeared to be working except for the virus' advancement. In the second case, the patient survived, due to having received more injections in larger doses. Afterwards, the poxes dried up and fell off with no visible signs of scarring.[24] The fact scarring had been lessened similarly constituted a significant achievement. Previously, the disease would leave pockmarks scarring the body.

He summarized his findings in a rather lengthy letter, finding many positives about the serum but also noting several drawbacks, mainly in its dosage.[25] He specifically pointed out, "As it is, I believe the use of the serum in these 2 cases has given good results."[26] Later, he commented, "It is my opinion that the vaccine serum will shorten the course of variola if given in the papular stage of eruption."[27] In closing, he stated, "Should other cases present, I will adopt the serum if possible."[28] Although the antitoxin had been used on only two advanced cases, the initial results had proven impressive, with Elliot willing to use it again.[29]

As will be recalled in his report about diphtheria, the same treatment used in making its serum might prove the same with smallpox. True to his previous statement, he had followed the concept as it applied to variola. On releasing his findings, they were published in the *Washington News*, *Philadelphia Record* and *New York Times*. The *News* and the *Record* articles wrote favorable accounts of the discovery.[30] The *News* wrote in bold type:

MARINE HOSPITAL SURGEON KINYOUN PROBABLY ON THE VERGE OF A VALUABLE DISCOVERY—TESTED IN THE PESTHOUSE.[31]

Similarly, the *Record* reported, "A new stage in that latest triumph of modern medicine, serum therapeutics, seems to have already been foreshadowed, if not attained, in the experiments of Dr. J.J. Kinyoun … with the antitoxin variola or smallpox."[32]

However, the *Times* was not convinced of its merits, rightfully stating that the serum had only been tried on two patients with marginal results.[33] The paper criticized the whole concept:

> It is not probable, however, that further experiments, made by Dr. Kinyoun or others, will lead to the production and use of an antitoxin serum, hostile to smallpox, that will greatly mitigate the severity of the disease, if applied in the early stages, and considerably reduce the mortality percentage for those who have failed to protect themselves by vaccinations and are attacked by it.[34]

Two cases did not make a cure, but stating such a possibility as an impossibility begs the bounds of logic. Others may have felt this way, too, because the germ theory combined with microbiology remained farfetched to many in 1895. In his 1896 annual report on the lab, he reported on the recent smallpox serum. He acknowledged research had all but ceased because the allocation from Congress had been spent.[35]

Most people probably acknowledged the germ theory as a potential cure for diseases, whereas others may not have been able to fathom the concept without seeing more proof. Although time and medical research would prevail, skepticism would remain problematic into the 20th century. As the *Record* correctly indicated with the phrase "modern medicine,"[36] science had become the driving force behind eradicating disease. Even so, the ways of old many times have been obstacles to the better ways of the future.

In time, the antitoxin would prove its worth and lead to its eventual eradication not only in America, but in other parts of the world. His treatment, which became known as the "Kinyoun Method,"[37] entailed pricking the skin on the upper arm several times, thereby allowing the vaccine to seep into the body. As reported by Dr. David M. Morens, senior advisor to the director of the National Institute of Allergy and Infectious Diseases (NIAID), the procedure to some extent mimicked the Chinese art of acupuncture, although there was no direct relationship. The method remained the treatment recommended by the U.S. Public Health Service up to 1961, until the advent of the bifurcated needle. Recently, several present-day medical researchers have come forward and acknowledged his treatment as the legitimate remedy in ending this once usually fatal virus.[38]

Dr. Walter Reed

At some point in his career, he met Walter Reed, who would become famous for his research on yellow fever.[39] He, too, had a keen interest in medical research, and in 1899, after the Spanish-American War, he went to Cuba to learn more about the illness that had killed many troops on the island. In 1900, he returned to Cuba as the head of a task force established by Sternberg with the purpose of studying it and other tropical maladies.[40] Kinyoun joined Reed on at least one of these fact-finding missions.[41]

Although Reed never found a cure for yellow fever, he proved mosquitoes to be the transferring agent. As part of his research, he used human volunteers—including himself—as guinea pigs to verify his theory. By eradicating the insects and their breeding areas, the contagion abated.[42]

Walter Reed died on November 23, 1902, from a ruptured appendix.[43] In a letter written on June 20, 1902, to Kinyoun, he revealed his possible appointment as the Army's next surgeon general, replacing Sternberg,[44] who stepped down from the position in 1902.[45] His premature death prevented this from happening. Reed and Kinyoun had become close friends in the 1890s. It has been reported that Reed looked upon him as a mentor, even though he was nine years older.[46]

More Discoveries and Other Assignments

As an example on how animal experimentation could have value, the *Miscellany* reported on March 2, in its *Washington Notes* section, about a procedure developed by Kinyoun for people with cleft lips.[47] The article read:

> Dr. Kinyoun, U.S.M.H. Service, suggested the use of sterilized bone pins with figure-of-eight sutures in the hare-lip, and cited some experiments made on rabbits, to prove the value of the method.[48]

At the Medical Society's meeting in Springfield, Illinois, he gave a presentation titled "The Management and Control of Infectious Diseases in Municipalities."[49] His former boss, Surgeon General John B. Hamilton, also attended and served as the society's permanent secretary.[50] Following this symposium, Wyman sent him to the Convention of Bacteriologists of the United States, Canada and Mexico held in June, at the Academy. He rounded out the year by representing the Service at a meeting of the American Public Health Association held at Denver, Colorado, in early October. Surgeon Preston H. Bailhache accompanied him.[51]

Afterwards, Bailhache wrote an extensive account of the meeting. The medical papers presented at the conference were numerous. Some of the more interesting topics included "The Mississippi River as a Sewer," "The Ventilation of Railway Coaches," "Disinfection in American Cities," "Medical Inspection of Schools," "Report of committee on disposal of the dead," "Disposal of the dead with special reference to the Prevalent Practice of Embalming," "Cremation or Earth Burial, Which?" "National Legislation for the Care of Public Health," "Report on the Abuse of Alcoholic Drink from a Sanitary Standpoint," "Baths, their necessity, their influence in economy, the dangers they present," "The Methods of Preventing Them," "Railroad hygiene," "Relation of Hygiene to Abortions and Stillbirths," "Influence of the Poorer Classes in the Cities—Education in Public-Health Matters," and "The Best Prophylaetic [sic] Against Typhus."[52]

Hygiene appeared at the center of all these presentations. The medical community had embraced the concept of microorganisms and bacteriology as a standard, combined with sanitation, as a way to limit the spread of disease. One topic was bathing, which in 19th-century America may not have been an everyday occurrence, if even weekly. Another paper commented that the poor were probably more susceptible to illness in larger cities, because of a lack of adequate sanitation services.[53]

In July, Kinyoun had forwarded medical information to the Venezuela legation in Washington. He received an acknowledgment from Jose Andrade at the Venezuelan embassy expressing gratitude for the material.[54] As a result, he would later receive the Order of Bolivar, the country's most prestigious award,[55] the belief being that he had mentored Eduardo Penny Andrade, who was an assistant at the Hygienic Laboratory and used the research back home. He wrote an extensive report in Kinyoun's 1895 annual report of the Hygienic Laboratory concerning bacillus typhus.[56]

Years later, Alice Kinyoun stated that her father had shared much of his European medical knowledge with Dr. Andrade, resulting in the saving of many lives in Venezuela.[57] Jose Andrade and Eduardo Penny Andrade may have been father and son, or one and the same person, in view of the close similarities between their names. Jose worked in the consular office, thereby allowing Eduardo to study at the lab, since he was a doctor.[58]

Safety of the Nation's Water Supply

Typhoid fever, also known as enteric fever, is a bacterium caused by the salmonella organism. The illness is usually transmitted by contaminated water containing human fecal matter and invades the intestines. Victims experience a high fever, severe abdominal pain, and extreme fatigue, and, if left untreated, will likely die within several weeks. It has also been referred to as dysentery because of similar characteristics.[59]

Towards year's end, he received another important assignment. Wyman formed a special committee consisting of Passed Assistant Surgeon C.E. Banks as the chairman, Kinyoun, and Assistant Surgeon W.J.S. Stewart as the recorder. This group had been brought about because of another outbreak of typhoid fever in late 1895. Dr. George M. Kober, with Washington's Health Department, reported on his findings, but his analysis had been limited by the lack of a proper research facility. Consequently, he had asked for Wyman's help and the lab's assistance. Wyman responded quickly and invoked the 1893 Quarantine Law, allowing the Service to intercede and act.[60]

The trio had been entrusted with examining the capital's water supply. Between September 24 and December 13, 135 inspections were conducted of the District's water. A fair amount of the area consisted of rural land. Many of the people relied on well water for drinking purposes, along with streams and the Potomac River.[61]

After conducting its investigations, he wrote an account of the committee's findings, titled "Report on the Water Supply of Washington, D. C."[62] His initial observation stated that the "Potomac water is not at all times free from sewage pollution."[63]

During this period, municipalities would frequently discharge waste into nearby rivers and streams; Kinyoun noted that "Harpers Ferry, Cumberland and Frederick"[64] disposed of their refuse by dumping it into the Potomac.[65]

Typhoid fever had been increasing, and in 1895 there were an estimated 500,000 cases that likely equated into 50,000 deaths. It had become imperative that action be taken to address the purity of the country's water supply. As the population continued to grow, with more people moving to the city, the most important health issue had become clean water. After extensive testing, bacteria had been found in all the water samples. Not all the bacteria proved to be bad, but within the samplings, more often than not, harmful levels had been found in sizable portions. For that reason, corrective measures had to be undertaken to abate this health hazard.[66]

It had been thought that sewage and bacteria would be diluted by the river on its way downstream away from the city. This proved not to be true because it would not necessarily dissipate in water. Another belief rested on the assumption that the water would purify itself over time. In an address before Washington's Board of Trade, Kinyoun debunked this notion. He stated that bacteria needs water to survive and, because of the hundreds of miles of water pouring into bodies like the Potomac, bacteria from the soil washed into many tributaries.[67]

Referring to Dr. Koch, he stated that a cubic centimeter of water containing in excess of 400 bacteria should be considered dangerous, whereas those having fewer than 200 could be considered safe. In fact, bacteria released upstream could survive up to 15 days. Moreover, several of the more communicable diseases, such as typhus, cholera, and diarrhea, have historically been waterborne. Residents of Hamburg, Germany once believed water would naturally cleanse itself. In 1892, though, cholera broke out, and in six weeks 10,000 people had perished as a result of this assumption.[68]

He stated there were two ways to correct the problem: "Own control of the watershed and abate the nuisances. This is not practical or feasible. The other is filtration of the water supply.... As used in several European cities...."[69] Kinyoun also recommended that farm wells be supervised, especially on dairy farms, where through the chain of transmission water enters the milk supply.[70] The doctor concluded: "The use of surface wells in the city should on general principle be condemned"[71] because they are, "as a rule constantly exposed to contamination."[72]

These recommendations represented aggressive measures to be considered that fortunately would come to pass. He predicted that if a filtering system consisting of sediment basins, beds and other procedures were utilized, then 95 percent of the diseases could be eliminated from the area's water.[73] Concerning sewers, he stated that they only serve a "secondary importance"[74] in cleaning water. Instead, efforts should be directed at purification first. Again, his European education and training had brought important sanitation methods to America. On his latest trip to Europe, he had studied municipal water purification.[75]

After the committee completed its study, Wyman acted swiftly and issued a directive to all the mayors in the country. He quoted the 1893 Quarantine Law as the basis of this empowerment. The letter asked all of them to report on their water supply, sewage disposal and other refuse removal as outlined on an attached questionnaire. The accompanying survey comprised nine sections totaling 25 questions.[76] Without any doubt, the safety and the ongoing monitoring and purification of the country's water supply had become a cornerstone of the public's health based on Kinyoun's report.

Vivisection

Vivisection is the practice of using live animals in scientific and medical research for the purpose of applying the results for a better understanding of a disease and to determine whether a potential cure would have a positive effect on the well-being of humans.[77]

In the preceding year, Kinyoun and Reed had opposed pending legislation limiting the practice of vivisection. They and others had officially opposed Senate Bill 1552, presented in large part through the efforts of the Humane Society. If passed, the legislation would have placed limitations on animal experimentation, citing such practices as cruel.[78]

In May, he sent a letter to Congress outlining his opposition. If it passed, the bill would not only limit research at the Hygienic Laboratory, but also the Medical Departments of the Army and Navy, along with the Bureau of Animal Industry. Proponents of the bill claimed the various laboratories associated with these departments had been performing horrific experiments on animals.[79]

Supporters alleged these procedures had been conducted in medical colleges and public schools. The doctor countered that these labs had been authorized by Congress, noting it had continued to fund these practices. Still, advocates now wanted to be present during experiments, with the ultimate goal of having the government abolish this form of research.[80]

He proceeded to defend the workings of the lab. "I feel it my duty, both to the Service and myself," he stated, "to call in question these statements with regard to the cruel manner in which the research work of the laboratories is performed."[81] Furthermore, he noted it would be unnecessary to refute every allegation because most of the lab's work was of public record. Specifically, research on those diseases requiring quarantine spoke for itself. Without animal research, the success in identifying, creating vaccines and eventually cures would have been impossible.[82]

Kinyoun refuted the proponents' arguments, asserting that scientific advancement to date had been achieved through "common experience,"[83] as opposed to "little, if any, benefits to the human race ... by these ... awful experiments."[84] He referred to these contentions as of questionable validity, since the record had proven otherwise as to their value. In support of his position, he went into great deal explaining the recent triumphs with diphtheria. As proof, he referenced many of the world's best doctors as authoritative sources in providing cures, naming Drs. Roux, Behring and Monod, along with Dr. William Welch at Johns Hopkins University. More importantly, though, he showed that if the vaccine had been present in the last five years, at least 150,000 lives could have been saved in the United States.[85]

Even with these facts, he reported that many supporters of the bill still disputed these findings. He had even appeared before an animal society attempting to impart the importance of the research.[86] But during his presentation, while outlining its success on diphtheria, he

> ... was told by several female antivivisectionists that they would sooner let a child die of diphtheria, than to save its life by the sacrifice of a guinea pig.[87]

In response, he commented, "I hope none of them were mothers."[88]

He revealed receiving two hate letters several years before after the press had printed an article about his experiments with cobra venom and its effect on cholera.[89] The first letter opened by saying, "You vile, merciless, rascally fiend. I judge by your name you are a nasty Frenchman, with no heart and without a God."[90] The writer called the lab a "place of torture ... for poor animals."[91] Kinyoun was of English ancestry, but the letter stated, "You will have to betake yourself to the vile and godless country from which you came or to hell to which you are destined."[92] In concluding, the author wrote, "I am a woman who despises brutes and all brutal actions."[93]

The second letter had even fewer niceties to say about him:

> Only the most damnable fiend cloaked in human form ever lifted the knife in vivisection. May the curse of an all-merciful God rest upon you. Laugh, sneerr; such as you do. But may every agony your hellish mind and hand inflicts be trebled upon yourself in this world and the one to come, and upon all like you. May your deathbed be such a scene of horror that all will forsake you. May God's curse be upon you.[94]

In wrapping up, he set forth several quotes from Welch, a renowned physician in his own right. Referring again to diphtheria, he referenced Welch, writing that in the more than 7,000 cases of the disease, the antitoxin treatment established repeatedly the effectiveness of its curative prowess. Its discovery derived entirely from the laboratory, implying the successful use of animals in research. The results were by no means accidental. All the steps undertaken in the process were documented.[95]

As his final comment, Kinyoun again quoted Welch:

> These studies and the resulting discoveries mark an epoch in the history of medicine. It should be forcibly brought home to those whose philozoic sentiments outweigh sentiments of true philanthropy [sic] that these discoveries which led to the saving of untold thousands of human lives have been gained by the sacrifice of lives of thousands of animals, and by no possibility could have been without experimentation upon animals.[96]

On May 19, Wyman forwarded Kinyoun's letter to the chairman for the Committee of the District of Columbia of the United States Senate for review and transmittal to Congress. Wyman sent a cover letter with it, also protesting the bill in his official capacity. He, too, highlighted the recent developments with the diphtheria antitoxin as proof of the necessity of using animals in research. In this case, horses had been used to develop the serum: they were injected with the virus, and then the animals' blood was drawn after they developed immunity to the disease. Because this procedure had not been developed prior to the 131,620 cases from 1891 to 1894, all told 51,820 people had died from it for a mortality rate of 39 percent. He stated that other statistics were available in support of these numbers.[97]

Wyman debunked a proposed amendment to the bill, apparently presented as a compromise.[98] The measure stated that it would "not affect experimental inoculation."[99] He countered by stating that "animals suffer as much from the after effects of experimental inoculation as from the minor operations connected with vivisection."[100] Further pointing out its inconsistency, he stated that if the law would prevent the bleeding of the horse in order to extract the antitoxin, then all would be prohibited in obtaining the end product, or antidote.[101] In concluding his letter, he made the following statement:

> Had this principle prevailed there would have been no discovery of the bacillus of cholera, upon which the suppression of that hitherto irrepressible disease has become a scientific and practical possibility. I may add that the quarantine methods of the present day, through which epidemic diseases are excluded from the United States by scientific disinfection, have their basis in these experiments.[102]

At the end of this discussion, one thing had become quite apparent. The Service, the lab and Kinyoun's discoveries had met their first public challenge as to the authenticity and need of bacteriology. What had been celebrated as wonder treatments in the press and accepted as undisputed truth in eradicating from civilization the ravages of the ages had fallen into question because of its success at the expense of innocent animals. In the end, the Service and scientific research survived this test of wills.

With all great advancements, there has always tended to be some skepticism about the veracity of the discovery. Sometimes, though, this doubt lies not in the result, but in the process, the question being whether the end costs too much. When this occurs, doubt can turn into denial, whereby the skeptics disavow truth. This almost occurred with the vivisection bill, where its proponents started denying the facts in order to support their point.

Personal Achievements

As previously mentioned, in appreciation of his work, he received word from the Venezuelan Republic of its desire to bestow upon him the Order of Bolivar. Missouri Senator Cockrell introduced Senate Bill 3214, allowing him to accept the award from the president of Venezuela.[103] The bill described the award as being "a gold medal of the fourth class of the Order of the Liberator, awarded in recognition of scientific services."[104] In December, the Senate approved the bill in the second session of the 54th Congress.[105] He likely received the medal because of Eduardo Penny Andrade, who had been stationed in Washington as part of the Venezuelan embassy.

The term "Liberator"[106] referred to Simon Bolivar, who from 1813 to 1822 led a liberation campaign in South America against the Spanish Empire, modeled after the recent American and French Revolutions. In 1822, he established the nation of Gran Columbia, encompassing much of the northern portion of the continent. He became known as the George Washington of South America. The country of Bolivia was subsequently named after him. The fourth grade means the honoree has the distinction of being an officer.[107]

On top of everything, he received his doctorate in philosophy from Georgetown University, while serving on its medical faculty.[108] The following month, he received a letter from J. Havens Richard, the president of Georgetown College (University).

The note served as an apology of sorts. He stated that although the doctor had been on the staff of the Medical Department since 1891 as a professor of Bacteriology and Special Pathology, he had never received an official confirmation of his positions. Richards begged forgiveness and as compensation appointed him the chair of these posts.[109] In closing, Richard wrote:

> I seize this opportunity also to express, in the name of the entire faculty and my own, the entire satisfaction and high gratification felt by us all on account of the distinguished ability and faithful zeal with which you have at all times discharged the duties incumbent upon you in the School.[110]

Chasing Public Germs

As the year unfolded, a review of sanitation in public places began to receive greater scrutiny by the Service. Kinyoun's lab became the cornerstone of this examination. As reported in the 1896 annual report, formaldehyde gas had been under review for a year and a half. Initially, the findings had not been impressive in comparison to other disinfectants. But on further review, significant progress had been made with the compound by German and French scientists, leading to a reconsideration of its value.[111]

Additional experimentation had shown "the powerful disinfecting properties of this agent."[112] Kinyoun's laboratory assistant, Passed Assistant Surgeon Geddings, had conducted numerous trials,[113] but the doctor held firm that further research would be needed, predicting "it will doubtless, revolutionize the system of disinfection as now practiced."[114] He went onto say that the gas could prove very useful in disinfecting apartments and their contents.[115]

Within the realm of sanitation, bank notes and railway cars surfaced as disease carriers. With the realization that diseases were spread from person to person and through contaminated surfaces, research into new hygienic measures became necessary. Paper currency, as opposed to gold and silver, was used in a sizable portion of the country's monetary exchanges, and railroads had become the major form of mass transportation. Thousands of people came into contact with one another daily through these modes, making their sanitation the next frontier in averting the spread of disease. With foreign ship travel and immigration having once been of great concern, a closer look at internal interchanges had become imperative.

Kinyoun advised how to disinfect bank notes, especially those potentially infected with smallpox. The formula comprised a 40-percent formaldehyde solution. He provided a sketch for a brass drawer to hold the solution and bank notes. The bills needed to be soaked in the mixture for at least two hours. The notes would need to be spread out in thin layers on a rack, not to exceed a depth of two bills. He advised that infected notes be bundled into stacks of 20 layered between saturated blunting paper slips and treated. On securely packaging them, they could be mailed by way of regular carriers.[116]

Railway disinfection offered a different challenge because of the sheer size of the cars. In mid–July, Wyman made an appeal to several railroad companies advising them of the lab's efforts to find a proper sanitizing element. He stated that the research not only included common germs, but those contagions subject to quarantine: smallpox, cholera, yellow fever, typhus and plague. Wyman explained that current measures caused damage to the coaches' furnishings and fabrics. To develop a better sanitizing agent, he asked the companies to provide fabric samples—to include bedding, carpet and upholstery—for testing.[117]

In September, he sent a letter thanking the companies for their participation and stating that the research had been successful. He reported that another experiment needed to be performed that would require the use of several coaches. Raising a new level of concern, he warned that tuberculosis and diphtheria were common passengers in their cars, warranting the additional research. As a courtesy, he invited the owners to attend the experiments. The treatment involved the use of formaldehyde gas, but he assured the companies there would not be any damage to the cars.[118]

Various Opinions

In August, Wyman directed him to attend the conference of the American Public Health Association as the Service's representative.[119] On learning of his son's attendance, the elder Kinyoun expressed his envy.[120] The summit convened in early October. As part of the proceedings, he spoke on railroad car sanitation, in particular the drinking water in the coaches.[121] He revealed the presence of "cases of diarrheal and enteric (typhoid) diseases ... significant enough that the presidents and other company officials of these companies would not drink the water they furnished to the passengers."[122] Further, the cars—along with any loose material and the furnishings—should be subjected to disinfection. In his final remarks, he stated that, as if things were not bad enough with the coaches, cases of diphtheria and tuberculosis had surfaced in the terminals.[123]

The common thread to his findings centered on the ever-growing exposure of people to one another, especially with the advent of rapid transportation systems and a burgeoning population. The greater the contact, the more likely the spread of disease. America had become mobile, but little had been done to ensure the proper implementation of protective sanitary measures of the carriers. As he well knew, only the ongoing cleaning of public places would protect individuals from the unseen maladies of their daily intermingling.

The following month, he again spoke publicly about the country's health standards. On this occasion, he revisited the topic of diphtheria.[124] As quoted in the *Washington Post* on November 30, he stated that there should be "compulsory use of the anti-toxin,"[125] as opposed to it being elective. He squarely pointed his finger at Congress, accusing it of being the culprit behind the contagion because it had not appropriated the necessary funds for the vaccine.[126]

Kinyoun had become outspoken in his opinions. As a result of his education and experience at the world's leading laboratories, he saw how lives could be saved and the spread of disease could be prevented through scientific applications. He had decided to do everything possible to change present medical thinking and usher in the ever-growing new ways of arresting death caused by bacteria and viruses. In particular, his use and expansion of the Hygienic Laboratory would hasten these important medical advancements.

VIII

The First Decade

Avocations

In his annual report on the lab, Kinyoun stated that the governments of Germany, France and England had established medical schools for their various military branches. He pointed out that the United States Army and Navy had recently been required to provide training classes for their new recruits. Concerning upgraded medical standards for incoming officers, the Secretary of the Treasury issued a directive on February 28 requiring them to take several entry courses, in particular bacteriology.[1]

But as to the Service, drawbacks existed because of its small size, along with the complexity and variance of its many duties. Instead, he proposed a medical school be established and made available throughout the branches of the agency, as opposed to being in one location. This would allow the courses to be more accessible.[2]

He also recommended a much broader curriculum for new officers comprising four areas of study:[3] "(1) laboratory instruction, (2) hospital and dispensary service, (3) immigration inspection service, (4) quarantine service."[4] Clearly, he had given the matter considerable thought, as evidenced by the proposed areas of training.

Commencing with laboratory instruction, it would be conducted at the Hygienic Laboratory for a term of three months.[5] The courses would instruct the officers on the "use of the microscope in clinical diagnosis, the principles of bacteriology, sanitary and clinical chemistry, plus the principles and practice of disinfection."[6] After completion, the officer would be better prepared to use this knowledge in "hospital work,"[7] the next round of instruction.[8]

He further directed that, upon completion, officers should be assigned to one of the agency's larger facilities to learn about hospitals. They should be placed in a ward for at least a year.[9] Instruction should focus on the "methods of sick call, medical and physical examinations, physical diagnosis, application of methods of accurate clinical diagnosis, case-history writing, treatment of cases, post mortem examinations, and reports."[10] After six months, the officer should study the surgical aspects of medicine, including operations, preparations, surgical assistance and dressings. Following this course work, one should study the agency's regulations, followed by a review of its business operations, combined with six months service in the dispensary.[11]

This would be followed by having the officer sent to the immigration center (Ellis Island) in New York, where he would be required to conduct inspections and examinations of immigrants. As part of the training, one should be placed in the center's hospital wards. They would receive hands-on experience with the wide range of diseases trying to make entry into the country, thereby gaining insight valuable for future quarantine duty.[12]

Lastly, Kinyoun proposed two forms of quarantine curriculum.[13] The first consisted of a three-month stint at a northern station, where the officer would learn about the "boarding, inspecting, disinfection of vessels (partial or complete), along with the detention and isolation of suspects."[14] This would be followed by a transfer to a southern station to learn about the boarding, inspecting and treatment of ships combined with the inspection of personnel, passengers and cargoes. The second plan offered a little more flexibility, whereby an officer would be given a six-month assignment to a station in the fall. Afterwards, he would be allowed additional time to complete quarantine training.[15]

In summarizing, he stated that these recommendations would require "radical changes."[16] Of interest, all training would start with the Hygienic Laboratory, his creation.[17] This requirement might appear self-serving, but in another respect it could be argued he simply wanted what was best for the agency. He and others had proven the germ theory to be fact, not fiction. Aligned with this, it would make perfect sense to have all the officers commence their studies at the lab, so as to fully understand how the science worked and interrelated with all the other operations of the Service.

He had previously advocated for the uniform regulation of the manufacture of serums and antitoxins by the federal government to ensure the safe production and distribution of these drugs.[18] Therefore, it would only be natural for him to promote training standards for new recruits. Once again, he had set forth his vision on how best to improve the system.

His advocating for a government medical school with a rigorous curriculum had a sound basis. The schooling would provide officers a thorough basis of instruction of the agency's operations and provide the newest forms of technological research. From another perspective, he was also promoting the standardization of medical courses. In his eyes, this would be for the betterment of not only future officers, but physicians and medical science as well.

Tidings and Advancement

In January, he received a letter from his father writing about the home front. Of particular interest, the elder Kinyoun continued to treat diphtheria patients with his son's antitoxin. He stated that some of the cases had been severe.[19] But by using the syringe "freely," the older doctor reported, he had "had but one result that of success": "I can use it with much confidence in all and any case," he wrote.[20] Regarding the syringe, he advised Joe that he would be keeping it until he retired. He instructed his son to send him a bill for the device.[21] Joe had initially forgotten to send it to his father,[22] but sometime later had forwarded the instrument.

In the 19th century, syringes had been designed for more than one application. They were large, and the apparatus consisted primarily of metal with variations containing glass. Today's device is much smaller and chiefly made of plastic.[23] Medical personnel do not use it multiple times on multiple patients for multiple sanitation reasons. Public health was still evolving, even in light of significant progress.

Kinyoun's responsibilities continued increasing until year's end. Wyman issued a directive to Surgeon Fairfax Irwin as chairman, Kinyoun, H.D. Geddings, and W.J.S. Stewart as recorder, appointing them to a board known as the sanitary board.[24] The panel had been established to assist the surgeon general with matters of his choosing. It could not act on its own, only on those matters referred by him. All reports would be in writing, signed by all members and submitted by the chairman combined with supportive information. It would operate as an appendage to the surgeon general, as both a governing entity and as an oversight commission.[25]

Bubonic Plague

Bubonic plague is a highly contagious bacterium that results in a painful death if left untreated without antibiotics. Throughout history, the name has been used to refer to numerous life-threatening maladies. Actual plague is referred to as bubonic, wherein it causes the lymph buboes to swell and turn black. Symptoms include vomiting, diarrhea, high fever, chills, disorientation and the expectoration of dark blood. It is transmitted by the bite of fleas found on rats and other rodents. In past ages, it has been called the Black Death and sometimes been confused with other deadly and highly infectious diseases.[26]

In March, Kinyoun wrote an article, published in *Miscellany*, about his findings in New York[27]; it was titled "The Viability of the Bubonic Plague."[28] In it, he stated his concurrence with Dr. J.H. Wilson, chief of the Bureau of Bacteriology in the health department of Brooklyn, on how to destroy the organism.[29] Although this may have seemed a passing comment, it bore important news, because now a method had been found to stop it. Beforehand, the disease always had unlimited sway as it decimated countless populations.

Interestingly, the *Correspondence* had printed an article the month before[30] titled "The Plague to Be Investigated."[31] The piece read more like an editorial than a general news story. Surprisingly, it mocked Wyman. The story described how a syndicate letter had been published in the media concerning disease.[32] Further, it had been submitted in part by a "female correspondent," who had "solemnly assured ... that this is a fact."[33] The first sentence read, "Dr. Walter Wyman, Supervising Surgeon-General of the Marine Hospital Service of the United States, has put his powerful mind on a special study of the bubonic plague, and that we will very shortly hear something in the way of some important discovery which will electrify the world."[34] Following this passage, the article took a direct swipe at him, stating

> If the veracious correspondent had informed us that Dr. Kinyoun of the laboratory was about to develop something it might have been credited in scientific circles, but if any human being ever heard of the much advertised WYMAN in any scientific capacity it would be a pleasant surprise to know of it.[35]

The writer proceeded to point out that the medical giants of the time—Dr. Koch and plague discovers Alexandre Yersin and Kitasato Shibasaburō—had studied the bacterium in its present habitats of Bombay, India, and China,[36] whereas the Service had not.[37] Wyman was described as "the head of the Marine-Hospital Service, who cleverly confronts an epidemic by gazing at the dispatches through the bottom of his glass at a 'high tea,' and giving the results ... to the admiring society reporter."[38] Ostensibly, he had been ignoring the mainstream press and possibly had been using the society pages to reveal new and promising developments at the agency. Kinyoun received praise and credit for his approach,[39] but the article continued to ridicule Wyman:[40]

> Great are the results produced by the proper distribution of the products of the Washington florists; and tremendous the effects brought about by careful attention to the social functions of the Capital!
>
> The code of morals which prevents country practitioners and obscure members of the profession in the city from advertising, does not seem to invade the sacred precincts, nor penetrate that luminous halo which surrounds the bureau officer at Washington, and in consequence we have syndicate letters galore, as a rule written a few weeks before the incoming of a new administration.[41]

The article read like a satire of Wyman and the government. He received the brunt of the admonishments possibly due to a previous altercation with the press. By calling it advertising, which many professions of the time forbade, the article almost imparts a question of ethical concern. Political and high-profile individuals have been known to court the media to serve their purposes. As head of the government's health agency, he may have done the same. However, in his case, it seemed to have backfired.

Besides the import of this scathing article, the study of plague and concern that it would reach the country had been underway for some time. Although not directly under the auspices of Kinyoun, its analysis had been assigned to Passed Assistant Surgeon H.D. Geddings, who also worked in the lab.[42] Geddings submitted a lengthy report on his findings, titled "Reports on the Bubonic Plague as Studied at the Pasteur Institute," as part of his 1897 annual report.[43] He had been sent to the Institute, like Kinyoun,[44] in hopes that he would learn the newest theories concerning this most feared disease.[45] At the Institute, he studied under Drs. Roux and Borel, whom he described as most obliging.[46]

Geddings retraced the organism's discovery by Kitasato and Yersin. He described it as a cocco-bacillus that was short, ovoid, thick, and spherical and about two micromillimeters in diameter. In postmortem examinations, the microbe had been found throughout the body, including tissues and organs, notably in the spleen, lymph glands, heart, blood and liver. In slower deaths, it would also manifest in the kidneys and lungs. It would enter the buboes, from whence it received its name. Testing showed how extremely quickly it caused death in several animals, especially rabbits, mice and guinea pigs. Rabbits and guinea pigs would usually succumb in 48–60 hours upon being injected with the bacterium; mice would die within 24 hours.[47]

Horses were used to perfect a serum. Upon injection, the animal would show various signs of distress, but in most cases it would overcome these reactions. He gave an elaborate account on the making of the serum and its care afterwards, particularly when sterilizing the equipment used in its administration, such as the syringe. If too much heat was applied, then it would destroy the antitoxin. In view of that, he provided heating levels on how to maintain its effectiveness.[48]

Two other valuable discoveries were witnessed by him. The first finding occurred through further experimentation with the production of horse serum. In this case, a toxin had been developed, which resulted in a breakthrough by way of a much safer process. Research showed that the toxin, or the chemical result of infecting the horse with the plague, could be used in place of the actual bacillus. In effect, the toxin created through this process could be called a simulated version of the disease. It would create the same immunity in the animal going forward, and in some cases the serum turned out to be of better quality and safer for the horse. In addition, this new method removed the scientists and the animal from direct contact with the plague. This alternate procedure limited its accidental spread in production.[49]

The second discovery resulted in the identification of plague through a scientific procedure, as opposed to the former method of visual observation. Again, science had trumped the ways of the past, allowing the trained physician the ability to identify the illness with an almost certainty. Additional studies would be conducted to perfect this finding, but at least the deep mysteries clouding the disease were coming to light and its diagnosis could be proven as fact, instead of speculation. Many illnesses mimic others initially, or mock the same symptoms, such as nausea, high fever and coughing. Only as a disease progresses do its peculiar characteristics become distinguishable from those of other maladies. Detecting the type of contagion early in its progression increases the probability of the patient's recovery. As a bonus, medical and government officials could better advise communities on making a proper diagnosis, leading to its early containment, thereby lessening the possibility of an epidemic.[50]

In June, Geddings sent another report, this time talking about the plague's ravages in Bombay, Hong Kong and Karachi, Pakistan. His account centered on five elements. These included the disease's mortality, types, and symptoms, the viability of the bacillus and serum therapy, and preventive inoculation. Under mortality, the death rate in India of those afflicted had ranged from 90 percent to 95 percent. However, it may have been less because the Hindus would not go to hospitals, even with "compulsory removal"[51] to these facilities for treatment. They even concealed deaths occurring among themselves. Consequently, this factor might have tended to further increase the number. But some individuals had received the serum thereby decreasing the death rate.[52]

Geddings reviewed the different known types of plague, which were bubonic, septicemia and pneumonic. His analysis traced the course of the infection, stating first that there remained some question on how it entered the body. He observed that, in India, people did not wear shoes and thus that it could invade by way of a cut or abrasion on the foot or leg. But in Hong Kong, where shoes were worn, the point of entry had been theorized to come from an insect or rodent bite, as evidenced on an individual's hands and arms. Several cases showed the illness may have originated in the lungs and intestines, but it remained unresolved on how it arrived in these organs. Another external source could be the general sanitary conditions of an environment; where surroundings were cluttered with garbage and filth, it appeared more often. One thing, though, seemed apparent: a red spot on the skin usually marked its entry point into the body.[53]

Although Yersin and Kitasato discovered the plague bacillus a few years before in 1894, there remained the question of its host and mode of infection. In time, the connection would be made between the flea and the black rat as the transmitters.[54] The same dilemma had faced yellow fever, but in 1898 Louis-Paul Simond, a French scientist, proved that plague was transmitted from the flea to rat, rat to rat, and rat to human.[55]

Geddings proceeded to analyze the plague's various symptomatic stages. He addressed not only its outward symptoms, but also internal ones, through postmortem examinations. The bubonic phase would exhibit gland swelling, or an enlarged bubo, accompanied by vomiting, delirium, a high fever and unconsciousness, followed by a transition into the septicemia phase that he called a merger of conditions. In septicemic cases, it would travel through the lungs and intestines, being less violent, with some patients recovering.[56]

In the converse, he noted that, upon becoming pneumonic, it "is at once the most insidious in its onset, the most difficult of diagnosis, and the most fatal in its results."[57] This final phase can be evidenced by a cough and labored breathing,[58] combined with a "dark-colored, or bloody expectoration."[59] Autopsies had revealed its presence in either one or both lungs. However, the overriding characteristic had been hemorrhaging throughout the body. Those areas most often bearing this trait included the spinal cord, kidneys and spleen.[60]

Concerning viability, it appeared to retain its virulence as long as moisture and heat were present. Furthermore, the sanitary conditions of the community weighed heavily as to its sustainability. He pointed out that European countries experienced it less because the cities were modern and had water purification systems along with waste removal, whereas Asian countries did not have such systems and services. Although overcrowding and filth alone cannot account for all the cases, these conditions remained a source of suspicion.[61]

The last area of his report addressed serum therapy and inoculations as a prevention. His conclusions about serums and inoculations boiled down to basically a work in progress. There were two serums, one developed by Dr. Yersin in Saigon and another formulated at the Pasteur Institute. Yersin's seemed to work the best, with a survival rate of 67 percent, whereas the Institute's experienced only a 50 percent survival rate. Regardless of the result, he stressed that either one should be applied; otherwise the morality rate would likely increase to 90 percent or higher.[62]

The next issue addressed was the serum's length of protection. In some cases, the plague could remain in individuals upwards of 42 days. Additional findings showed that physicians and medical personnel should receive another inoculation no later than 32 to 35 days after receiving their first one.[63] In other words, no one knew for sure how long the immunity would last. At least research established the treatment's durability, so previously inoculated individuals knew to get a booster.

Two other serious problems affected the serum's success: the local population's resistance to being vaccinated and its short supply.[64] Concerning locals, whom he termed "natives,"[65] the epidemic had occurred primarily within this group. Because of religious beliefs, customs and general suspiciousness many people had refused treatment, even after becoming ill.[66] This had led critics to "sneer"[67] at efforts to bring the situation under control.[68] The other issue had been supply. There had not been enough of it produced to meet the demand. Geddings concluded by acknowledging progress, but stated that much more needed to be done.[69] His final sentence best summarized the situation:

> The study is at once fascinating and discouraging, for new difficulties constantly arise to take the place of those which have been overcome by laborious effort.[70]

These reports brought forth several new elements in combating disease. First, one must be able through research to distinguish one illness from another, as had been achieved with plague. Second, vaccination prior to an outbreak and then administration of an antitoxin serum to those who became infected proved to be critical elements in saving people through these preventive and curative measures. But the most important aspect of these procedures centered on its further spread, and this could only be accomplished by the implementation of these two elements. The other problem—almost as destructive as the disease—rested on changing cultural attitudes, especially when people remained unwilling to accept the benefits of medicine.

Another unfortunate factor rested on the inability to detect how the disease transmitted to people. Researchers had come close to unraveling this question, and if they had dug more deeply into the issue of filth and overcrowding, it might have become more apparent. As evidenced in Europe during the Dark Ages, overcrowded populations lacked proper sanitation facilities, making them very susceptible to the plague. Eventually, the flea and the black rat became the identified culprits. These organisms freely breed among garbage and poor sanitation conditions. The tiny flea riding on the rat had always been the carrier of the Black Death. Ironically, as this new era of research was underway, another little insect—the mosquito—would be identified by Dr. Walter Reed as the agent spreading yellow fever.[71]

Kinyoun praised Geddings' findings and stated that they confirmed his earlier conclusions about the plague. He acknowledged that the bacillus had now become his most feared contagion, especially in light of its rapid spread throughout Asia and ever increasing proximity to the United States.[72] In less than two years, he would be confronted with this insidious germ as it invaded the shores of San Francisco.[73]

Formaldehyde and Cuba

One of the most important new disinfection compounds had been brought to Kinyoun's attention when he returned to Berlin in 1894.[74] The element had been developed by Von Hoffman and had been named "Formalin"[75] or "Formaldehyde."[76] The base ingredient of the compound came from alcohol. On his return, he started experimenting with the agent, and the initial results proved to be of considerable value. With the help of Geddings, testing centered on its use as a germicide, addressing proper strength, its penetration in fabrics, rooms, books, mail and on ships. Research included its operation, duration of treatment, combination with steam, use in lamps and lastly neutralization after application.[77] As part of his 1897 annual report, he included his two papers on the subject:[78] "Formaldehyde as a Disinfecting Agent and Its Application"[79] and "The Disinfection of the Railway Coach."[80]

These experiments analyzed the substance extensively and provided the proper guidelines for its use in almost all foreseeable situations. The most significant discovery centered on its proven worth as the next generation of disinfectants. In most cases, the disinfecting process would require a 12-hour application. However, when used to clean fabrics, books and bedding, broader measures were required to assure its effectiveness. Combining formaldehyde with steam increased its penetration. Similarly, by using formaldehyde lamps first in suspected areas, it increased the initial containment of the disease before opening up a room and preparing the contents for treatment.[81]

During this period, yellow fever remained a major concern. In experimental testing, formaldehyde had proven successful in disinfecting the holds of ships, with one exception—wooden boats. This type of vessel, in comparison to iron ships, retained moisture in its numerous compartments, limiting the gas's penetration. In those cases, sulfur dioxide remained useful.[82] At the end of his report, Kinyoun commented, "I would state that formaldehyde is one of our best disinfecting agents, if not the best.... While not fulfilling all the requirements of an ideal disinfecting agent, it is equal, if not superior, to our other agents."[83] To the contrary, as the late 20th century would demonstrate, formaldehyde would also prove to be carcinogenic, thereby dangerous to people and animals.[84]

As part of his research, he had been to Tampa, Florida, observing its effect in sanitizing railway cars. Wyman shortened his visit, though, and ordered him to Havana. He would meet with Dr. Burgess, the American Sanitary Inspector at the port, regarding baggage sent to America. The trip had been arranged as part of the Service's preparations for the upcoming quarantine season, the spring and summer months when tropical diseases usually flourished and spread. While in Havana, Kinyoun was to educate Burgess as to this new disinfecting agent. Wyman ordered him to write a report outlining those procedures needed to guarantee that cargo from Havana would be free of infectious organisms.[85]

On his return, he submitted a lengthy account covering more than the use of formaldehyde in sanitizing baggage. He described how the island had become afflicted with an epidemic of smallpox, along with yellow fever. Smallpox had already claimed upwards of 4,000 inhabitants. Apparently the disease had been imported by Spanish troops sent to quell the Cuban War of Independence that started in 1895, eventually leading to the Spanish-American War of 1898. He reported that the disease had primarily spread among the civilian population. The soldiers had not experienced many cases, probably because of their vaccinations. It continued to spread among the local population because of their fear of inoculations.[86] Aversion to hospitals added to the spread: once infected, people would not seek medical assistance at a hospital,[87] which they called "lazaretto," or "a place in which to die."[88]

He reported that it affected the "poorer classes, in overcrowded and unsanitary dwellings."[89] Contributing to its spread had been an increase in the rural people living on the streets as war refugees in deplorable and filthy conditions. Compounding the situation was the lack of good hospitals, with most being used by the Spanish Army. So far, the epidemic had been raging in Havana and Pinar del Rio. The local government had enacted various ordinances in hopes of reversing the situation. These measures included requiring everyone to be vaccinated and prohibiting cemetery visits because the bodies, although buried, could still be infectious.[90]

Besides smallpox, yellow fever had also been running its course on the island. Houses with cases of the fever had been marked with a yellow flag displaying the letter Y for *viruela*. Many people, especially children, ignored the warning and would freely enter the structures. Adding to its spread, hospitals did not segregate patients from those with other infectious diseases. He pointed out that in one instance, patients with yellow fever, dysentery, malaria and smallpox had been placed in the same ward. This created an incubator for these maladies to spread among the convalescents, a situation whereby the sick would likely go from bad to worse, leading to their ultimate death.[91]

In light of these horrifying conditions, Kinyoun and Burgess worked towards implementing new measures to prevent these contagions from reaching America's ports. Kinyoun stated that the epidemics would remain for some time. The best way to address this problem centered on vaccination of the populace, as ordered by Dr. A.J. Porter and to be performed by Dr. Burgess. Another precaution required the crews of ships to be inspected and vaccinated, if this had not been previously done. Cubans wanting to go to the United States had to either be quarantined for 12 days prior to their departure or agree to be vaccinated before arriving. It was recommended that ship crews be vaccinated before going ashore. In order for them to enter American ports, they would need to have a smallpox certificate confirming their inoculation.[92]

Within the course of his visit, issues arose with the vaccine. First, its potency had been shown to decrease over time. Kinyoun recommended using another version of the serum, derived from the glycerinated lymph. Next, the current supply proved insufficient to accommodate the population, requiring a larger inventory. Another problem arose concerning baggage. It needed to be sanitized, and for this process Burgess would use formalin. The fumigation process, however, would be conducted aboard the ships, as opposed to on land, thereby preventing its further spread. For those infected areas in the city, he advised using formaldehyde lamps.[93]

The last item in his report discussed yellow fever. Kinyoun had detected its presence in a mild form after inspecting several areas of Havana. Although it was not an epidemic, the approach of warmer weather meant its occurrence would increase measurably. He revealed that some of the sugar warehouses were full of smallpox and yellow fever patients. Upon examining the harbor's wharves, he found them very unsanitary, creating a major problem for the transfer of ship cargoes to land for further transfer internally or to awaiting ships. The doctor recommend using a floating wharf, where cargo could be transferred and properly disinfected before being allowed on shore or transferred to departing vessels.[94]

In completing his report, he acknowledged that although problems persisted, they were not totally insurmountable. Measures could be put in place rendering passengers and cargo safe before arriving in the United States. Of course, disinfecting procedures needed to be maintained to accomplish this task. Cuban officials would also be instrumental in guaranteeing the success of these efforts. Unfortunately, this could prove to be difficult with the civil war ranging in the country.[95]

IX

Abroad Again

Double Assignments

On July 29, Kinyoun received dual assignments from Wyman directing him to attend the 2nd International Conference on the Hygiene of Railroads and Vessels in Brussels, Belgium, as a delegate of the United States. Afterwards, he would proceed to the International Conference on Leprosy in Berlin, Germany. While in Europe, he was instructed to visit various laboratories and acquaint himself with recent advances in the study of infectious disease.

2nd International Conference on the Hygiene of Railways and Vessels
September 6–8, 1897

An international conference is a grouping of delegates assembled for the purpose of establishing common standards and acceptable practices; a general discussion of common issues in science, medicine and law; codification of agreed upon principles into international law to be ratified by governments with the common goal of establishing a uniform basis of understanding to be followed by nations,[1] sometimes referred to as cognitive norms,[2] or without ratification of the conference's findings.[3]

Kinyoun's first conference dealt with railroad and ship sanitation. On his return home, he wrote a paper about the findings presented at the symposium.[4] There were 150 attendees representing 11 countries. All of the delegates were from Europe or the United States, and many served as official representatives of their respective homelands, since, unlike in America, the governments owned the railroads.[5]

A distinction should be drawn between the two forms of ownership. First, except for Russia, many of the European countries were much smaller in size, Europe being roughly equal in size to the United States though comprised of many nations. Furthermore, not all of these governments were democracies, but instead autocratic empires, where the state either owned or controlled public services for monetary, political and military reasons. In the United States, the private sector either owned or controlled the railroads. The only exception in Europe to government ownership of the railroads was Great Britain.[6]

The agenda for the conference comprised three areas[7]: "Organization of the medical service, Guaranties of the efficiency of the employees and Hygienic precepts and measures."[8] Most of these topics concerned railroads, with numerous papers presented on each section. The European delegates all agreed that the railways should be government controlled, thereby ensuring better operations, especially medical and military matters.[9]

DEPARTMENT OF STATE,
WASHINGTON.

August 23, 1897.

To the

Diplomatic and Consular Officers

Of the United States.

Gentlemen:

I take pleasure in introducing to you Dr. J. J. Kinyoun, Passed Assistant Surgeon, United States Marine Hospital Service, who is about to proceed abroad as a delegate to the International Conference of Hygiene and Sanitary Service on Railways and Shipboard to be held at Brussels, and as a delegate to the International Conference on the Leprosy question to be held at Berlin.

I cordially bespeak for Dr. Kinyoun your official courtesies.

Respectfully yours,

John Sherman

Letter of introduction by John Sherman to diplomatic and consular officers of the United States introducing Dr. J. J. Kinyoun, "Passed Assistant Surgeon," and announcing his appointment as a delegate to the International Conference of Hygiene and Sanitary Service on Railways and Shipboard and the International Conference on Leprosy, August 23, 1897.

Most of the papers reviewed the sanitary measures used towards passengers, cars, stations, cargo and the shipment of animals.[10] All of these procedures had the combined purpose of preventing "the spread of infectious disease."[11] Belgium had established purification points on its lines, where coaches could be sanitized before being granted further passage.[12]

Concerning the sanitation of ships, only two delegates presented papers on the topic. Dr. Gatewood made one of the addresses.[13] The other, written by the

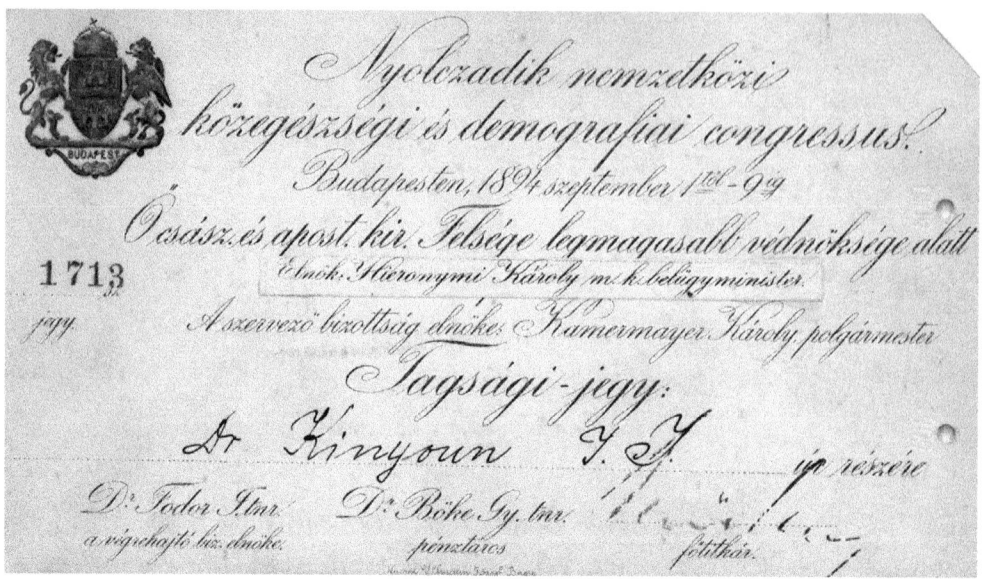

Ticket to International Congress for Dr. Kinyoun, Budapest, September 1–9 (issued in 1897, but apparently reused from 1894).

Westminster and London medical health officer, was titled "Medical inspections of the canal boats."[14] Afterwards, no one responded to the presentation.[15] This led to an interesting comment from Kinyoun: "There were but few persons present who were in any way interested in maritime hygiene or appeared to know anything about it."[16]

The United States and Europe comprised two very dissimilar bodies of land. The North American continent resided thousands of miles away with different health and territory issues. Its coastline alone came close to equaling Europe's. In addition, many European countries had little or, in some cases, no coastline. Therefore, the issue of diseases entering their territory by sea may have been of less concern than entry by railroads.

The conference ended with an agreement to revisit the topic at the 3rd International Conference to be held at Paris in 1900. The doctor reported that one delegate from each country attending this conference would be selected to attend the next one.[17] In terms of the meeting's overall value, he related:

> As a conference dealing with the subjects of international concern it has not been, in my humble opinion, a great success so far as it relates to the United States and Great Britain.[18]

Afterwards, he thought maybe it fulfilled the needs of those individuals wanting a general railroad conference.[19] To the contrary, he wrote that the same had already been achieved and should remain under the jurisdiction[20] of the presumably ongoing "International Congress of Hygiene and Demography."[21] On a positive note, he noted that while procedures improving the European railroads should be applauded, other improvements awaited attention.[22]

In a postscript to his letter, he did not spare words as to his true feelings about the conference. As an honorary secretary, he had to follow a certain formal decorum as a co-author of the summit's affairs.[23] But after attending a few sessions, he described it as a lot of "Talk, Talk."[24] Everyone spoke in different languages, which no one could understand.[25]

The proceedings did not overly impress him; all they spoke about, he complained, was whether medical personnel should be considered as consultants or employees of the railroad. Furthermore, most of the discussion centered on the railways being owned by the government and using them for military purposes. Instead, Kinyoun believed railroads should be used for the well-being of the passengers.[26]

The biggest European fallacy was the belief that railroads served a national military purpose. In fact, since most of the countries had different rail gauges,[27] the railroads remained intrastate, meaning the lines could not cross into a neighboring country.[28] This factor limited any military practicality as far as invading or transporting troops into another territory. In the United States, in contrast, all railroads operated on the same gauge, allowing for commercial and military continuity across all the states.[29] At its conclusion, he again criticized the conference because in essence the whole setting had been slanted towards European wants with little consideration paid to America's needs.[30]

International Leprosy Conference
October 12–14, 1897

Leprosy, a bacterium, is also known as Hansen's Disease, named after G.A. Hansen from Norway, who discovered it in 1873. The disease afflicts the skin, leading to ulcers and lesions resulting in a lack of sensation. Leprosy is a chronic condition, which, if detected and treated early, can be controlled. On occasion, its symptoms have mirrored those of tuberculosis. There are two types of the illness: lepromatous and tuberculoid. Death rarely results from either form.[31]

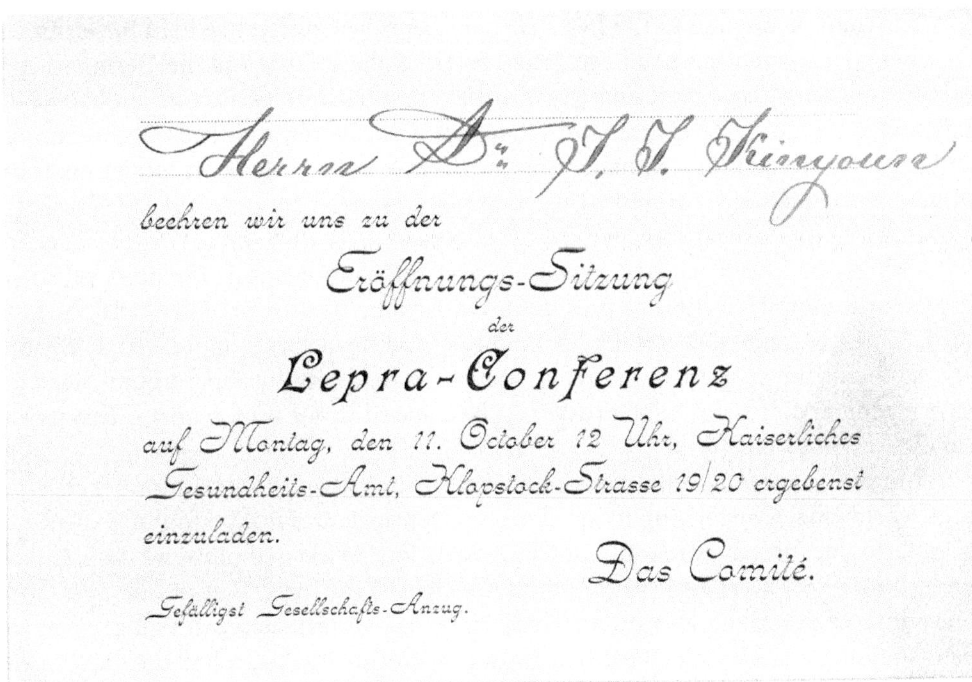

Herrn Dr. J. J. Kinyoun
beehren wir uns zu der
Eröffnungs-Sitzung
der
Lepra-Conferenz
auf Montag, den 11. October 12 Uhr, Kaiserliches Gesundheits-Amt, Klopstock-Strasse 19/20 ergebenst einzuladen.
Das Comité.
Gefälligst Gesellschafts-Anzug.

Leprosy conference invitation to Dr. J. J. Kinyoun.

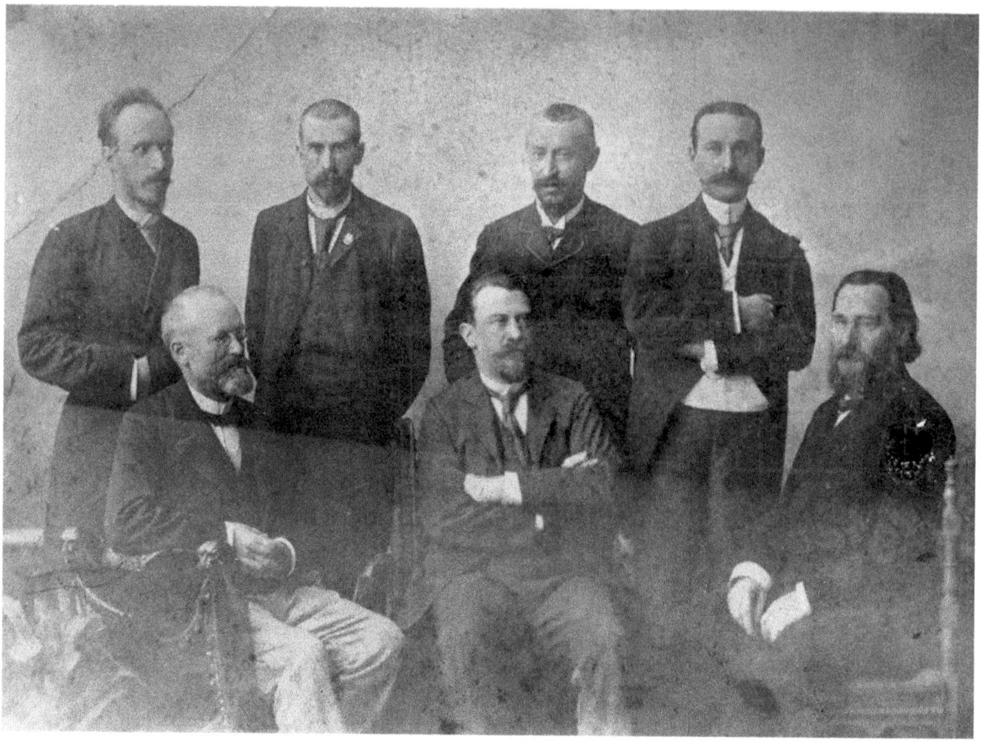

Photograph of Budapest group: Drs. Roux, Metchnikoff, Nocan S. (?), Nuttal (George Henry Falkiner) & etc.

Kinyoun proceeded to the International Leprosy Conference held in Berlin in October. The convention had been called by Dr. Robert Koch and the German Leprosy Commission. Delegates from 19 countries attended with two acting as observers, England and France. Dr. Hansen, the bacterium's discoverer, attended the conference and reported his findings on managing the disease in Norway. A sizable number of private individuals were present. The assemblage focused on three items:[32] "(1) General considerations regarding leprosy; (2) etiology and pathology; (3) prophylaxis."[33]

Officers had been selected to preside over the congregation. The body selected Professor Rudolph Virchow as president, Dr. Armaur as vice-president and Professor E. Ehlers as general secretary. Six honorary secretaries were appointed, Kinyoun among them. The purpose of the group was not to read lengthy papers, but instead to have a general discussion on leprosy.[34] As best stated in the final report, "This was a conference, not a congress."[35]

Initial discussions centered on the susceptibility, origins and number of victims worldwide. Concerning its spread, a consensus could not be found, except its origination occurred more often in individuals in a weakened physical state, those undernourished, poor, or living in filth. Few denied the infectious nature of it, and one conferee described its similarities to tuberculosis. The delegates all seemed to deny that their country was the disease's source. Worldwide, India had the most cases at 130,000, followed by Japan with 20,000; there were 160,000 documented cases in total, from 27 countries.[36]

The attendees agreed leprosy originated from a bacillus appearing as a rod-shaped organism reproduced in chains. Various theories examined how it entered the body, ranging from the skin, air, mucus and other pathways. Hereditary transmission, though, was ruled out as a cause. There appeared to be no effective treatment for the illness, although efforts had been undertaken to find a cure. At present, the most reliable remedy against its spread was a clean living environment. Out of 17 nations attending the conference, most had "no legal measures"[37] on its containment, and in a majority of these countries the illness had been increasing.

As the conference's end, the delegates approved several measures. First, everyone except the French agreed[38] that leprosy should be considered a "menace,"[39] and that if an individual contracted it, then the person should be isolated to prevent its spreading. Isolation had been the main point of contention, because in some countries, such as India, where 300,000,000 people lived, isolation could lead to possible social unrest, even in light of 130,000 cases. The point being, this number in comparison to the whole population would be considered minute. Second, some participants believed an international leprosy commission should be created as an oversight body. The majority concluded otherwise, stating that the conference had not been entrusted with the authority for such a course of action by their governments. Instead, their purpose had solely been to address those actions to be taken upon its detection.[40]

The initial resolution called for "compulsory notification and isolation of every case."[41] But because of objections from the French delegation, the final version resulted in a watered-down version, allowing for a "wide latitude of discretion in dealing with individual cases."[42] Consequently, without a uniform mandate, and absent an obligation of countries to be informative and initiate protective measures, the conference provided little substance.

In closing, the honorary secretaries set forth the general conclusions of the conferees in a summarized report.[43] The report's first item acknowledged Hansen's discovery of the disease[44] and referred to it as the "bacillus leprae."[45] Next, it stated that how the organism originated and infected the body remained a mystery. Suspicions abounded, though, with most believing that it likely entered through the body's skin or mucus. Added to this, it tended to occur more often in the poor, although it had also been found in the higher circles of society. Lastly, a link between its occurrence and heredity had been discredited. And, unfortunately, an effective serum had not been developed for its treatment.[46]

In concluding their report, the secretaries issued the following statement of findings:

> (1) In such countries where leprosy forms foci or has a great extension, we have in isolation the best means of preventing the spread of the disease.
> (2) The system of obligatory notification, of observation and isolation as carried out in Norway, is recommended to all nations with local-self government and a sufficient number of physicians.
> (3) It should be left to the local authorities, after consultation with the medical authorities, to take such measures as are applicable to the special social conditions of the districts.[47]

Kinyoun offered an addendum to the report. He stated that the extent of the disease in the United Sates remained for the most part unknown. Therefore, he advised immediate steps be taken to determine its full extent. On learning the true nature of its progression, corrective action could be instituted in cooperation with the states and federal government.[48]

Other Investigations

Other areas of investigation in 1897 included malaria, tuberculosis, typhoid fever and yellow fever. Several years before, a study had been conducted concerning the water of the District of Columbia. The report showed malaria present throughout the capital region. Recently, the belief had developed that the disease spread through the air, as opposed to through water. This idea received an immediate debunking. Several cases had proven otherwise. In North Carolina and Tennessee many individuals had become ill. Yet after drinking water was boiled, incidences of malaria decreased considerably. This demonstrated that water was the main conduit and not the air. To be certain, though, Kinyoun and the lab initiated further studies in hopes of defining its pathways.[49]

A recent paper on yellow fever by Dr. Sanarelli of Montevideo created a stir within the profession. He claimed to have discovered its cause. Though his findings resulted in initial praise, questions soon arose as to several ambiguities. Kinyoun wanted to embrace the findings, but set forth eight questions that in his opinion needed answering before he could accept the results. Each question conflicted to some degree with Sanarelli's finding in view of existing knowledge about the illness. The doctor made known that until these questions could be answered, he would not accept the paper's finding. The Hygienic Laboratory would conduct its own investigation, without delay, in hopes of proving the paper right.[50]

Research on typhoid fever expanded in hopes of establishing a better diagnosis. Dr. Eduardo Penny Andrade, an assistant at the lab, published an account of his results on this subject. He presented numerous conclusions derived from multiple sources, including Ehrlich and Metchnikoff in trying to isolate the bacillus. Over time, he had been able to separate typhoid fever from colon bacilli in contaminated water. Through the use of a Petri dish and allowing for upwards of three days, the organism became distinct. Once again, another breakthrough had been achieved at the Hygienic Laboratory. Although requiring more research, it represented a significant factor in identifying infections separately and showing water to be the actual dispersal agent.[51]

The Lab

In the 1897 summary of the laboratory's needs, Kinyoun laid out his grand vision as in previous years, but this time on a different scale. Before revealing his plan, he noted that the lab had turned 10 years old. During this period, it had grown in size, depth and stature; it had moved beyond administering to the ills of sailors to addressing the nation's health and quarantine system.[52]

Because of this factor, he advocated it becoming a public health laboratory and a separate governmental entity.[53] He stated there had been "growing sentiment among health officials and sanitarians that the General Government should do more than it has been doing in the domain of public medicine."[54] It should increase its focus on "the investigation into the cause, the prevalence and prevention of disease."[55] Others supported this concept, including the health boards of numerous local governments and states.[56]

Previously, local and state governments had been suspicious of national efforts as an impingement of their respective rights to govern. Nonetheless, he argued that this former impediment of states' rights had decreased considerably in recent years. The reason for this change in attitude stemmed from greater harmony between these layers of government and a better handling by municipal health authorities that before had been lacking.[57]

He stated that this change had turned into a "common consent"[58] between the federal and state governments,[59] whereby "certain prerogatives"[60] now belong to the federal government, whereas before these implied or inherent powers had been entrusted to local and state governments in the case of epidemics.[61] Kinyoun remarked that unfortunately this had occurred less often than it should, mainly in the absence of a plan, national in character, outlining when such authority should be activated by the government.[62] In the past, he noted:

> As a rule, the investigations relating to medical subjects have been made during or at the close of an epidemic, and as soon as the danger had apparently ceased the inquiry ceased. This, as said before, is believed to have been caused by the antagonism of the local authorities, and not because there was no necessity for inquiry.[63]

Kinyoun noted how many believed the federal government should not only have the independent authority to act or investigate,[64] but also look "into the nature, origin, and prevention of contagious epidemics and … other matters relating to public health."[65] And it should have the right to act on an international basis, as well.[66] These statements represented particularly radical views and concepts for late 19th-century America. For one, he pressed for matters of public health to be within the exclusive province of the federal government. He went further by stating that the government's outreach should extend to other countries outside the nation's jurisdiction.[67]

Precedent existed for his proposition, because the Service did require ships leaving foreign ports for the United States to be certified as to the absence of suspected contagions. On the other hand, except for the Quarantine Act of 1893, federal intrusion had been reserved in exercising this authority. Before it had treaded lightly in hopes of not arousing a state's ire.

In concluding his report, he stated that a national laboratory should be created without delay and that it should be under the jurisdiction of the Marine Hospital Service.[68] Its primary purpose should be "the study of the etiology, pathology, and prophylaxis of the acute infectious diseases, viz, yellow fever, cholera, smallpox and plague, etc."[69] In simple terms, the facility should research the cause, cure and prevention of the most serious maladies.

Kinyoun referenced his 1896 report, where he first set forth the substantive provisions for a research commission, while citing yellow fever as the most infectious of the major diseases. He pointed out that the illness had only received special attention twice in the last 20 years. But if a commission had been created for ongoing research, then most likely this illness might have been mitigated by now. Moreover, there would not be a timeline requiring a result, because science should not be measured by time, but instead by a positive outcome achieved over time. This would allow researchers to concentrate more on the cure, rather than on an abstract deadline.[70]

His proposals were sweeping, adding a new perspective on advancing medical research into the 20th century. And through his own intuition, he had been instrumental in developing new serums and techniques treating and combating the world's deadliest diseases. For several years, he had advocated for increased space, a separate building and a larger role for the Service.[71] These constituted ambitious statements for a passed assistant surgeon who remained outranked by many of his peers in the agency. He may have acted alone, and then again he may have had the blessing and encouragement of Surgeon General Wyman. The answer to this question has remained elusive, but could be answered either way, because Kinyoun had proven before to be outspoken in his opinions.

In a few years, his recommendations would begin to take hold and bear fruit, although he would not be there to oversee the changes.[72] The important thing, though, was his continual requests aimed at trying to improve his creation, the Hygienic Laboratory.[73] What he had accomplished amounted to a new beginning in the evolution of modern American medical research. Within the year, part of his recommendations became a reality when the United States Army appointed Dr. Walter Reed head of the Yellow Fever Commission to study its cause with the outbreak of the Spanish-American War.[74]

X

War and the Third Pandemic

The Spanish-American War: Yellow Journalism and the Age of Imperialism

Prior to 1895, tensions between Spain and America had been gradually increasing over Cuba. The United States had been developing important economic and trading ties with the island. But civil unrest had been occurring over the last few years because of Spain's rule.[1]

While this unfolded, yellow journalism had come to life under the craftsmanship of William Randolph Hearst of the *New York Journal* and the *San Francisco Examiner*, along with Joseph Pulitzer of the *New York World*.[2] The phrase meant any news reported in a highly sensational, fabricated, or mongering manner for the purpose of selling newspapers, influencing public opinion and manipulating government policy.[3] In a sense, it could be called the capitalism of the First Amendment, whereby the voice of the press had lost its innocence and constitutional purpose for the sake of self-serving manipulation and greed. It had become an age of extravagance, not only for big business, but for the shear purpose of adulterated power.

In 1895, an insurgency occurred in Cuba, leading Spain to bolster its military presence causing it to crack down on the insurgents. Spanish General Valeriano Weyler imposed harsh measures to suppress the uprising. Hearst and Pulitzer responded by firing up their papers' rhetoric supporting the island's independence and pressed for American intervention. President William McKinley did favor the colony's freedom, but not at the expense of war. Wanting to avert such an event, he dispatched Stewart L. Woodford to Spain in hopes of arranging a diplomatic solution. Stewart reached an accord with its new prime minister, Praxedes Sagasta, that gave Cuba autonomy on January 1, 1898.[4]

Within days of Cuba receiving its self-rule, unrest broke out in Havana at the hands of Spanish officers supposedly in protest over repeated newspaper commentaries against General Weyler. In response, the USS *Maine* was sent to Havana as a show of force and to protect American interests. On January 25, the ship entered Havana harbor and laid anchor. It had become the nation's second battleship and the first ship bearing the state's name. The U.S. government also dispatched ships to Hong Kong and the coast of Spain in anticipation of hostilities. As a precaution, it beefed up its naval presence in the Gulf of Mexico and Key West.[5]

Mysteriously, on February 15 at 1:40 a.m., the *Maine* experienced a massive explosion resulting in its sinking and the loss of 266 men out of a crew of 355. American outrage became immediate, and the press blamed its destruction on Spain. The navy conducted an official inquiry and concluded that an external explosion caused the ship's magazine to explode, indicating sabotage. Consequently, the press accused Spain of sabotage. The country's public opinion soon joined the war movement prompted in part by the Hearst and Pulitzer newspapers.[6]

McKinley had been against war, but with the *Maine* incident and the rantings of the press, he had little choice but to ask Congress on April 11 for permission to deploy troops to intervene in Cuba. Although not an outright declaration of war, Congress authorized the president to issue an ultimatum to Spain requiring it grant Cuban independence and withdraw its troops from the island. He signed the decree on April 23. Spain refused and immediately declared war on the United Sates. On April 25, Congress followed suit and passed a declaration war, leading to the Spanish-American War.[7]

Kinyoun at War, Yellow Fever and Montauk

Yellow Fever is a virus which occurs primarily in the tropics and transmitted by the mosquito. The disease is characterized by a high fever, jaundice and dark-colored vomiting attributed to intestinal bleeding. If the disease is left untreated, death can occur.[8]

Upon hearing about the war and the nation's call to arms, Kinyoun sent the following letter to the president:

> Sir:
>
> In obedience to your call for volunteers for national defense, I have the honor to tender you my services to be employed in any capacity in maintaining and defending our national honor.
> I am, sir,
>
> Very respectfully,
> Your obedient servant,
> J. J. Kinyoun
> Passed Assistant Surgeon, M.H.S.[9]

He forwarded the letter to Wyman, asking him to deliver it to the president.[10] On May 12, he received a reply from Dr. Sternberg, the surgeon general of the Army. Sternberg replied that it had been filed for future reference.[11] While being pigeonholed, within a few months he would be summoned to assist with the return of the army's troops from Cuba.[12]

The war proved to be short-lived and ended on August 12,[13] when Spain and the United States signed a "Protocol of Peace."[14] This agreement would be followed by a formal peace treaty eight months later,[15] the "Treaty of Paris."[16] Under its terms, Spain ceded Puerto Rico, Guam and the Philippines to the United States with Cuba becoming a free sovereign.[17] With the war's end, America became recognized as a world power and an emerging empire with the acquisition of Spain's former colonies.

During the conflict, the dark shadow of disease had raised its ugly head. Yellow fever had broken out among the troops on both sides.[18] The army dispatched Dr.

Walter Reed to the island hoping he could determine its origin. His efforts proved unsuccessful. Many authorities thought the illness was infectious. To the contrary, in 1881 Dr. Carlos Finlay had set forth the theory it might be spread by mosquitoes, as opposed to contact among humans. His theory would soon be proven right.[19]

In May 1900, Reed returned to the island, accompanied by a task force of doctors, called the Yellow Fever Commission, entrusted with the job of conducting an official investigation. Its objective was to find the source of the illness. Within a year, he and his team, especially due to the efforts of Dr. Henry Carter, concluded that the mosquito was the carrier. As a result, he received immense credit for the discovery, as opposed to Finlay and Carter. Reed, though, did acknowledge Finlay as the true discover of the cause and gave Carter credit, too, even though he wrote the official report announcing the actual connection. To its credit, the commission found ways to eradicate the virus by controlling the mosquito population and its habitats.[20]

With the war over, the troops began returning home. Unfortunately, the question of how yellow fever spread would not be finalized until 1901.[21] As a precaution, quarantine measures needed to be put in place. During this period, a series of letters were exchanged between Wyman; W.H. Francis, secretary-treasurer of the Kensington Engine Works, Ltd.; and Kinyoun concerning the purchase and transport of heavy disinfection equipment to various sites. Delivery locations for these utensils included Montauk, New York; the Marine Hospital in Baltimore; Santiago, Cuba; and several other cities.[22]

With the Service's gearing up for the troops' return, equipment became part of the sanitation process in preventing the introduction of yellow fever and other tropical illnesses. To everyone's dismay, Francis telegraphed Wyman, informing him of a major problem in delivering the equipment. He stated that none of his employees would go to Montauk. They feared contracting the "fever."[23] As a concession, he could provide one man, but only on a temporary basis.[24]

Other components were ordered throughout this period. Kinyoun, too, made requisitions. In his case, he purchased formalin retorts and apparatuses for several ports.[25] By these acquisitions, the seriousness of the situation could be clearly seen through these letters. In August, he received an order relieving him of duty at the lab and directing him to Montauk, where Wyman asked him to oversee the sanitation operations on the disinfectant barge *Protector*.[26] Montauk had been chosen as the most logical place to screen the returning troops. Situated on the far eastern point of Long Island, it served as a good location away from any major population and provided a better site to contain an outbreak.[27]

During his stay, he witnessed a unique part of history and in all probability came face to face with Theodore "Teddy" Roosevelt, Jr., one of the political giants in early 20th-century America. Roosevelt and his men would be quarantined at Montauk for 30 days.[28] Photographs have shown Teddy and Kinyoun at the station, but not together.[29]

Although undocumented in any official reports of the Service, Kinyoun and his family visited Havana sometime after the sinking of the battleship *Maine*. Family pictures show him in a rowboat alongside the ship hovering next to its sunken deck. After it exploded, the hull settled back into the shallow water of its moorings.

The harbor, while able to accommodate large ships, was not a deep channel port. The pictures showed daughter Alice in the boat along with her father. To this day, the family possesses two relics from the battleship that she picked up off the deck slightly covered in water. The first is a shell fragment, and the second is a portion of the brass trim from the captain's quarters.[30]

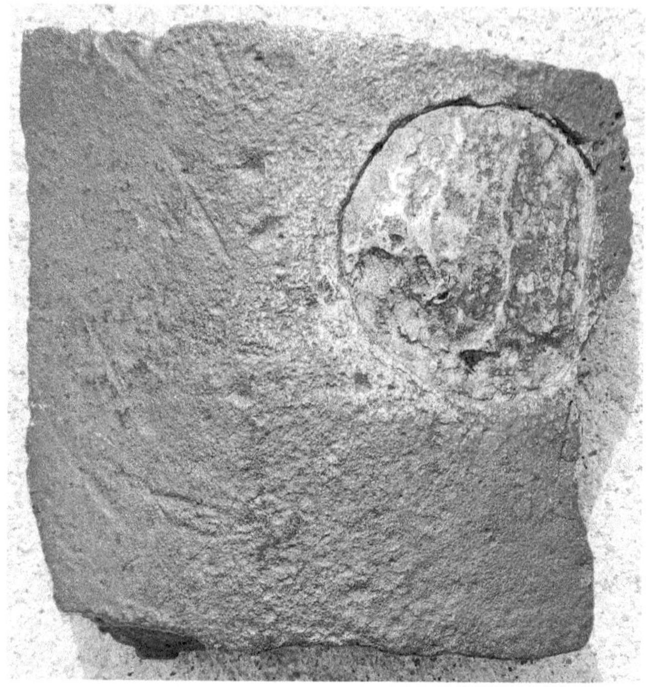

USS *Maine* shell fragment taken from ship's deck by Alice Kinyoun Houts.

Approach of the Black Death

As 1897 drew to a close, the presence of bubonic plague continued to raise its ugly face throughout the Far East, decimating millions in its wake while creeping from country to country.[31] Since 1855, in a remote part of China, the Black Death once again reemerged. This particular outbreak became known as the Third Pandemic. It started in the Yunnan Province, where a revolt had commenced leading to Chinese troops being sent into the region. The province rested on the southwest border of the Himalayan Mountains bordering Tibet, India and Myanmar.[32] The plague's first known existence had originated centuries before in this part of the Himalayas.[33]

On returning home, the soldiers soon became stricken with it. Over time it simmered beneath the surface before exploding on to the population in 1894, starting in Canton. Eventually, it transformed into the pneumonic version of the bacterium causing widespread loss of life reminiscent of the earlier Great Plagues. By 1898, it had invaded Hong Kong and much of India.[34] It now poised ready to spread around the world, and this time it gazed at the West Coast of the United States on account of the major international trading routes between Asia and America.

In light of this major outbreak, the annual report of the Marine Hospital Service for 1898 contained numerous reports concerning its outbreak, which had likely reached Kinyoun.[35] Under a separate section titled "PLAGUE,"[36] the Third Pandemic's spread received considerable mention. The greatest concern was its appearance in Bombay, India, followed by reports of its presence in a score of other cities.[37]

It 1896, it arrived in Bombay. By September 1897, officials were documenting anywhere from 40 to 50 deaths a week, increasing to 60 by October, culminating in

83 a week from November to December. This trend continued into the early part of March 1898. From December 7, 1897, to June 21, 1898, there were 14,351 deaths. But authorities suspected the figure to be much higher because many of the cases had been concealed by the local population.[38]

In analyzing the statistics between the European and the indigenous residents, the former fared better than the latter. Of a total population of 11,290 Europeans, 22 had died, or less than .02 percent. The local population of 821,764 had seen 18,638 deaths, or 2.3 percent of the population, a sizable contrast between the groups.[39]

Several reasons may have contributed to this variance. Possibly, a few of the Europeans had some immunity to the illness, since their continent had been exposed to the malady centuries ago. Second, the variance may have stemmed from the difference in basic sanitation habits between the groups, with the Europeans utilizing better practices on a more regular basis. In comparison, Bombay's population probably lacked modern hygiene measures. India had long been known for the overcrowding in its major cities leading to poor sanitation and, in turn, the spread of disease.[40]

Some of the indigenous groups experienced the plague on a lesser scale. Although not totally invulnerable, the Mohammedans and Parsees appeared largely free of the illness. The same held true for various Hindu sects, except the Jains, who were greatly afflicted during this bout. To combat further spreading, the English sent numerous physicians to the country and imposed strict quarantine measures.[41] They instituted the "Ward System,"[42] a network where the city had been sectioned off into grids with troops guarding all entry and departure points, only allowing passage to those individuals passing a medical inspection by a health officer.[43] Additionally, "all the houses in the section were searched for the sick and dead."[44]

Unfortunately for Bombay, the death toll had become staggering. Between October 1896 and April 1897, there were more than 20,000 victims. But when other parts of the city were counted, the number likely exceeded 70,000. In the summer months of 1898, it started to taper off, but by August it had reappeared at a rate of 103 deaths per week, rising to 210 a week by early October 1898. With the numbers increasing, officials felt certain that there would be another epidemic from 1898 to 1899. As proof of this fear, a report listed 14 other cities experiencing plague.[45] These included "Broah, Surat, Thana, Satara, Sholopore, Belgaum, Dharwar, Kathiawar, Baroda, Karachi, Kohlapore, Sachin, Bhor and Cutch."[46] Within this group alone, 840 people had died in a single week.[47]

In mapping out the plague, it was found to be occurring in almost every corner of the country. In November 1897, Poona had become its center, spreading to the rail line located between Madras and Sholopore, 500 miles from Bombay. It next appeared 1,800 miles to the north of Bombay in Hardwar, neighboring a pilgrimage site close to the Himalayas. South of Bombay, it had erupted in the towns of Goa, a Portuguese settlement, and at Hubli.[48]

The death rate continued to rise, especially in Poona, where out of 6,000 cases, 4,300 had perished. For those receiving hospital treatment, fatalities were 66 percent. Those not receiving help had a morality rate of 80.50 percent.[49] These figures represented phenomenal amounts, approaching tolls not seen since the plagues of early

Christianity and the Middle Ages. There appeared to be no end in sight to its spread and when it would run its course.

It continued to flare up elsewhere in India. To the south, Karachi saw a reoccurrence in September 1897; the disease then disappeared, but reemerged at an even greater level by May 1898. At this time, cases totaled 1,007, resulting in 740 deaths, until its decline June. Bombay again saw it reappear in January 1898, with unabated devastation. To make matters worse, by the end of January 1898, it had spread to five additional cities: "Hyderabad, Sarati, Kashegeon, Dhoti and Warligeon."[50] Others followed, and by May 1898, it had claimed 1,022 lives out of 1,369 cases.[51]

The problem with its reoccurrence centered on one thing, its potency. In each instance, it had become stronger, more infectious and deadlier. Over time, this factor had been shown to be a unique trademark of the malady. It will make an initial introduction into a region and lie dormant, only to reappear with greater intensity. In many cases, the bacterium will transition from the bubonic form into the pneumonic version. Upon this conversion, it becomes almost impossible to contain, resulting in countless deaths within the course of a day after exposure.[52]

By April, it had reached Calcutta. In a detailed report by Ambassador P.F. Patterson, the United States consul-general to the city, he stated early cases had been viewed with suspicion and after further examination proved to be bubonic. Out of 25 cases, 12 had perished.[53] He noted that with Calcutta having a population of 800,000,[54] it had so far been "Plague sporadic."[55]

While the numbers of cases may have seemed relatively small in comparison to the entire population, panic had stricken the city because of the quarantine. These actions greatly disturbed the population because it interfered with their customs. In particular, the possibility of troops searching zenanas, or women's rooms, caused major concern. The people objected to house inspections, the separation of their families and the segregation of victims. Many inhabitants were more afraid of being detained in the city than being infected with the contagion. The Bengal legislative council provided some calm after remarks made by the lieutenant governor regarding the mildness of the outbreak.[56]

India would not be alone in trying to cope with the epidemic. Reports circulated about the disease breaking out in other countries. From January to July 1898, the Service received countless updates on its whereabouts. It appeared in Egypt, Djiddah, and southeastern Europe, where officials feared it would further spread because of the upcoming religious pilgrimages to places like Hedjaz.[57]

The consul to the United States in Amoy, China, Mr. A. Burlingame Johnson, informed Wyman of the plague's continual spread throughout the country. Besides Amoy being plague-ridden, so were the towns of Canton, and the ports at Tainan, Taiwan and Taipei. In all of these cities, it had become epidemic with 2,338 cases documented from April 29 to June 15, 1898, with 1,483 dead. From other areas, incoming accounts indicated it had become pneumonic, resulting in the death of thousands.[58]

Johnson also reported a ship had had 20 deaths a day while heading towards San Francisco. He further reported that the daily toll in Amoy averaged 100.[59] In another passage, though, he predicted that "the spread of the epidemic will be checked, as the hot sun is fatal to the plague germs."[60] Such a connection did exist between plague cases and the weather, but the science of the time did not totally support this conclusion.[61]

In July, two other ships reported carrying plague, the *Carthage* and the *Glenturret*. The *Carthage* had arrived at Aden coming from Bombay bearing seven cases; the ill were transferred to Woosung. The captain of the *Glenturret* later confirmed the death of all the victims. Having stopped in Shanghai, the ship became quarantined with shore contact banned by the authorities. No further cases occurred on the vessel.[62]

In another part of the world, Consul-General Frank C. Partridge, stationed in Tangier, expressed his concern in an April communiqué about annual pilgrimage to Mecca associated with the increased shipment of goatskins to the United States. Sometime before, cholera had been present in this material, but it had since disappeared, allowing for renewed shipping. However, the plague had now broken out in Djiddah, and the fear rose it would manifest itself within animal skins from Moorish traders coming into America, just as cholera had done before. At the same time, the pilgrims going to Mecca potentially could become infected with the disease and introduce it back to Morocco, where it could harbor in goatskins bound for export.[63]

Because of this possibility, the diplomatic corps had put pressure on the Moroccan government to stop the pilgrimage. The year before, the same situation had occurred, and on that occasion the Moroccan government had canceled the holy journey to Mecca. Nonetheless, this year the grand vizier refused, pointing out[64]:

> ... the pilgrimage is one of the great essential precepts of religion and ordained by divine law, and neither the Makhzen [Moorish Government] nor anybody can interfere with the shra so as to deny the divine ordinances being followed by their adherents ... although they [the Moors] may be fully aware that one of them going thither will never return, and that death would result to all of them, yet they would desire it and seek it, willingly spending their money and scarifying themselves in observing the divine law in joy and gladness.[65]

But even in light of this response, the grand vizier would be willing to allow "a quarantine station for returning pilgrims."[66] With this news, the consular office imposed restrictions at Moorish ports on returning pilgrims, citing as the reason that returning travelers might bring it back to Morocco. Because of this concern and its association with animal pelts, Italy imposed a prohibition on all hides coming from Morocco and the Barbary states.[67]

Other nations followed suit, not as to the importation of hides, but in allowing its citizens to participate in the pilgrimage. Russia issued its prohibition in February 1898, stating that Persia was doing the same and therefore that quarantines would be established at Persian ports in the Persian Gulf. France, too, had set in motion restraints in hopes of preventing the plague from surfacing in Algeria and Tunis. All of these countries feared it would be contracted during the annual holy trip, thereby necessitating the implementation of these restrictive measures.[68]

Secretary of State Gage made an official request upon the Ottoman Empire "for a strict enforcement of the sanitary regulations to prevent the spread of bubonic plague."[69] He stated that the United States hoped the Ottoman government would

> ... be more efficient in the enforcement of its sanitary regulations upon receiving the conjoint recommendations of the several powers.[70]

Constantinople, the capital of the Ottoman Empire, sat at the strategic trading crossroads between Asia and Southern Europe, North Africa and the Middle East on the Bosporus Strait between the Black and the Mediterranean Seas. If this intersection of civilization remained open, absent quarantine protections, then the whole of this merging land mass would be once again open to the passage of plague. Gage's letter to the Ottoman government stressed the importance of proper sanitation guidelines in what could be perceived as an almost critical assessment of its procedures. Apparently, other nations had expressed the same concerns to the Empire. After all, the Justinian Plague of AD 542–543 and the medieval plague occurring in AD 1346 had both passed near and through these straits before decimating all of Europe and much of Northern Africa.

Though everything seemed dire, a serum had been developed showing some promise. Waldemar Mordecai Wolff Haffkine, who had relocated to Bombay, invented a vaccine that had proved effective in roughly 50 percent of those individuals receiving it. Haffkine had studied with Élie Metchnikoff at the Pasteur Institute in 1889. To prove the value of his serum, he had injected himself with the plague bacterium after being inoculated with his vaccine. Prior to inventing the serum, he had previously made a serum for use against cholera.[71]

At a lecture in Poona, India, he shared his findings about its value. He described an experiment involving 20 rats, with only 10 receiving the vaccine. Next, he placed an infected rat within the group. As a result of the 10 not being inoculated, nine contracted the disease and died. Among the 10 that had received the vaccine, only one became ill. Between the groups, one had a 90 percent prevention rate and the other had a 90 percent death rate.[72]

Haffkine shared statistics from four towns where his serum had been used on the local population. In Lower Daumaun, there were 2,197 inoculations, with 6,033 not receiving the vaccine. Within these groups, just 36 of those injected with the serum subsequently died after becoming infected with the disease. In the unvaccinated group, 1,482 ended up dying. The comparisons between the groups proved to be eye-opening.[73]

The other three cities had similar outcomes. The vaccine showed great promise, even with an average success rate of 50 percent.[74] To the contrary, against the "pulmonary forms"[75] of the disease—the pneumonic strain was known for causing the greatest number of deaths—it had not yet proven successful. To his credit, though, the vaccine proved to be a positive preventive measure.[76]

The plague continued to traverse the world, especially from the East. It would only be a matter of time before it reached the shores of America. But until it ran its course in India, China and other countries, the number of deaths became almost unbelievable. In these two countries alone, the death toll had crested at 12,000,000. As seen in India, once it left the big cities, like Bombay, it soon spread into the countryside, killing millions.[77]

Kinyoun had not been directly involved with the emerging pandemic, but he assuredly had become aware of its ever-expanding outreach through all the correspondence flowing through the Service.[78] Even though preoccupied at the lab with other matters, the plague ominously made its path towards him, not only from a medical standpoint, but a personal one as well.

XI

1899: The Year of Great Upheaval

Encirclement

As 1899 unfolded, Kinyoun's future would soon be overcome by the darkening approach of bubonic plague, as it moved ever so assuredly around the globe. Within six months it would be knocking on America's West Coast. The encirclement of the planet by this most feared of all maladies had been occurring very slowing since the 1850s. By 1896, it exploded upon the world's stage, moving from port to port and from city to city. Not unlike days of old when it swept across Europe with unimaginable carnage, this time it had conquered much of the Far East leaving only the United States in its sights.[1]

By August, 220,907 plague cases had been reported in Bombay, resulting in the deaths of 164,083 people. Worldwide it had become staggering, with 13 countries reporting its presence: Russia, Persia, Austria, French Ivory Coast, Arabia, Egypt, Portugal, Madagascar, Turkey, Singapore, Japan, Formosa and Brazil. It had now become a pandemic. From all accounts, it seemed unstoppable with its main transporter being seafaring vessels.[2]

Dr. Stuart Eldridge, the country's chief sanitary inspector who had been stationed in Yokohama, Japan, wrote an extensive account about the plague's passage on ships traveling between eastern ports and those bound for the United States. He set forth inspection procedures to detect the disease by examining the crews and passengers before boarding.[3] The process involved "a thorough palpation of the neck, maxillae, groins, and region of the thigh, immediately below the latter: the tongue, facial expression, and general condition."[4] Any individual bearing the slightest trait of infection should be detained for a more complete examination.[5]

He pointed out that on a ship arriving in Yokohama from China, all of the steerage passengers received the inspection. Women suspected of carrying a disease were removed to a separate place for a private exam. Head counts were maintained on all individuals[6] going through the process by way of a "mechanical apparatus,"[7] and double-checked by two individuals. Any disparity between the figures required a recount. While physical examinations were conducted, an inspection would be made of the ship's interior, assessing its sanitation and looking for afflicted individuals hidden on board as stowaways. Lastly, the baggage would be inspected and, if all right, labeled clear.[8]

Eldridge stated that if any ship had previously been carrying a suspected case, then it would be noted as part of the screening process. In such event, the information would be forwarded to the quarantine officials stationed at the port of arrival. As an additional precaution, all the passengers' health certificates would be transmitted to the port, thereby giving them a basis upon which to assess each individual's condition upon their arrival.[9]

The biggest problem existed in fully implementing these measures. The main impediment rested in the lack of disinfecting equipment needed to sanitize ships. He related that although the Imperial Japanese Government had agreed to quarantine precautions, they appeared to be less than Eldridge had anticipated and not compliant with American law. Another problem lay in the large amount of steerage passengers, making it difficult to handle the volume. Even with these limitations, the inspector applauded Ambassador Buck in his efforts to have the Japanese absorb the responsibility of decontaminating vessels.[10]

But even with this assistance it appeared limited to the "graver infectious diseases … such as cholera and plague."[11] As to smallpox, they did not pay as much attention. As part of the Japanese process, people showing signs of infection would be required to take a bath, sometimes containing an antiseptic.[12] Afterwards, they would be given an "aseptic robe"[13] to wear while their clothing was cleaned by high-pressured steam, followed by the disinfection of their luggage. Next, the crew and passengers would be quarantined for seven days (plague) or five days (cholera).[14]

Although the disinfecting process seemed thorough, Eldridge noted deficiencies. First, it needed to be faster, possibly implying more ships could be processed and released for passage. Second, he could have been suggesting that the sooner infected passengers were uncovered, the greater the likelihood of containing the contagion. He also criticized the lack of proper equipment, such as barges and launches used in transporting people and their belongings to shore for processing. Overall, the procedures needed significant improvement to be effective.[15]

He examined several instances of ships having been stopped between October 21, 1898, and April 18, 1899, because of smallpox. A trend became apparent. Although the procedures on paper had a sound basis, the practical application of these measures had become difficult. The main impediments were official oversight between countries, improper equipment and the lack of consistency. Because of these factors, it sometimes became impossible to establish a truly safe screen from one country to the other.[16] And with plague running amok not only worldwide, but especially in the Far East, it appeared only a matter of time before it reached America.

On April 17, 1899, a steerage passenger on the *Gaelic* exhibited symptoms of plague while in route from Hong Kong to Shanghai before journeying to San Francisco. The ship's surgeon made the discovery. By nightfall the victim had died, which led to the body being tossed in the ocean. The ship next proceeded to the port of Woosung, whereupon the steerage compartment was fumigated with sulfur and the victim's personal effects destroyed. The vessel proceeded to Nagasaki, arriving on April 21, and remained at the quarantine station for seven days.[17]

On May 26, the *Nippon Maru*, a Japanese ship, embarked from Nagasaki, after first departing from Hong Kong, towards her ultimate destination of San Francisco.

Shortly after its departure, a Chinese steerage passenger became ill and succumbed within an hour. The ship's surgeon had examined the individual beforehand, noting he had appeared healthy at the time. The victim's friends stated that the person had a history of seizures, indicating heart trouble. Oddly enough, the body had not shown any outward signs of plague, especially the glands that would usually become dark in color.[18]

As a precaution, the steamship proceeded to a quarantine station where doctors removed a portion of the deceased's glands for examination. The next day, they confirmed it as plague. Afterwards, the authorities cremated the body. This resulted in the ship being disinfected, including the passengers, crew and baggage. After a seven-day quarantine, the *Nippon Maru* proceeded on its original course.[19]

Between Yokohama and Honolulu another death occurred, arousing more concerns. An investigation proved it to be plague. Mysteriously, while sailing into San Francisco harbor, two bodies had been purportedly thrown overboard.[20] In Eldridge's report, he stated that tests had been conducted on "the bodies of two passengers drowned in the bay."[21] A later investigation raised the question of whether the passengers having plague were thrown overboard to cover up the true cause of their death.[22]

Eldridge appeared to have some reservations about the matter, writing:

> Although, in the presence of so tremendous, imminent, and little understood a danger as plague. We can scarcely be too severe or minute in our precautions. I knowing the uncertainty of purely bacteriological diagnosis in the hands of others than thoroughly trained experts, may be pardoned for some skepticism as to the actual infection of the *Nippon Maru*.[23]

In other words, he had doubts as to its presence. Maybe, for some unknown reason, he did not accept the previous findings. But this seemed to contradict the second sentence, wherein he basically stated that one can never be too careful when it comes to such a vicious illness. He admitted in the first sentence that little is known about its ravages, but in the third reversed himself again by asserting his suspicion about its presence, unless certified by an expert. It raises the question: who would this expert be, if not him?

It would seem he might know in light of his broad experience. But why the double-talk? One will never know for sure. In all honesty, Eldridge could have been simply qualifying his position scientifically, so that a better understanding could be had before announcing its presence on the country's doorstep. To publicize such a possibility, without firm proof, could be catastrophic from a public relations standpoint—let alone from a medical perspective—and lead to widespread panic.

Eventually, the *Nippon Maru* would be identified as the probable original carrier of bubonic plague to America.[24] During the next two years, Kinyoun would become embroiled in one of the most horrific cover-ups in the nation's history. The campaign to deny and conceal its presence would in short order destroy his career and leave him an obscure figure as one of the major leaders in the country's evolution in advancing modern medicine.

The *Nippon Maru* would not be alone in transporting the plague, because on June 23, another Japanese vessel named the *America Maru* began its journey from Hong Kong to San Francisco. In route, a Chinese crewman showed signs of it even after being cleared by quarantine inspectors at Kobe. The ship was placed under quarantine when the symptoms became more pronounced and tissue tests confirmed the disease. Unfortunately, the man succumbed to the illness the following evening. The same day, a Japanese sailor showed similar symptoms.[25]

While in Yokohama, Eldridge viewed patients at the quarantine station, courtesy of its director, Dr. Hoshino, an American trained physician. During his observations, he examined a Japanese and a Chinese patient, both sick with what he thought to be plague. In the former, the disease appeared more advanced, with the latter being in its early stages. He also noted that the *City of Peking*, an American ship, had a Chinese steerage passenger with the contagion, who subsequently died.[26]

In concluding his report, he set forth a compilation of all the vessels inspected from July 1, 1898, to June 30, 1899. All told, he had examined 165 ships sailing from the Far East to America.[27] It represented a tally of ships, people and their baggage reviewed during this period. He ended by stating that he had sent "193 formal official letters"[28] along with "932 official forms,"[29] totaling 1,125 documents in conjunction with the inspections.[30] In passing, he remarked that the task had been by "no means trifling."[31]

In reviewing it, several conclusions can be drawn that reveal maybe why the plague had had such ease in its travels. First, although conscious efforts had been made to inspect and isolate suspected carriers, the system lacked cohesiveness among ports and nations, especially from the disease's launching pad in the Far East. Eldridge repeatedly demonstrated his understanding of the sanitation process, but related difficulties in having a truly effective dragnet to effectively contain it. Moreover, governments lacked the necessary disinfecting apparatus, had inadequate inspection procedures and lacked official oversight from port to port.

In the course of his tenure, Eldridge oversaw a staggering number of inspections involving 39,194 people. Many of these individuals came from the steerage classes, or those huddled in the crowded bowels of ships. They could not afford the more expensive accommodations of passage and therefore had been relegated to often dingy, tight and unsanitary living spaces, conducive to the spread of disease.

Although his numbers appeared impressive, the figures reveal a darker side to the inspection process. With this said, and the large number of passengers examined, only 375 of them had been vaccinated, or one hundredth of a percent of the total. The same held true for the 22,260 pieces of baggage inspected, with only 2,840 being treated, or 13 percent of the total.

Understandably, some passengers may have been already vaccinated, but probably a distinct minority. The disinfecting of baggage showed a greater effort, but live organisms migrate, not physical property. Personal effects can be tainted and operate as conduits, but the organism must have something to live on in order to continue to multiply and spread. In time, without fuel, such as water, or a host, the organism will die, thereby leaving baggage devoid of further infection. If the procedures had been reversed, whereby more people, or all passengers, had been vaccinated, as opposed to the baggage, especially the apparently more susceptible steerage passengers, then possibly the plague could have been averted from its impeding course.

A Falling Out?

On January 10, 1899, Kinyoun received a directive from Wyman stating that because of his position on the sanitary board, he needed to be available to attend board meetings. Accordingly, prior orders allowing him the freedom to oversee vaccination centers and inspect railway cars had been revoked. If he believed a situation warranted his presence, then he would have to secure special permission before leaving Washington.[32]

Afterwards, it appeared he had published Wyman's directive in his monthly report of the Hygienic Laboratory, sparking what appeared as a sharp response from his supervisor. In a letter dated February 4,[33] Wyman wrote, "Your attention is called to an inaccurate statement concerning the investigations relating to car sanitation and vaccine establishments."[34] He stated that his letter of January 10 did not terminate these previous orders, but only those portions allowing him to leave the city at his discretion.[35] In concluding, Wyman stated:

> ... you were specifically instructed that in the event it became necessary for you to make any investigations requiring your absence from Washington, to report the fact and await special authority in each case from the Supervising Surgeon-General, M.H.S.[36]

For some reason, the letter of January 10 had caused a misunderstanding between them, possibly signaling a strained relationship. Although the correspondence may have been a routine way of clarification, Wyman's response appeared curt. Kinyoun's publication of its contents may have caused him some embarrassment. Obviously he had either misread the order or wanted to make a stand about what he may have felt as a curtailment of his professional freedom. He may have thought Wyman to be interfering in his job.

On the other hand, Wyman, who up to this point had held Kinyoun in high regard, needed him close at hand, especially for his participation and medical insight on the sanitary board. As both these men well knew, the plague could be arriving very soon. Wyman may have felt compelled to keep his subordinate close in case immediate action would be required, either because of the plague, or in the event some other pestilence reared its head.

Letters

Between March 6 and March 21, a series of letters were exchanged among an assortment of Kinyoun family members, including Joe, Lizzie, Mrs. Nathan W. Perry and the Kinyoun children.[37] Although not of major historical importance, they do shed light on their various personalities and reveal the household's daily happenings. In particular, they offer a glimpse of his children.

The first letter disclosed that Lizzie had taken a trip to visit family in Charlotte, North Carolina. Joe had remained home with the children, and Lizzie's mother had moved in to assist with their care. Kinyoun wrote to her and gave an update on everyone's activities. He related how Conrad had had a nut stuck in his tooth and Dr.

Donnelley had been able to remove the particle. Alice was supposed to see the doctor, but he had kept her home because there had been two cases of diphtheria reported in the office. He concluded by conveying his well wishes to her and Aunt Julia.[38]

A second letter to Lizzie offered an interesting look into several windows of his world. Addressed to "Sweetheart,"[39] he wrote:

> I would have dropped you a line yesterday had I not been so busy with my boys. The course is now so nearly finished and there is yet so much to do that we will have to have night sessions just like Congress.[40]

This reference probably referred to his teaching a course at the lab for new enlistees and younger officers. The subject possibly dealt with bacteriology, or with some particular research.

In another passage, and a bit amusingly, he wrote that "Joe Perry"[41] had been asking for a duck for some time, so the doctor fixed it for the Sunday dinner.[42] Afterwards, Joe commented, "he was quite disappointed that it came without the 'fur' being on it."[43] Apparently he had misunderstood the true nature of his son's request: he wanted a live duck for a pet, as opposed to a duck for his dinner.

The letter talked about Alice's vision being nearsighted and necessitating an eye exam with Dr. Suiter. In addition, he reported that he thought Connie had been finally weaned. In her absence, he had taken Connie to be "kodaked [sic],"[44] but he was still waiting on the photographer to finish the images. As for happenings, he advised her that the Medical Society would be having a meeting and he intended to write a paper on meningitis for the gathering.[45] Ever the scientist, he wrote that he had almost completed building a "disinfecting shed"[46] at the Bureau.[47]

In a letter to Lizzie from her mother, affectingly signed "Momma Perry,"[48] it talked about the doctor and his class. It stated he would leave early in the morning to teach his course, with the family rarely seeing him. Because the class had been running behind in covering all the material, it necessitated make-up sessions at night.[49] Mrs. Perry had enclosed a letter signed "Alice Eccles Kinyoun."[50] Allie had written it on behalf of herself and her younger brothers Perry and Connie. She wrote how they missed her and they send their love and kisses to her.[51] Mrs. Perry had also expressed how much the children missed her. Even so, the children were doing well.[52]

Upheaval

On April 27, Kinyoun received two orders from Dr. Wyman.[53] The first instructed him to appear before Surgeon Charles E. Banks, chairman of the board of examiners on May 16, at 10:00 a.m. for the purpose of determining his promotion to surgeon.[54] The second relieved him as director of the Hygienic Laboratory with orders to assume charge of the San Francisco Quarantine Station no later than June 1. He would be relieving Surgeon S.D. Brooks. What's more, the order directed that he turn over all public property of the lab to Passed Assistant Surgeon Milton J. Rosenau.[55]

After roughly 12 years as the director, the lab's founder had been dismissed from his position. The assignment appeared to be a total surprise. Several reasons support this conclusion.

First, Wyman did not appear as one who would necessarily reveal his plans prior to issuing an order. He had been described as having

> ... a great penchant for detail, and management expert will be gratified to know.... Doctor Wyman developed a manual of procedure for use at Service Headquarters ... and reduced to writing almost every procedural step in handling correspondence, accounts, appointments and separation of personnel ... and other administrative operations.[56]

The manual provided a guidepost, whereby

> individual responsibility and authority in the Headquarters organization were set down in detail from routine transactions to matters involving policy, and supervisory personnel were held accountable for the application of its provisions.[57]

From these references it can be determined that he was a stickler for details and viewed as a procedural adherent not necessarily willing to compromise. Another statement commented, "He was a cautious person, very careful not to commit himself on any subject until he was completely sure of his ground."[58]

As to his bearing on matters, one account stated:

> Doctor Wyman's approach was one of persuasion. Although, he was tenacious in his opinions and judgments, his attitude was not that of demanding acceptance.[59]

Wyman had impressive credentials. Originally from St. Louis, he graduated from Amherst College with a BA in 1870 and earned his medical degree from St. Louis Medical College in 1873. The next two years he worked at City Hospital in St. Louis as an assistant physician followed by a year in private practice before joining the Marine Hospital Service in 1876, as an assistant surgeon overseeing hospitals. He moved to Washington, D.C., in December 1888[60] after being appointed "Chief of the Quarantine Division."[61] On June 1, 1891, he succeeded John B. Hamilton as supervisory surgeon-general and remained in the position until his death on November 21, 1911. He remained single his entire life.[62]

The aforementioned descriptions shed some light on the real Wyman. Being described as "cautious"[63] seemed to fit his profile. He held a rank of considerable weight and bearing that affected every citizen. Wyman had to be careful because he worked in a new realm of science that contained many uncertaintics. But he seemed to carry a protective guard by not committing himself to a stance until he knew for certain the result based on the best available facts. As the next two years would unfold, this aspect of his personality would have an adverse effect on Kinyoun and his efforts battling plague in San Francisco.

He appeared to be a meticulous organizer who strongly believed in a proper order for everything. It would probably go without saying he would be persuasive. In light of his standing and authority, he would need to be an advocate in order to convince the Washington political hierarchy to support and fund the Service. This would be especially true with the new discoveries in microbiology and educating politicians on how unseen living organisms can cause sickness and death. Simply put, he needed to be a politician, too. This can be observed by the statement, "his attitude was not that of demanding acceptance."[64] In other words, he could be very aggressive in his point of view—but not unflinching—because he well knew he lived in a give-and-take environment as a government bureaucrat.

Besides these observations, Wyman and Kinyoun may have grown apart, as possibly evidenced in those letters dated January 10 and February 4. In the first, Wyman curtailed Kinyoun's activities, and in the second he admonished him for misinterpreting his previous order and maybe for publishing it in the lab's regular report. Being procedurally oriented, he had fired back a terse response to his director. Another factor may have been the doctor's ongoing requests in his annual reports about ways to improve the lab's operations and ways to improve the bureau. These may in time have irritated his supervisor.

Another factor, noted by several authorities, could be the rise of Dr. Milton J. Rosenau. Born 1869 in Philadelphia, he graduated from the University of Pennsylvania with his medical degree. Afterwards, he studied public health, along with sanitation, in Vienna, Berlin and Paris. In 1890, he joined the Service and worked with Kinyoun periodically at the lab. With plague approaching, based on repeated reports of its breakout from China, Wyman had sent him to San Francisco in 1896. His job would be to oversee the quarantine station on Angel Island located in the bay in preparation for its possible arrival.[65]

On March 2, Rosenau assumed his new position in San Francisco, and as his first order of business he commenced the sanitation of baggage[66] belonging to "Chinese immigrants,"[67] as directed by Wyman. A wire had been sent to other Pacific coast quarantine stations with the same instructions. Rosenau reached out to the San Francisco Board of Health offering his assistance and putting them on notice of how he intended to act upon the discovery of any suspicious cases of cholera, diphtheria, or plague.[68]

He proceeded to refit the facilities at Angel Island with bathhouses and other equipment to hasten the disinfection process. Moreover, the inspection of all immigrants would be conducted at the island. Within a short period, he started having confrontations with the local officials. They soon raised their hackles, stating that all things quarantine were their sole responsibility. Once again, "states' rights" reappeared, challenging Rosenau's federal authority. Fortunately for him, President McKinley intervened based on the Quarantine Act of 1893, establishing him as the lead official in charge.[69]

During the mid–1890s, Kinyoun's role seemed to diminish as one of Wyman's top officers. His job had taken on more of a mundane role, inspecting railway cars, teaching classes, and setting up exhibits.[70] All of these tasks could have been conducted by someone else. It appeared Roseau had gained favor with Wyman over Kinyoun. Even though Wyman probably still held him in some high regard, things may have changed between the two men.

Even his possible promotion could be viewed as a slap. The same day he received it, Wyman ordered him to San Francisco and to turn over the Hygienic Laboratory to Rosenau. But first, Rosenau would proceed to Havana, Cuba, to activate its quarantine station.[71] Ironically, Kinyoun had recently promulgated the requirements and procedures for setting up the stations at Havana and San Juan.

Rosenau had experience operating a quarantine facility, so sending him to Cuba made sense. But afterwards, the question arose why he would not have been better suited to return to San Francisco and assume the operations at the Angel Island station? With plague coming, it seemed wiser to return him to his prior position, as opposed to sending Kinyoun, who, although experienced, had not been in this role for quite a while. The next question was whether Wyman had made these changes to protect Rosenau by placing him in charge of the lab, as a safe harbor? We will probably never know, but it begs the question. Until Rosenau completed his assignment in Cuba, Dr. E.K. Sprague would run the lab.[72]

Something had happened with his career. Sometimes, subordinates receive more notoriety than their superiors, which can lead to conflict. Maybe this factor had developed between the two. Promotions have always been looked upon with favor, but in Kinyoun's case, it appeared more like a demotion. And now, he had been ordered into a potentially hostile situation, as experienced by Rosenau in his dealings with the local quarantine officials. Up to this time, there had not been any confirmed plague cases, though there may have been some rumblings of it among Chinese immigrants.

No matter what the reason for the transfer, whether real or merely coincidental, within a few short years their relationship would end. Again, there would not be a clear reason. But Wyman would never mention Kinyoun's name going forward.[73]

Farewell Dr. Kinyoun

The removal of Dr. Kinyoun did not sit well with the Washington, D.C., medical community. In tribute to their colleague, they held a farewell dinner.[74] The invitation read:

COMPLIMENTARY DINNER
To
J. J. KINYOUN, M. D., Ph. D.
ON THE OCCASION OF HIS DEPARTURE FOR
San Francisco, Cal.
By
Members of the Medical Profession
AS A MARK OF ESTEEM AND IN RECOGNITION OF HIS PROFESSIONAL ATTAINMENTS AND PUBLIC SERVICES
Washington, D. C.
May 20th, 1899 AT RAUSCHER'S[75]

The evening's program had been printed on the invitation's backside, under the heading "Toasts and Responses."[76] The master of ceremonies, or "Toastmaster," would be Dr. Joseph Taber Johnson.[77] Four other physicians would pay tribute to Kinyoun: first as a "Sanitarian," by Dr. W.C. Woodward[78]; second as a "Bacteriologist and Pathologist," by Dr. W.W. Johnston[79]; third his "Relation to the General Practitioner," by Dr. I.S. Stone[80]; and lastly as "Director of the Hygienic Laboratory," by Dr. George M. Kober.[81] The final speaker would be Kinyoun.[82]

Under each title, a quote had been set forth by a noted person exemplifying the doctor's personality and character.[83] The passage beneath Dr. Johnson read, "Look, he's winding up the watch of his wit; By and by it will strike."[84] Dr. Johnston's read,

"Science is **** like virtue, its own exceeding great reward. *Charles Kingsley.*"[85] Dr. Kober's, though, probably summed up the man best with, "Then on! Where duty leads, Thy course be onward still.— *Heber.*"[86] Other guests probably offered additional accolades in addition a fair number of humorous stories.

During the course of the evening, Dr. Johnston stated that "no city, especially the National Capital, could afford to lose men of Dr. Kinyoun's attainments."[87] Dr. Kober openly criticized the transfer, by remarking:

> It seems a pity that this modest, unassuming scientist should be divorced from a laboratory which already has accomplished so much and promises still more for the future usefulness of this branch of the public service.[88]

The invitation list was extensive and included a "Who's Who" of not only the Washington, D.C., medical community, but other prominent physicians. Dr. John F. Moran must have been placed in charge of acceptances and regrets. Several days before, he received three letters from invitees expressing their apologies for their unavailability. The first decline came from G. Burkwell with the surgeon general's office in the War Department, explaining he would be absent because of vacation.[89] Another one came from Dr. William H. Welch with the Medical Department at Johns Hopkins University in Baltimore, Maryland. Kinyoun and Welch had known each other for many years and shared a mutual respect. Unfortunately, he had scheduled a meeting out of town on the same date.[90] Welch asked him to tell the honoree:

> I should have liked to join in this well merited tribute to the excellent scientific work and the many admirable personal qualities of Dr. Kinyoun. Kindly express to him my congratulations upon this pleasant testimonial from the members of the medical profession and convey all my best wishes for his continued successes and prosperity in his new fields of activity.[91]

But the most interesting response came from Wyman. It stated he would be leaving for the Cape Charles quarantine station on Saturday for a scheduled inspection the following day. He wrote that a steamer needed to be put in place along with other duties, thereby making his presence impossible.[92] He concluded by writing, "It would have given me great pleasure to have been able to accept the kind invitation, and to show my presence at the dinner my high appreciation of Dr. Kinyoun."[93]

It would have been unlikely he wanted to attend the dinner. Several members within the medical profession had already voiced their disapproval of the doctor's departure. Wyman well may have anticipated criticism at the event, as that expressed by Drs. Johnston and Kober. Maybe his plans could not be changed, or maybe it afforded him a convenient opportunity to be absent. And maybe, too, it would have given him "great pleasure,"[94] not so much in attending, but in seeing it as Kinyoun's leaving.

Two days after the dinner, Wyman sent him a directive informing him that his travel arrangements from Washington, D.C., to San Francisco had been completed for his transfer. Interestingly, in Wyman's dinner regret, dated May 17, he told Dr. Moran he was leaving on the upcoming Saturday, the same day as the party. However, his letter to Kinyoun on Monday, May 22, had been sent from his office in the capital,[95] meaning he may not have left and thereby could have attended the event.

As further evidence, he had asked the doctor to confirm receipt of his order.

By comparing these dates, it would appear he never intended to attend the dinner. By requesting Kinyoun's acknowledgment to his office in Washington, it certainly implied he had not left for Cape Charles.

As a follow-up to his pending promotion to the rank of surgeon, Wyman sent him a letter dated May 29 reporting that he had received a passing score of 80 percent, qualifying for the new grade.[96] It was a bittersweet moment as he and his family packed their bags for California. Becoming surgeon was the highest rank obtainable within the Service, outside of becoming the supervisory-surgeon general, but in Kinyoun's case, the reward may have felt more like a Pyrrhic victory. Something seemed amiss in his life after so many years of success. As time would soon prove, it would be his undoing, causing him to become an obscurity within the medical and scientific world. But, it was now on to "California, or Bust," as the "49ers" had said a half-century before as they crossed the Great Plains to the Golden State in search of riches and fame.

XII

Angel Island

The Nippon Maru

Kinyoun and the family moved to Angel Island sometime in early June. On the agenda of his farewell dinner, Dr. Kober best described Kinyoun, stating, "Then on! Then on! Where duty leads, Thy course be onward still."[1] Nothing could be more accurate of Kinyoun, who had now been asked to give up his passion, the lab, and become a quarantine officer. In the end, this change would tarnish him and ultimately finish his career with the Service.

As if on a collision course with him, the *Nippon Maru* fatefully journeyed towards San Francisco as well. The ship had made two previous trips to America. It was considered one of the best of its kind, sleek and fitted with many amenities. Nevertheless, its arrival on June 27 would greatly change life in this burgeoning metropolis and set it upon a most dramatic course for the next two years. Kinyoun's life, too, would change, and neither he nor San Francisco would be for the better.[2]

While the ship had been identified as a plague carrier,[3] reports have indicated that the *Australia* may have been the first transporter a year later.[4] It is possible, however, that the *Nippon Maru* may have actually planted the contagion the previous year. As reported by Dr. Eldridge, the ship had undergone considerable scrutiny from port to port, as a potential harbor of plague. Shortly after its departure from Nagasaki, an adolescent Chinese passenger in steerage became ill and died. After reviewing a portion of the victim's glands, the illness proved to be plague. Following a thorough disinfection and a seven-day quarantine, the *Nippon Maru* received clearance and proceeded to Honolulu.[5]

During its passage, another passenger mysteriously passed away. Dr. Deas, the ship's doctor, kept the body and, on arriving in Hawaii, had it examined by Dr. Alvarez, the territory's bacteriologist. When his findings pointed to it being plague, Sanitary Inspector Dr. D.A. Carmichael sent a letter to Wyman and to someone at Angel Island, presumably Kinyoun, advising them of the situation.[6]

With this finding, the port authorities denied the ship docking permission. After considerable discussion by local authorities, they placed the *Nippon Maru* in quarantine for seven days. But after four days, for reasons unknown, the ship received approval to proceed onward to San Francisco. But during the voyage, a previously sick steerage passenger succumbed on June 25. Because her symptoms appeared to be plague, the body was thrown overboard. Back in Honolulu, the cultures taken from

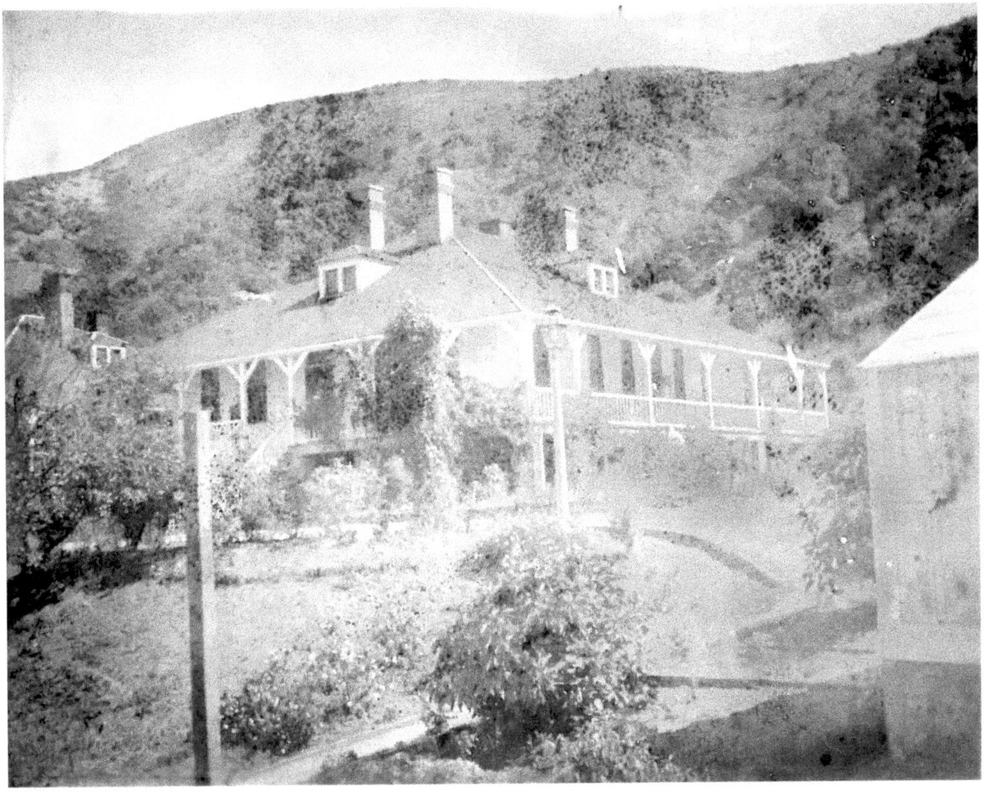

Angel Island, 1899.

the deceased Chinese man proved to be positive. The findings were reported in the *Examiner* on June 26, a day before the ship's arrival.[7]

Unfortunately, news of the *Nippon Maru* and its plague-ridden journey caused quite a stir in San Francisco. Public officials became alarmed at its impending arrival, while others set upon a course of total denial, claiming plague could never gain a foothold. Others claimed that even if it did enter, it would be confined to the Chinese and not the city's Caucasian population. Tensions started to flare, and contradictions abounded with great regularity.[8] The play had now been written for this great medical-political drama. All that remained was for the curtain to rise on Act I.

As the ship entered the city's harbor, two more passengers died under suspicious circumstances, purportedly resulting in their bodies being thrown overboard with another report stating that the bodies had been burned in the ship's furnaces. Other accounts stated that the two had drowned, because, being stowaways, they had jumped ship to evade capture and deportation.[9] Whatever the case, it had now landed in the city, for better or for worse.

The Stage

Sometime around June 12, Kinyoun arrived at his new post. On the same date, he received a letter from Treasury Secretary Gage appointing him the "Custodian

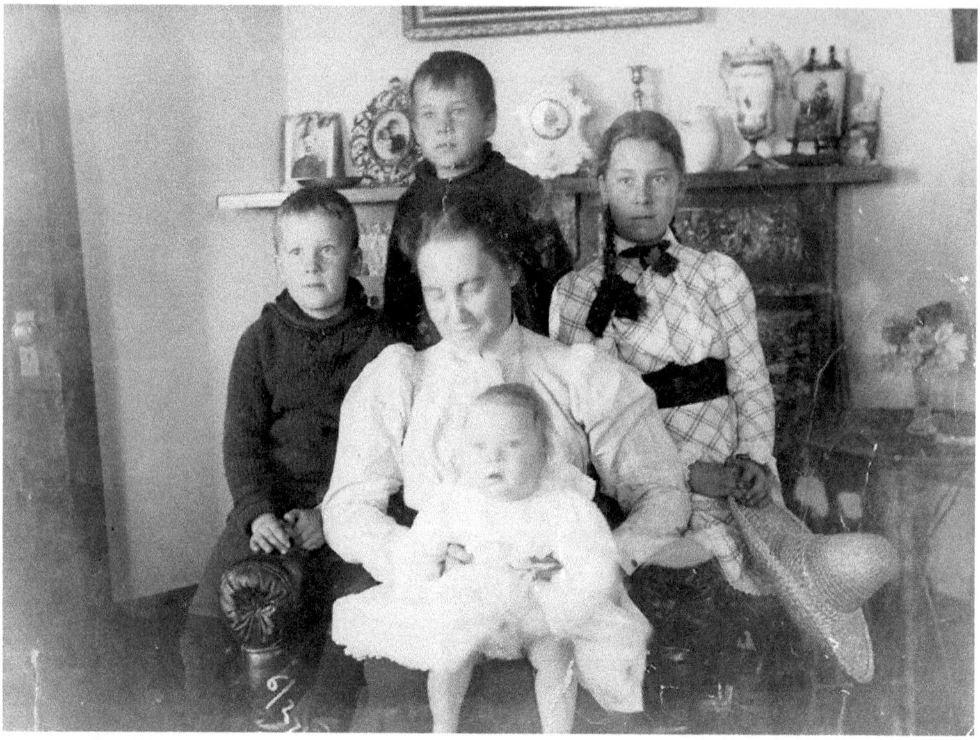

Kinyoun family, Angel Island: Perry, Conrad, and Alice (left to right) behind John in Lizzie's lap.

(without compensation)"[10] of the Angel Island facility. Vice Surgeon Brooks was to be relieved of command and Kinyoun to "assume custody"[11] of the premises. Two days later, Gage sent another letter. It appointed him the quarantine officer for San Francisco's port.[12]

The island would not be considered an ideal home, especially for a young family. It was the largest of three islets in the Bay. In its early days, it had been a hunting and fishing site for the Coast Miwok Indians. The first Europeans to visit were the Spaniards in 1775, aboard the ship *San Carlos*. During the Civil War and Spanish-American War, it served as a military base. In the late 19th century, it received the name Fort McDowell. By 1891, the Marine Hospital Service had established a quarantine station to regulate and inspect immigrants arriving from Asia and other places.[13] During its operation, close to 1,000,000 people passed through the facility, earning it the nickname "The Ellis Island of the West."[14]

As the Kinyouns settled into their new surroundings, they would soon learn about the very complex nature of San Francisco. The city had long been known for its rowdiness, beginning with the Californian Gold Rush of 1849. Although it had been 50 years since its rugged start, other factors had intervened during this period adding to its unique composition and occasional volatility.[15]

Early on, the town had seen an influx of Asian immigrants, especially the Chinese and to a lesser extent the Japanese. They had come to America seeking new opportunities and offered themselves as inexpensive labor. They were greatly utilized in the construction of the transcontinental railroad. As their numbers grew, concern arose as to their ever-increasing presence. Starting in 1882, Congress passed a succession of exclusionary laws limiting Asians, followed by a curtailment of their civil liberties and ability to freely assimilate into communities. This eventually led to their confinement into separate neighborhoods, commonly called "China Towns."[16]

San Francisco would be no exception in placing restrictions on its Asian populace, leading to the creation of its Chinatown, where the Chinese and others of Asian descent had been relegated for living quarters. Chinese children could not attend the same schools as white children. Riots would break out with the white community. The whites soon blamed the Chinese for a whole host of social and economic ills ranging from prostitution and drugs, as evidenced by opium dens, along with the spread of disease because of their living conditions.[17]

Another facet resided in the city's questionable political system and commercial entities. San Francisco had become the largest port on the West Coast, followed by Seattle and Los Angeles. Unlike the East Coast of the United States, which had numerous harbors due to its geography, the western seaboard had a limited number of major ports, thereby making competition intense. Combined with America's new geographical holdings in Asia, these ports saw the opportunity for expanded trade opportunities.[18]

Probably the greatest factor fueling competition had been the explosive population growth in Los Angeles and Seattle during the preceding decade. Between 1890 and 1900, the population of San Francisco had grown 14.6 percent, while Los Angeles had grown by 103.3 percent and Seattle by 88.3 percent. In 1900, San Francisco had a population of 342,782, Los Angeles 102,837, and Seattle 80,671.[19] Although San Francisco held a commanding lead, the other cities, if their present growth rate continued, would be in striking distance of surpassing it by the end of the next decade, if not sooner. Therefore, the Golden Gate had cause for alarm and could ill afford any adverse publicity that might impede its position as the leading commercial center on the West Coast.

Two other factors played heavily on the demeanor of the city: yellow journalism and politics. These elements created a contentious backdrop, not only as to the inner workings of San Francisco, but the state's political machinery, as well. As previously noted, one of the primary causes for the country's plunge into the Spanish-America War was the highly prejudicial, or "yellow,"[20] journalistic reporting of the time. The practice had dawned under the craftsmanship of William Randolph Hearst and Joseph Pulitzer, with Hearst being in San Francisco.[21]

The political climate of the port also weighed heavily on what happened in the city. It had been long considered a rough-and-tumble town, even though it began showing signs of refinement and sophistication. But power had become concentrated in the industrialists, select politicians and political bodies at all levels of the government. Even before Kinyoun arrived, his predecessor, Dr. Milton Rosenau, had faced issues over the question of federal versus state control of quarantine and port matters.[22]

The biggest political player in the upcoming crisis would be California Governor Henry T. Gage, a Republican. Gage assumed office on January 4, 1899, five months before Kinyoun's arrival. Heretofore, he had been a successful attorney and represented the Southern Pacific Railroad. He welcomed the country's expansion in Asia, touting California's trade with the Orient, and would be known for his adherence to the patronage system.

He could be very forcible in his ways. Early in his administration, he had been characterized by a newspaper cartoon portraying him with a leash around his neck being held by Collis P. Huntington, one of the state's four railroad barons. The cartoon portrayed the governor as a political puppet of the railroad.[23] Huntington, along with Mark Hopkins, Charles Crocker and Leland Stanford founded of the Central Pacific Railroad and would be referred to as the "Big Four."[24] Gage, infuriated by the cartoon, managed to secure the passage of a state censorship bill, curtailing the press's freedom when writing about politicians and politics.[25]

Within short order, Gage would become directly involved in denying the existence of bubonic plague. Before the crisis, he had appointed a new San Francisco Health Board. The newly elected mayor, James D. Phelan, a Democrat, had an automatic seat on the five-member body accompanied by four members of the medical profession. Phelan, a reformer, wanted to change the city charter, granting the mayor greater authority in political appointments in hopes of limiting the present patronage system. Membership on the board had been dictated in part because of the poor relationship established between Rosenau and the local quarantine officials during his tenure as quarantine officer.[26] As a result, the political stage had been significantly transformed, leading to an inevitable future confrontation. Unfortunately for Kinyoun, he would soon experience its wrath.

The new board consisted of the city's new health officer, Dr. William M. Lawlor; Dr. J.H. Barbat; and his brother, Dr. W.F. Barbat, the newly appointed city bacteriologist. As one of its first acts, Gage recommended the appointment of Dr. J.E. Cohn as the state's quarantine officer for the city. These appointments had been made prior to Kinyoun's arrival. This board would control the appointment of roughly 240 jobs, thereby making this body extremely powerful.[27] It represented political patronage at its best. By this move, everyone knew their boss and owed them allegiance.

Another important element within this setting centered on the acceptance of microbiology and the spread of infectious germs. Although Kinyoun and other medical authorities had proven these theories as fact, that did not mean everyone, even in the medical profession, had accepted these findings. Doubt also existed in San Francisco as to the merits of this new science. William Lawlor, the city's health officer, headed up the list of non-plague believers, which would prove detrimental in the unfolding crisis. As reported on July 7, 1899, by the *Examiner*, Dr. W.P. Burke openly stated his disbelief in such a theory upon the quarantining of the *Nippon Maru*.[28]

Others had expressed the same misgivings. And yet some believed it to be a purely Asiatic illness, not to be contracted by the white population. Nor did the city's chief bacteriologist, Dr. Barbat, seem concerned about it entering the city. His reasoned that because of the climate being healthy, it would be unlikely to take root.[29] Such was the mindset of many when it came to bubonic plague.

June 27th

On June 27, the *Nippon Maru* steamed into San Francisco Harbor. It ominously bared the quarantine flag, announcing the presence of plague. Kinyoun acted without delay, ordering the vessel into isolation. On its arrival, he inspected it several times and interviewed the captain, along with its medical officer Dr. Deas. The passengers were removed and placed in confinement for 14 days. Next, the boat and its contents received a thorough disinfecting. Afterwards, he sent it to the Pacific Mail Company's dock for unloading and then had it anchored a mile offshore.[30]

The following day, nine Japanese stowaways were found, who had been smuggled on board, apparently upon the ship's departure at Yokohama. Further intrigue resulted when the other two stowaways, who had purportedly either jumped, been thrown overboard, or burned in the ship's furnaces, surfaced bobbling in the bay wearing life jackets bearing the ship's name. Dr. Hill, the San Francisco coroner, examined their remains and removed their glands for study. In his opinion, they had drowned, but the tissue samples also showed trademarks of plague.[31]

Even with these developments, the vessel's galley prepared a lovely cuisine for the detained passengers, ranging from "Leg of Mutton, Braine Cutlets, to Pork with Apple Sauce."[32] Of some humor: two entrées on the menu had been altered. Someone had marked through the word *anchovy* in "Boiled Rock Cod with Anchovy Sauce"[33] and replaced it with the word "Plague."[34] And in the entry for "Turkey and Fresh Oyster,"[35] the word *oyster* had been scratched out and changed to "Bacillus."[36] Apparently, someone either had a sense of humor or had decided to mock the situation.

Lawlor became incensed over the plague situation, criticizing Kinyoun for letting the two stowaways slip through the quarantine process, when in fact they had left the ship before it arrived at Angel Island. Because of his condemnation, the press opened its initial barrages at Kinyoun, setting in motion a war of words. Later, Barbat concluded from his bacteriological exam that while they had drowned, they likely had the plague as well.[37]

The question of who had authority added to the brewing firestorm. Being a bureaucrat, Kinyoun shook the proverbial political tree with his federal empowerments, thereby setting the stage for future confrontations. His predecessor, Rosenau, had apparently done the same thing.

Kinyoun had quickly exerted federal control over the *Nippon Maru*. Compounding the matter, when Dr. Chalmers sought to inspect the vessel, he denied him access, unless he wanted to be placed into quarantine afterwards. This humiliated Chalmers, especially in his role as California's top quarantine officer. Adding additional fire to the situation, he released the ship on June 29, after only two days. His reasoning was that it had been thoroughly fumigated according to the prescribed regulations of the Service and therefore could be released. The following day, the ship proceeded to the Pacific Mail's dock for mooring in San Francisco.[38]

On learning of this development, Chalmers ordered the vessel to move away from the shore, but the captain refused, causing a stalemate of sorts. The day before, the health board had threatened any passenger with arrest and fine if they left the ship. This action struck a blow to Kinyoun by denying him access to the specimen glands for examination. This was a mistake on their part, since he had the only laboratory sufficiently equipped to make a complete determination of the illness. Nevertheless, Barbat released his findings confirming it to be plague.[39]

Even with this revelation, a tug-of-war persisted between the local officials, the press and the *Nippon Maru* about who was in charge. Hearst's *Examiner* pressed Kinyoun, questioning whether he had adequately complied with proper containment processes. It alleged that the state's measures might be better than the Service's. At the same time, the owners of the ship became caught in the middle of this debate. They eventually gave into the state and agreed to the ship's removal from the Pacific Mail's dock and have it fumigated again as demanded by Chon, the city's new state representative for quarantine affairs. He and Lawlor visited the vessel and oversaw its disinfection. Afterwards, they proceeded to Angel Island and demanded to see the passengers still in confinement. Kinyoun denied them permission to land. On July 2, Cohn released the ship, allowing its departure.[40]

On July 11, after the passengers had been held for 14 days, Kinyoun announced that they would be released and free to leave the island at noon the next day. The incident had ended without anyone else coming down with the illness.[41] He had been in San Francisco for only a month and already a ruckus had occurred over those matters concerning the city's health and safety.

With this impasse ended, several important questions remained. Had Kinyoun properly handled the quarantine? Had the press and state officials complicated or unnecessarily interfered in the matter? And the most important question: had plague gotten ashore?

Concerning the first question, it could be described as mixed, with one side responding that he did perform his duty to the letter of the law and others, like the press and Chon, finding fault in how he released the *Nippon Maru* from quarantine after two days. He had thoroughly disinfected the ship as prescribed by the Service and the 1893 Federal Quarantine Act. Moreover, he had conducted countless fumigations and disinfections of ships over the preceding decade, and the passengers remained in quarantine for 14 days. It could be argued that if anyone knew the proper procedures it would have been him. But because of the ongoing issue of state versus federal authority, Chon felt compelled to sanitize the vessel a second time, which caused considerable damage to the passengers' personal effects still on board.

Concerning the second question, it became obvious from the start that the press and state complicated the matter by their interference and meddling. First, the press—specifically the *Examiner*—took the side of the state and criticized Kinyoun. A more objective alternative would have been to determine the facts first, as opposed to creating a sense of suspense, fear and outrage.

In Kinyoun's defense, *The Wasp*, a weekly publication published for the Pacific Coast, strongly criticized the California and San Francisco officials for interfering in the matter. It stated, "They have always been a nuisance and can never be anything else. They are the result of petty political upheavals and generally represent the insolence or rapacity of a little brief authority."[42] The publication commented how the city stood as the eminent commercial trading center for Asia.[43] But, because of incidents like the roughhousing of the *Nippon Maru*, these "officials have made us the laughing stock of the world."[44] It expressed its support for federal supervision of all matters relating to quarantine.[45] In unambiguous prose, it opined:

> It is ridiculous that these incompetent State officials should be allowed to menace the prosperity of a seaport by imposing their own regulations on foreign shipping.[46]

The paper encouraged the ship's owners, Toyo Kisen Kaisha, to sue the state board of health for the damage caused to the vessel and its contents, especially since it already had been cleansed and released from quarantine. It pointed out that the second fumigation had been haphazard, resulting in harm to the ship's freight and furnishings.[47]

In its opinion, the state should have allowed Kinyoun to examine the gland specimens from the two stowaways found floating in the harbor because of the superior laboratory facilities at Angel Island. It reported that he had the scientific equipment to make a definitive analysis of the tissue samples.[48] Equally important, he had the knowledge in light of his European travels and research. Underscoring his handling of the affair, the paper wrote:

> Dr. Kinyoun, of the Marine Hospital service [sic] made short work of the plague hunters of the State Board of Health. To use a sporting expression, it was a complete knockout in round one. The position taken by Dr. Kinyoun in the controversy was a masterly one.[49]

The article criticized Barbat, in not using the island's laboratory, writing that "no competent scientists should begin an experiment of so delicate a nature without the appliances for carrying it through."[50] It metaphorically commented that

> a scientist undertaking to cultivate germs of bubonic plague, for the purpose of discovering whether the city is threatened with a great scourge, is not supposed to conduct his operations as if he were getting ready to cultivate potatoes.[51]

The third question has become the most perplexing. Nonetheless, it holds the key to what would happen over the next nine months. Had in fact the plague somehow gotten ashore from the *Nippon Maru*? The best guess would be, maybe. The ship had a history of carrying infected passengers. Although disinfecting procedures and quarantine measures had followed its course to America, possibly the bacterium managed to escape the effects of sanitation.

It had been docked at the Pacific Mail from June 29–July 1. The crew did not leave, and no one became sick. It is not to say an infected rat (if any remained alive from the fumigations) could not have escaped to shore. The Board of Health took possession of it on July 1, and towed it out to sea for a second fumigation. Even after 14 days of impoundment, none of the passengers came down with the disease.[52] One possibility could have rested in the dead stowaways floating in the harbor. This would have been doubtful for several reasons. Although Barbat thought they had plague, the size of San Francisco Bay would have surely diluted the contagion. Other possibilities abounded, but none of any substantive merit.

One may wonder why this question should even be asked. Yet something happened between the arrival of the *Nippon Maru* on June 27, 1899, and the first confirmed case of bubonic plague on March 6, 1900.[53] In a pamphlet written by Dr. R.A. Forrest to Judge Kelley on November 17, 1900, titled *Echoes of the Plague Scare in San Francisco*,[54] he revealed that cases of plague had started showing up in Chinatown after the ship's arrival. He acknowledged that these may have been rumors, but in January 1900 he reported that several important members of the Chinese community had confirmed its presence. Evidently, they had been hiding victims through false death certificates, secret burials and abandoning bodies.[55]

Somehow, whether it had been aboard the *Nippon Maru* or some other vessel, the plague had arrived prior to its documented appearance. Many ships traveled along the same route from Asia to San Francisco during this period and had suspicious illnesses among passengers. It could have been any one of them. Three such suspects were the *America Maru*, the *City of Peking* and the *Australia*.[56] Each ship had been a plague carrier before its arrival in San Francisco with the *America Maru* and the *City of Peking* arriving on July 16. Although both had been quarantined and disinfected at Yokohama by Dr. Eldridge, either may have been the transporter.[57]

The *Australia* has received the major credit in being the malady's first carrier in early January 1900. The shipped docked close to Chinatown, near its sewer lines emptying into the bay. Dead rats had been reported in large amounts throughout the Chinese community, suggesting plague being transmitted by their cousins arriving off the ship.[58] Adding credence to this possibility were reports of 11 plague cases involving Chinese, occurring between January and June 1900.[59] Therefore, it seemed the malady might have already gained a foothold.

All of these theories to answering the third question have a sound basis. In a lengthy account by Kinyoun in August 1901, published in the *Occidental Medical Times*, he stated that the plague had been in San Francisco as early as November 1898. In support of his position, he revealed the existence of medical records from two doctors who had treated potential cases involving Chinese. The results had been conclusive, and the Chinese called it the "black fever."[60] Moreover, in a confidential file belonging to Wyman, he acknowledged the plague's existence as early as 1898, claiming the Chinese had hid the illness from health officials.[61] He had inherited a cesspool surrounding the contagion's existence. Regardless of who, or how, or when, one way or another it had arrived and had become his problem.

Fears

Shortly after Kinyoun's difficulties with the *Nippon Maru*, Wyman decided to set in motion more vigilant inspection procedures. His actions stemmed not only from the plague's appearance in San Francisco, but more out of fears of its ever-growing presence throughout the Far East in the Philippines, Hong Kong and Hawaii. Acting out of his own concern, he appointed Passed Assistant Surgeon J.C. Perry to the Hong Kong consular office as a medical attaché.[62]

The Philippines and Hawaii had become important as America's newest possessions the year before. The army had large contingents of troops stationed in these territories, which would be returning home soon. Therefore, stronger measures needed to be taken in order to prevent the plague's entrance into the country by way of its troops. And with these new acquisitions being so close to infected areas, it became critical to establish proper screening and disinfection measures. Accordingly, Hong

Kong would serve as the staging point for this undertaking, since it represented the epicenter of the pandemic.[63]

Perry arrived on August 23, and his orders from Wyman could not have been clearer: "Your detail by order of President is to protect Philippines as well as United States."[64] From the start, he had an almost impossible task. On November 18, he submitted a report describing the situation and his efforts in trying to contain it and ensure compliance. His account left little doubt as to the futility of his task.[65]

First off, there was a lack of buildings to detain and disinfect Chinese passengers. Second, British colonial law did not allow for their detention. Complicating matters, only one steamship line, the Pacific Mail, had the proper equipment. What's more, the company would not allow passengers from other lines to be treated, although discussions had been initiated in hopes of overcoming this obstacle. Even worse, Hong Kong did not have a quarantine station or any disinfecting equipment, and the primary sanitizing agent, formalin, could not be acquired in sufficient amounts. The situation appeared hopeless, and although individuals would be treated, their baggage would be omitted from the process. The worst of the matter occurred when examined individuals were allowed to associate with those who had not been inspected, thereby negating the remediation process by potential re-exposure.[66]

His report did compliment the sanitation equipment and procedures used by the Pacific Mail in Hong Kong, thereby making it the only saving grace for an otherwise dangerous situation. The underlying problem with the whole process was not so much in who had what equipment, but who was being disinfected. Towards the end of his report, Perry made a startling revelation, quite possibly showing how plague spread. On the surface the sentence appeared benign suggesting its containment.[67] However, to the contrary, he may have unknowingly revealed how terribly flawed the process had become, when he wrote,

> The inspection of all passengers is done on board the ships a few hours before they sail. All Asiatic steerage and crew are carefully and individually examined....[68]

The key phrase was "All Asiatic."[69] In other words, only this class of passengers received a thorough inspection and disinfection, meaning that the remaining passengers, being predominantly white or of higher social and economic stature, may not have been required to go through the process. This further would mean that these passengers could have in fact been more prone to transport the deadly malady than passengers of oriental descent. As will be recalled, the citizens of San Francisco, as echoed in its press, thought plague to be a disease only of the Chinese and not its white populace.[70]

To see the error in this assumption, one would only have to read the history books about the early plague epidemics of the 6th, 14th and 17th centuries in Europe, where it ravaged the world's Caucasian population. From time immemorial, civilizations have placed heavy emphasis on race and ethnicity as the culprits for the spread of disease. Tragically, and with certain foolhardiness, this remained the case in 1900 in America and much of the world.[71]

In support of this factor, Perry set forth a chart documenting the disinfections conducted on 99 ships, along with the crews, passengers, steerage passengers and their baggage. He broke his summary down into two categories—people and ships sailing to U.S. ports and those sailing to Philippine ports. On the surface, his report appeared thorough and orderly, but on further examination it bared very ominous findings.[72]

As to those traveling to America, a shocking disparity could be seen between the inspection of cabin and steerage passengers. Out 38 ships processed, a total of 2,327 individuals were screened, consisting of 191 cabin and 2,254 steerage passengers. As for 61 ships departing for the Philippines, 2,706 passengers were inspected, consisting of 395 regular and 2,311 steerage classes. The numbers also showed that a total of 3,627 crewmembers bound for America had been examined, as well as 2,761 bound for the Philippines. Obviously great care had been exerted in reviewing those individuals of a lesser class, being the crew and steerage passengers.[73]

The problem with these statistics lay in their overemphasis of the common class traveler, predominantly Asian, who did not have the monetary means to afford a higher-class ticket. And because of the low fare, these people had been cast to the bowels of ships, which harbored unsanitary conditions easily leading to the spread of diseases, especially plague. Regular cabin passengers were passed over the most. Again, the probable logic behind this practice stemmed from the age-old prejudices towards Asians, more pointedly the Chinese, as being unsanitary people and hence disease carriers.[74]

But nothing could be further from the truth in regards to this obvious course of conduct. Travelers of European ancestry were just as prone to be or become carriers of plague and other maladies, regardless of their race and ethnicity. This was what Perry's accounting demonstrated: these people had been waived through the process, and for all intents and purposes the contagion could have arrived on California's shore more so from individuals of European origin than those from the Orient. It is not to say that the crews and steerage passengers did not bring the disease, because evidence does point in this direction. What is being said is that travelers of European ancestry may well have been infected by steerage members. However, because they received less scrutiny, this could have led to them being the primary transporting agents of it to America, as opposed to Asians, thereby, in theory, possibly making the Europeans the true culprits.

Another overlooked consideration could be in the sanitation of the ships. It appeared that the lower level of these vessels had become breeding grounds for all types of pestilence because of poor sanitary practices within the ship's quarters. If these areas had been well cleaned, then probably the billets would not have been a source of so much illness. Since these people paid less, they received unsanitary and diminutive spaces in which to reside during voyages. As a result, these living quarters became incubators for the world's worst scourges.

Possibly some very simple cleaning measures could have saved countless lives and contained the spread of these malaises. Kinyoun had noted in his earlier experiences that many times poor habitat conditions could be attributed to unsanitary lifestyles of the voyagers, as opposed to the premises. Overall, nothing could have probably been done to correct the matter because many cultures did not know about common sanitation measures and would not comply with them because of their customs. It must be remembered, too, that sanitation and the understanding of microorganisms and their pathogenic cycles remained somewhat of an unknown at this point in history.

Either way, the plague continued to encircle the world. Perry tried the best he could to contain the situation from spreading, even though some of his efforts may have been misdirected in its containment. A lot of his problem dealt with a lack of uniformity among all the transport lines. As a breakthrough, companies with disinfecting capabilities began to allow others to use their facilities. But other hurdles lay ahead, such as making sure all ports used formalin in the decontamination process. Several ports had started vaccinating passengers before boarding, which proved beneficial as well. However, no matter what, the disease continued to creep towards the country's western coast, and initial indications showed it had already become established, regardless of who made the delivery.[75]

Wyman Enraged

On September 1, Kinyoun sent Wyman his first official report on Angel Island. It represented compilations of what needed to be done to make the facility a first-rate quarantine station.[76] In his conclusion, he mentioned a forewarning from his predecessor, Dr. Brooks, concerning the "considerable annoyance still caused by the State and city quarantine officers."[77] He stated that they would board ships even though it had become a purely federal right of jurisdiction. Apparently, the matter had been brought before the state courts for resolution with a decision pending. He reminded Wyman of his own recent run-in with these officials with the *Nippon Maru*. As a reminder, he pointed out it had been a prior carrier of the plague before entering San Francisco.[78]

A week before submitting his formal report on the state of conditions at Angel Island, Kinyoun again appraised Wyman as to the ongoing intrusions affecting his duties as the quarantine officer.[79] In response, the surgeon general wrote to Secretary Gage about the obstructionism by state and city representatives. He stated that in May 1897 a similar incident occurred and one as far back as 1896, when Rosenau was the quarantine officer[80] trying to enforce the Quarantine Act of 1893. The Service had placed an officer in the port at the time because of the state's and the city's inability to comply with the act's provisions.[81]

Because of this failure, the federal government had to intercede on its own behalf to make sure proper sanitary protocols were in place. This may have explained the reoccurring interference by these governmental bodies because of the federal intervention. And considering the state's patronage system, where the appointees earned their income from inspection fees, its oversight could be expected to be contested and ignored by them.

Wyman reminded Gage that he, along with President McKinley, had approved Kinyoun's detail to San Francisco. To date, the state and local quarantine officials continued to usurp the right of the federal authority to handle all things pertaining to the inspection, disinfection and quarantining of people and the vessels carrying them. It

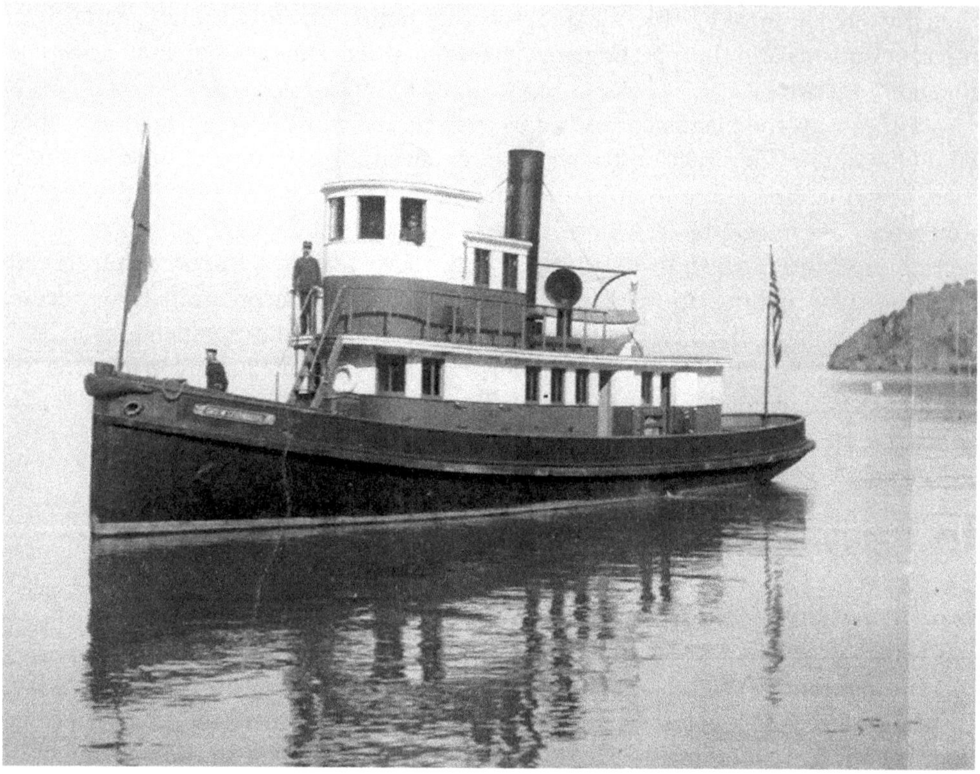

UMHS Quarantine scuttle *Gen Stenberg* bearing quarantine flag on bow and United States flag on stern, San Francisco Bay, 1890.

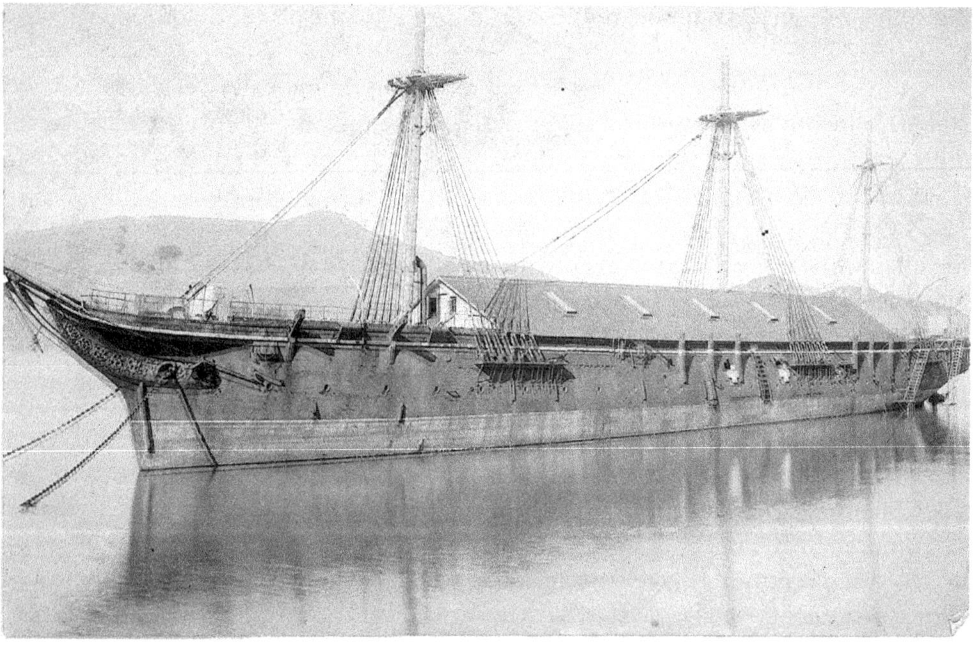

Asian junk, San Francisco Bay, 1900.

had become so bad that ships entering the harbor ignored the right of the quarantine officer to inspect their ships.[82]

He also advised Gage about the pending litigation in state court brought by the quarantine officer in San Francisco addressing the issue mentioned in Kinyoun's report. It stated that the suit had been brought to quell the state's activity. So far, the state courts had ruled in favor of its inspection rights, though he allowed how on appeal it would likely be overturned in favor of the Service.[83] By the lawsuit, it could be surmised that the state and city were not about to stop their meddling because of the fees they needed to support the system.

If the state and local officials had initially complied with the 1893 Quarantine Act, then in all probability Wyman might not have sent Rosenau to San Francisco in 1896. Consequently, neither he, nor Kinyoun, would have been present when the *Nippon Maru* entered the bay, with or without the plague. If they had been compliant, then they would have been running the port and collecting their inspections fees without interruption. It could be said that the lack of proper quarantine measures, combined with a heavily laden and reliant political patronage system, proved to be the system's own worst enemy.

Exemplifying the gravity of the situation, Wyman stated that uninvited state and local officials would board ships at the same time an inspection was being administered by federal authorities—a direct violation of the statute.[84] He further commented, "There can only be one quarantine officer."[85] In support of his position, he quoted a section of the statue, which read:

> No person except the quarantine officer, his employees, United States customs officers, or agents of the vessel, shall be permitted to board any vessel subject to quarantine inspection until after the vessel has been inspected by the quarantine officer and given its discharge.[86]

He pointed out that, with the plague running rampant in Asia and with large numbers of American troops returning from this part of the world, Kinyoun and his staff had more than enough to handle without these ongoing intrusions. Wyman noted that under the law, the Service could not levy fines and penalties for those obstructing its operations.[87] As a counterbalance, he recommended using guards from the "Revenue-Cutter Service"[88] in stopping the future boarding of ships by unauthorized officials.[89] In response to his appeal, Gage sent a dispatch to the customs collector in San Francisco advising him to provide Kinyoun with guards, so he could conduct his duties without further interference.[90]

Before concluding his report to the secretary, Wyman noted that he had included various newspaper articles by the *Sacramento Record-Union* and the *San Francisco Chronicle*.[91] He stated that the writings offered a glimpse into "public sentiment in California with regard to this matter."[92] One could assume the contents may not have been totally favorable as to the Service. Moreover, with Secretary Gage adding federal muscle into the equation, things most certainly would continue to be confrontational in the public's eyes. Kinyoun would soon experience how the poisonous pen of the press would infect the truth.

XIII

Y. Pestis

The Monkey

With the monkey's death, his worst fear had come true. Several days before, he had inoculated several guinea pigs, rats and a monkey with tissue samples from a suspected plague victim. The rats and guinea pigs had died several days before, but the monkey was the last, confirming his suspicions that it had perished from the dreaded malady.[1]

Kinyoun had been hoping the pestilence would not reappear, as he had surmised it had in June of the previous year. If anything, he wanted to leave this place and return to the Hygienic Laboratory. His predecessor, Dr. Rosenau, had switched roles with him, leaving him with the unwanted chore of confronting the world's deadliest contagion.[2]

During the previous summer, when a suspected case of the plague had appeared, the press, along with the commercial and political interests in San Francisco, had become quite outspoken about its existence to the point of denying its presence. He soon became a target of these various groups, questioning among other things his medical expertise.[3]

With the monkey's death, he knew his worst nightmare had just unfolded. Two of his assistants asked him to run the tests again, but he declined, knowing full well it to be *Y. pestis*. Subsequent tests done in Washington at the Service's laboratory would later confirm the results.[4] He knew that with it being plague, there would be little time to spare to contain it.

A hailstorm quickly erupted, putting him at the center of the uproar and eventually making him the scourge of the city.

Plague

On March 6, the remains of Chick Gin, who had been living in the basement at the Globe Hotel on 1001 DuPont Street, were reported to authorities. Ironically, he had been found in the room of a Chinese undertaker. Assistant Police Surgeon Frank P. Wilson suspected that the man had died from bubonic plague. He referred the matter to Assistant City Physician Dr. Wilfred H. Kellogg, the city's bacteriologist, who in turn, on March 7, informed Surgeon James M. Gassaway, the Service's chief officer in San Francisco.[5] Wyman soon learned about it and contacted Gassaway about the situation.[6]

At the same time, City Health Officer A.P. O'Brien closed off Chinatown with a police barricade and started to search all houses looking for additional cases. After several days, the search had been completed, finding nothing. Accordingly, O'Brien lifted the quarantine. With this news, the press hailed the plague as a fake.[7]

After the meeting, he cabled Wyman and reported that gland specimens from the victim had been given to Kinyoun for testing. In response, Wyman recommended that Gassaway inform the local health board that all Chinatown residents not exposed to the contagion should be treated with the Haffkine vaccine.[8]

Wyman sent 25,000 vials to vaccinate people. Coincidentally, the supply equaled the population of Chinatown. He directed Gassaway to tell the local board that this procedure would assist in abating the plague's spread and hopefully avert an epidemic. He stated that there would be sporadic reoccurrences over the course of a year, which could be easily contained. Wyman told him to apprise Kinyoun of his dispatch.[9]

On March 8, six more suspected cases appeared in Chinatown.[10] On the same day, Kinyoun received specimens of the victim from the Globe Hotel and started inoculating animals. Simultaneously, the Chinese Six Companies commenced an investigation into the victim's history, provided by the Chinese consul.[11]

On March 11, Gassaway wired Wyman telling him the guinea pigs and the rat inoculated by Kinyoun had died and the monkey was very sick. He further stated that a second meeting had been scheduled with the local health board, Mayor Phelan, the press, the president of the commercial entities and the Chinese consul-general concerning the unfolding state of affairs. Three days later, he reported that the monkey died, thereby confirming the presence of plague in San Francisco.[12] He further reported that, besides the inoculation, Kinyoun had utilized the procedure called necropsy, or autopsy, in making the diagnosis.[13]

In response, O'Brien reinstated the quarantine of Chinatown, leading to more outcries from the newspapers. The local health board now required an autopsy on all bodies of suspected plague victims and a certification by a Caucasian doctor as to the cause of death before burial. To prevent its spread, the local health board had secured 30 inspectors to comb through Chinatown and direct the occupants to clean their living quarters. Compounding matters, the local board did not have any money for the task.[14]

Over the next few days, there appeared to be a lull in the crisis. However, it would be short-lived, with the detection of two new suspected cases that Kinyoun determined to be negative. For the present, the situation remained unchanged, except for the recruitment of 150 inspectors, consisting of medical and lay personnel to commence the cleanup and house-to-house inspections in Chinatown. The city had agreed to fund the operation. Gassaway reported that Kinyoun was now overseeing inoculations.[15]

After a period of relative calm, the situation dramatically escalated on March 21, with the placing of guards at exit points throughout San Francisco for Chinese leaving by sea or rail. Gassaway informed Wyman that the Chinese appeared to be transporting infected members to different communities in order to avoid detection. It further appeared that bodies were being hoarded to prevent the true cause of death from being discovered. This practice occurred as a way to circumvent the requirement of a burial certificate because any delay made a diagnosis more difficult after several days of decomposition. At the same time, houses and sewers were being cleaned with bichloride and sulfur dioxide.[16]

The situation reached the national level late on March 21, when the Associated Press sent a cable to the Service stating that plague existed in the city. The report announced that there had been four deaths and the matter had been kept confidential, while attempting to contain it. It noted the news had been "suppressed by the authorities until to-day"[17] because they wanted to make sure their findings were conclusive to the cause of death before going public. The release stated that Kellogg and Kinyoun, "after a most careful examination of the bacilli from glands of the victims … confirmed plague as the cause of death."[18]

The following day, *Scripps-McRae* released a statement from Dr. Williamson, the local health board's president. His statement was direct and to the point: Chinatown had plague, the Chinese were hiding the sick and the press had been covering up its existence. Consequently, Mexican ports banned entry from San Francisco, in effect a reverse quarantine, to be followed by others. In support of his conclusion, he stated President Montgomery from the University of California's medical department and Professor Orphlus from Cooper Medical College had verified his findings after examining specimens.[19]

Gassaway wired Wyman about Williamson's statement, commenting that it had been issued because of "the persistent lampooning of newspapers and public protest."[20] It had been made in part as a political response to those trying to misrepresent the true nature of the crisis.

This became evident on March 25, when the San Francisco *Chronicle* responded to Williamson by calling it the "criminal plague fake."[21] It decried "Dr. Williamson and the rest of the dollar-marked crew that comprised Mayor Phelan's gang of health officers."[22] Showing the real motivation behind its article, the paper stated, "The business men ... of the city ... have suffered by the gang's plague scare."[23] As time would show, the anti-plague factions' clamor would increase in intensity, drowning out anyone remotely suggesting its existence.

On the heels of his statement, things calmed down briefly, but new concerns arose, leaving to question whether anyone had a firm grasp on the situation. As the month ended, Kinyoun reported two more cases. He conducted autopsies on both and wired Wyman stating that the cases had been reported as pneumonia but were actually plague.[24]

Efforts to cleanse Chinatown commenced, but the local health board lacked the funds and experience to do a thorough job.[25] Reports continued about other cases and the Chinese hiding bodies from the authorities.[26] Kinyoun stressed the urgency in handling the matter, advising Wyman:

> Expect there will be further spread. Every condition favorable among this population. Requires quick action. No time to lose. Further information soon as obtained. Confidential.[27]

On March 27, *The Chronicle* printed "Phelan Fears His Specter," reporting that he sent a letter to the eastern press saying that although there had been a case of plague on March 6, the city remained free of any additional cases.[28] The paper called him "a petty political wire-puller."[29] It called the plague a fake and alleged that more health inspectors had been seen in taverns than in Chinatown. The mayor had wanted to defuse the situation, but it backfired. In another article, it lambasted Williamson and the local health board for recklessly spending its funding and needing more city money for the cleanup. It stated that no plague had existed from the beginning.[30]

Kinyoun knew the situation would get worse because of Chinatown's condition. The area had been well known for its filth and lack of sanitation. Trash and garbage permeated the streets with the sewers serving as passageways between residences, along with these avenues being repositories for human waste. Because of these connecting tributaries, those infected or dead could be channeled through these mazes for hiding, removal out of the city, or dumping into the sewers, in which case they ended up in the bay. On top of these problems, the channels made great breeding grounds for rats.[31]

Other corpses would be buried under houses. Kinyoun heard about this practice and would go out at night to dig up bodies. He would take the remains back to the island's lab for testing. In later years, his daughter Alice stated that he did this on several occasions and feared for his life if caught by the Chinese.[32] Several times, he had been offered bribes, threatened and warned that the Service's patrol boats would be attacked.[33]

The Habitat

The Chinese easily could be blamed because their habitat had been well known for its poor sanitation. People lived upon people. The housing resembled shantytowns in many areas. Opium, prostitution and other vices dotted the landscape. This environment had likely not been their choice for a community. They had been forced into this setting because of segregation.[34]

Although the Chinese had never been directly enslaved, they had been relegated to a lesser status in the United States by way of the Chinese Exclusion Act and other immigration laws in the 1880s and 1890s.[35] In San Francisco, the Chinese lived separate from the rest of the population. This did not occur by accident, but through efforts of the white population.

They became resistant when everyone started blaming them for the supposed plague. Later, when vaccinations became a requirement, they reacted bitterly and refused the treatment. Quarantining the population drew louder protests and fears.[36] It had only been a few months since the plague had cast its shadow on Honolulu in December 1899. Hawaiian officials decided to burn those infected parts of its Chinatown. However, the flames got out of control, resulting in its total destruction. More than 6,000 houses were destroyed, leaving most of the residents, not only homeless, but also destitute. Concerns of a similar recurrence in their neighborhood weighed heavily on them.[37]

Ironically, Honolulu may have contracted the plague from San Francisco, coming from the *Coptic*, when it arrived in September 1899. The city's first alleged plague cases had previously been documented as arriving on the *Nippon Maru on* June 27, 1899. Even Wyman would later acknowledge that the plague may well have been in the port as early as 1896, when Surgeon Rosenau served as the quarantine officer.

Regardless of the time of arrival, the Chinese viewed the quarantine as causing them greater exposure to the disease by the barricades. They had been intimidated, physically beaten and discriminated against since their arrival in the city. Now they had been sequestered into the malady's likely incubator, their own backyard. Consequently, they feverishly covered up the plague, hoping to avoid the white man's incursions once again into their lives.

The Situation Worsens

On April 1, Texas issued new quarantine directives. Although not mentioning California, the action had been taken as a protective response.[38]

While everything seemed to be moving in an orderly fashion with inspections and the cleaning process, Kinyoun advised Wyman on April 26 of another case, which he later confirmed as plague. He stated that the new case had no connection with the March 6 victim, thereby raising concern it had spread.[39] On May 13, he cabled Wyman about the discovery of two more cases, with one originating near the Sacramento River. Later, he confirmed that one of the victims, a Chinese girl, had died of plague, evidenced by a large bubo in her femur.[40]

The victim had been misdiagnosed by a white physician as having typhoid fever. He now called the plague epidemic because the two confirmed cases occurred in isolated locations demonstrating its moving to other locations.[41] Kinyoun asked Wyman to keep the matter confidential, "on account of vicious local press attacks."[42] As a precaution, the local health board would advise the merchants and press about the new cases.[43]

Kinyoun asked about attending the announcement and committing the Service to any type of assistance. He called the "situation very serious"[44] and said it would "require almost superhuman effort."[45] Its abatement would require controlling 25,000 inhabitants at a cost upwards of $100,000. However, he advised, if depopulation would be required, then the amount could exceed $1,000,000. In concluding, he reported that the portable sulfur furnace had arrived and been given to the local health board for its sanitation efforts.[46]

A sense of urgency can be seen in this wire. He referred to the situation as epidemic, and with the impending press release, one could sense his anxiety. Most importantly, he sought direction from Wyman on how to proceed, thereby showing his actions were on behalf of him.

Wyman promptly replied to him. First, he directed him to be present at the meeting and determine assistance needs. Second, he was to be advised immediately of the meeting's outcome. Third, he cautioned that no funds could be advanced by the Service unless authorized by a higher official.[47] And lastly, he stated that the 1890 quarantine law could be used as an option.[48]

In another telegram, he related that the Chinese consul-general in San Francisco would be approached and asked "to use his influence to have the Chinese comply cheerfully with necessary measures and consult with you [Kinyoun] as the representative of the United States Government [sic]."[49] With this statement, he officially assumed management of the situation.

Wyman next ordered areas suspected of infection to be cordoned off with guards placed at all railroad stations and ferries preventing any Chinese from exiting. In effect, this order quarantined these individuals. The cable directed the completion of house inspections and the use of Haffkine vaccine. Further, he directed the removal of questionable cases from their houses to a facility in Chinatown, or extradition to Angel Island. He ordered the killing of all rats, inspection of railroads outside California and establishment of "a disinfecting corps."[50]

He told Wyman that five plague cases had been reported to date and part of the group's discussions centered on preparations for an epidemic. He stated that no one wanted to release any information to the press because of a potential backlash.[51]

Kinyoun informed Wyman about his assessment of the meeting, which had included members of the Chinese Six Companies.[52] The Chinese Six Companies formed in 1882, comprising the six mayoral Chinese districts in California. Having roots back to 1875, its purpose centered on promoting morals, limiting Chinese immigration and curtailing prostitution, so as not to increase resentment by white Americans. The group also acted as a legal guardian of Chinese liberties by employing attorneys to defend any infringement by the white population.[53]

After the meeting, the participants agreed to reconvene and refine plans on how to proceed in approaching the Chinese about mitigating the plague. Kinyoun thought that once the house inspections commenced, there would be a mass exit. The local health board remained committed to doing the work and believed it could secure the necessary funds for the task. As far as guarding the transportation points, he believed only the Service could handle the job. He asked Wyman whether he should go to Stockton for an inspection, since one plague fatality had come from the town.[54] Wyman approved the request and directed him to visit other neighboring communities, saying he would send additional officers as help. In closing, the surgeon general stated he would be shipping 20,000 vials of the Haffkine vaccine within two days.[55]

From May 18–19, a total of 17 telegrams were exchanged between Kinyoun, Wyman and others, reflecting the gravity of the situation.[56] Wyman instructed him to hire two assistants at a fee of $200 a month to conduct train inspections. These individuals were to be placed at the Oregon and Reno, Nevada, borders.[57] He directed Assistant Surgeon Cofer, in Los Angeles, to hire two other inspectors to monitor the Southern and Santa Fe lines at the Arizona border.[58] Next, he notified Dr. Harris, the Quarantine Office at Eureka, California,[59] and the quarantine officer in Hoquiam, Washington, to inspect all Chinese coming from San Francisco.[60] The following day, he ordered Dr. Foster at Port Townsend, Washington, to screen not only all Chinese, but their luggage, too.[61] Because of the magnitude of the brewing crisis, Wyman directed three additional surgeons from the Service to report to Kinyoun.[62] He even wired Dr. Roux at the Pasteur Institute for guidance.[63]

In another dispatch, Kinyoun reported that the whites had been telling people not to receive the Haffkine vaccine, thereby hindering the abatement efforts.[64] Wyman replied, asking whether a few whites being inoculated might help persuade the Chinese.[65] He answered that when inspectors try to enter Chinatown to conduct house inspections they are barred from entering. With this development, he requested permission to impose the 1890 quarantine law.[66] Wyman cautioned him to act with "tact and discretion in enforcing inoculations of Chinese and be not too precipitate or harsh."[67]

He directed the inspectors at the Oregon and Nevada borders to deny passage to Chinese and Japanese without a Marine Hospital Service health certificate.[68] Wyman also ordered trains crossing the border at Yuma and The Needles to be inspected and to deny passage to those from these groups who did not possess a certificate.[69] Next, he proceeded to alert the health officers of Texas[70] and Louisiana about the plague and that the Service had taken steps to prevent these nationalities from leaving the state.[71]

On May 20, Kinyoun provided Wyman an update. The inspections were ongoing, but the Chinese continued to deny access to their homes. In a different vein, Japanese residents had started taking the vaccine, so they could depart, but only one Chinese had been inoculated. So far, the Chinese remained amicable to him, although not to the local board of health. He met with the Chinese consular official and other Chinese representatives, who questioned the law restricting travel. Afterwards, he reported that they might file a lawsuit challenging the local health board's and the Service's actions restricting the Chinese.[72] Kinyoun asked for "full power"[73] to coordinate transportation limitations. Again, he stated that the press refused to print the truth about the plague.[74]

The following day, Wyman wrote to the Secretary of Treasury, asking that President McKinley be briefed about the plague. He requested that the president authorize the Treasury Department to establish regulations to contain its spread, as authorized by the 1890 Quarantine Act.[75] The president agreed to the request.[76] Wyman informed Kinyoun, stating that regulations would be forthcoming by 10:00 p.m. The order directed that regulations be written limiting the travel of Asians, absent a health certificate.[77]

On imposing the regulations, Wyman sent out two supplemental directives. The first went to Kinyoun, informing him of its contents and directives.[78] The second constituted an all points order to Marine Hospital officers located at those exit and entry points in California, Nevada, Arizona and Oregon, thereby effectively sealing off the California border. It directed them to inspect all trains departing California. Every Chinese and Japanese individual wanting to leave was to be thoroughly scrutinized and a determination made about where they had been living or visiting. Upon detection, any person having plague was to be barred from leaving the state.[79]

On May 22, Treasury Secretary Gage implemented the regulations advising all officers of the Service, local and state health boards and other parties of authority.[80] The caption read:

INTERSTATE QUARANTINE REGULATIONS TO PREVENT THE SPREAD OF PLAGUE IN THE UNITED STATES[81]

The secretary stated its issuance had been authorized pursuant to the 1890 Quarantine Act and applied to all territories of the United States. The law contained three sections outlining how government and other officials would proceed going forward.[82] The first section directed that the surgeon general "would forbid the sale or donation of transportation … to Asiatics or other races particularly liable to the disease."[83] The second section forbade all transporters or carriers from granting passage to anyone suspected of having it.[84] And the third section stated that any body of a plague victim would not be allowed transport "except in a hermetically sealed coffin" approved by a representative of the Service or the local board of health.[85]

Afterwards, Kinyoun sent several wires to Wyman seeking help from the U.S. marshal in the inspection process.[86] He reported that 18 Chinese had been vaccinated, along with 250 Japanese, noting their cooperation. The blockade around Chinatown appeared to be holding, but house and business inspections remained elusive. Regarding actions by the state board of health, it had issued a press statement asserting that there were no plague cases.[87] Lastly, he wrote about rumors of pending legal action aimed at challenging the regulation.[88]

At this point, Wyman requested a full accounting of Kinyoun's actions. He inquired as to the veracity of reports about the Chinese being forcibly inoculated as reported in the *New York Herald*.[89] The doctor responded that the board of health had only conducted voluntary vaccinations, but the press had been fabricating reports.[90]

Of special note, the local board of health's Secretary H.L. Nichols, M. D., sent Kinyoun a letter with a copy of a resolution it passed confirming the plague's manifestation. It directed the city's public services—police, city physician, plumbing inspector and sanitary inspector—to assist in coordinating the plague's containment. It expressed the desire to work with the state board of health in Sacramento to join its efforts to work with him and the Service.[91]

The plague had now become a matter of national concern with the issuance of these regulations. No longer did it remain a California problem because it affected the well-being of the entire nation. The right of the state in this matter had been superseded by the federal government.

The real tug-of-war over which body politic had jurisdiction would explode onto the forefront of daily life in California. The doctor would become the chief villain in this battle of the brow, even though he had been adhering to Wyman's directives.

The Injunction

On May 23, Kinyoun advised Wyman of an injunction.[92] On learning of the development, Wyman informed the attorney general that he had notified the Treasury Department of the suit's likelihood. The district attorney in San Francisco had been directed to intercede on behalf of the government and Kinyoun.[93]

Because of this new turn of events, he pointed out that the railroads would probably stop selling tickets to destinations outside the state.[94] He asked Wyman's assistance in setting up an internment camp on Angel Island for suspected plague carriers.[95]

On the 24th, Kinyoun wired Wyman that the injunction had been filed and that he had been briefing the district attorney on the government's actions. He recommended that all departure points from California be quarantined to prevent the plague's spread throughout the country.[96] Wyman responded, asking who filed the injunction and for a summary of its major points.[97]

He answered it had been brought by the Chinese Six Companies representing the Chinese, with the Japanese purportedly joining as plaintiffs.[98] Titled *Wong Wai vs. Williamson ET AL.*,[99] the injunction had been brought against the local board of health, Board President Williamson, and Kinyoun, representing the Marine Hospital Service, as an agent of the United States.[100] He summarized its contents to Wyman:

> Claims are that the Federal Government has exceeded its authority in prohibiting free passage of Chinese within the State, claiming the 1890 Act applies only to interstate traffic, and therefore has no power in the premises. Also demand to be relieved of restriction imposed by board of health (local), claiming that there is no plague in San Francisco.[101]

On May 25, Kinyoun reported that Judge Morrow had accepted the application for injunction and had decided he would not immediately rule on its imposition. In the meantime, house inspections were continuing, as well as those being conducted through the rail and shipping carriers. However, a deceased Chinese suspected of having beriberi had likely died of plague.[102]

As both sides waited for Morrow to review the petition, Kinyoun proceeded to enforce the Treasury quarantine regulations and apprised Wyman about other plague matters. He suggested that the Service stress the importance of Haffkine as a way to curb the Chinese's negative perception of the treatment. By not taking the vaccine, all Chinese and Japanese would be subject to a 15-day quarantine before being allowed to depart the city.[103]

Wyman asked Kinyoun if the restrictions on the Japanese could be lessened, especially if they had not resided or associated with anyone in Chinatown.[104] In response, he cautioned against such a measure, stating that while he had made some exceptions, under the present circumstances it would be best to require a certificate attesting that they had not been in contact with any Chinese. He allowed that he might be willing to do the same for those Chinese who had not been in contact with Chinatown and its residents.[105]

On May 26, another problem arose. Threats had been received by Kinyoun stating that the boats used by the Service to patrol the harbor were going to be sunk and the launches destroyed. With this development, he requested assistance from the Secretary of the Navy.[106] The Navy agreed, and he would be placed in charge of overseeing the operations.[107] Revenue cutters would be at his disposal to intercept transports.[108] The doctor explained that the patrols were needed more at night when Chinese would try to slip out of Chinatown with their dead.[109]

Morrow's Ruling

On May 28, Morrow ruled in favor of the injunction.[110] The order prohibited all attempts to inoculate Wong Wai and any other Chinese with Haffkine. And all Chinese were to have the right of free passage to and from the city and within the state. The suit had been brought by Mr. Wong Ai, a Chinese man seeking to leave the quarantined area without being inoculated. The suit had the support of the Chinese Six Companies, along with other interested parties, and represented a major challenge to the government's quarantine.[111]

Following his order, Morrow issued a lengthy opinion. He first reviewed the allegations by the complainant, consisting of the required vaccination of Haffkine prophylactic before the issuance of a health certificate. Morrow next addressed the drug's questionable value coupled with the risk of death, the absence of plague, restraint of travel, infringement of personal liberty, too broad an application to a class of 25,000 Asians, and a denial of equal protection as guaranteed by the United States Constitution.[112]

With the complainant's counsel having presented its evidence in support of the injunction, the judge had asked the respondents to show cause, or offer their set of facts, as to why the restraining order should not be issued as prayed by the complaints. The only piece of evidence introduced by the Service consisted of a cable sent by Wyman to Kinyoun on May 21 directing him to proceed with quarantine measures pursuant to the 1890 Act, authorized by President McKinley.[113] The submission of this document alone failed to demonstrate any scientific facts of the plague's presence that had been the basis of its actions. He ruled that the government could not claim it as law without being accountable under the Constitution.

Morrow found numerous faults with the quarantine, starting with the question of authority. He appeared to sidestep this question and pointed to the Municipal Charter, Articles II and X for guidance. Article II, he allowed, created the legislative body of the county and city, called the board of supervisors. Article X established the city's health department under the supervision of the board of health with sweeping jurisdiction over all things pertaining to the public's health. Because of this structure, he reasoned, the board of supervisors should have been the body to have drafted and issued the regulations concerning the purported contagion.[114]

His ensuing finding centered on the breath of the quarantine and its effect on Chinese residents, as opposed to any other class of people. All told, he reasoned, San Francisco had a population of 350,000 residents with 25,000 being either Chinese or of Asiatic descent. Not all Chinese lived in Chinatown, and these individuals had been allowed to freely move about without a vaccination. He found that not a single block, street, or house had been identified as being contaminated by the local board of health or the board of supervisors, his point being that the quarantine unjustly classified the Chinese and Japanese as carriers of the disease when not all of them lived in Chinatown. Accordingly, their confinement as a class based on race proved to be discriminatory and denied these individuals the right of equal protection.[115]

Morrow reviewed the facts presented by the petitioners. The respondents were the local board of health and the Service, which had not presented sufficient facts in their defense. In particular, they had not mentioned the fact that the Chinese had steadfastly refused to allow inspections of their premises. They consistently had gone to great lengths to hide victims, circumventing attempts at containment. The Service had acted because the local board of health had not acted, and the state board had refused because it was controlled by the state's political system and its governor.

The Service knew the imminent danger of leaving the malady unchecked. The naysayers, though, should have known what recently had happened in China and India, leading to countless millions of deaths. Understand that judicial review, as a rule, cannot examine those facts beyond the presented evidence. But in extraordinary situations, equitable cognizance should be brought into consideration for the better good.

Morrow did present several legitimate constitutional points. He conceded laws that enacted for the public good and welfare have been generally viewed as prudent legislative acts within the police powers of the state. When such edicts cannot be justified, they become subject to the court's review. In those cases where personal liberty and property have been infringed, then such instances can be viewed as arbitrary and capricious. Accordingly, the law cannot be allowed to stand in light of such an intrusion upon one's civil liberties. Solely categorizing one class of individuals as being more prone to the plague than another, without supporting evidence, becomes wholly unacceptable[116] even though San Francisco could segregate one race from another in a separate neighborhood, such as Chinatown.

He questioned those parts of the regulations issued by the Service stating that people exposed to the illness should not receive Haffkine, since it was not intended as a preventive measure after exposure, but only before. He reasoned that its use after exposure could prove life-threatening to the recipient. Citing Wyman, he stated that if one has been exposed, then the serum should be administered, instead of Haffkine. Since the Chinese had been confined to the infected area, it had no value as a vaccine in preventing the disease's spread, but to the contrary could cause great individual harm. Therefore, he ruled that it had no value, as claimed by Wyman.[117]

Afterwards, he addressed Kinyoun's sole piece of evidence in support of the Service's authority: the wire he had received from Wyman directing him to proceed under the 1890 Quarantine Act. Morrow recited the law in question before giving his opinion as to its application and relevance to the case. He noted that the statute was quite broad in allowing the Secretary of the Treasury to supervise the surgeon general in establishing regulations and ordinances when the president deemed it in the best interest of the country to curtail and prevent the spread of yellow fever, smallpox, cholera and the plague.[118] With this said, he stated:

> the statute is open to interpretation that the promulgation of rules and regulations to prevent the spread of the disease ... is made to depend upon the fact that it has been made to appear to satisfaction of the President that the disease exists.[119]

He reasoned that if this were the case, then the question became open to review, and he argued that the president had not made such a statement as to the plague's existence. In his opinion, this element of the law had not been satisfied by the respondents. It appeared Wyman had not presented satisfactory evidence of its existence.

All he had done was quote authority under the statute without offering any findings of fact. In addition, the ruling criticized him for only requiring a certificate from Kinyoun to allow people to leave Chinatown.[120] Morrow found that no compelling reason existed for the restriction.

Morrow stated that the directives issued to Kinyoun lacked any firm substantive basis to uphold the quarantine, again citing their violation of the petitioner's right to equal protection. He set forth several cases in support of his position, where Chinese had been discriminated against because of their race. In these cases, the police power had exceeded its authority and restraints had been imposed in favor of the aggrieved parties.[121]

Reaction

Immediately after Morrow's ruling, Kinyoun wired the state board of health about the judge's findings, adding that the Service had ceased inspections in Chinatown. Ironically, the state board now wanted the city board of health to impose a quarantine on all the Chinese. He reported that apparently the city's business interests along with other parties had now realized the seriousness of the situation. Before ending the telegram, he reported that observation of the Chinese would remain in effect for those departing by rail, even though a health certificate had been banned by the court's ruling.[122]

Following this, he telegraphed Wyman a synopsis of Morrow's opinion. He stated that the district attorney had not told the Service about the court's ruling fearing it could spark further action by the "General Government"[123] and neighboring states. He also recommended that all inspections end.[124] Kinyoun ended his cable, writing, "As Bureau has all the facts concerning situation, will wait instructions. Rush answer."[125]

Wyman quickly responded and offered several countermeasures along with several questions. First, he told him to meet with the district attorney and formulate a course of action. He recommended that the local board of health announce the plague's existence. Absent its willingness, he instructed him to go find a case. On finding one, he should proceed to quarantine the area. In the meantime, he would confer with his superiors in Washington.[126]

Kinyoun responded that he had instructed the border inspectors to cease further inspections and await new orders. In other news, he reported that the local health board had put before the city supervisors a resolution proclaiming the plague's presence. Though it would not place a cordon around Chinatown because of the judge's restraining order, he reported that the state board of health would act accordingly, if the local board acted.[127]

On a positive note, the supervisors had made arrangements to meet with the merchants and local health board. The state board wanted him to delay any actions. It wanted the Justice Department to have the district attorney seek a modification or dissolution of the order based on the judge's failure to properly weigh the evidence of plague and the issue of inoculations.[128]

On May 29, the board of supervisors passed a resolution empowering the local health board to institute a quarantine around Chinatown[129] and establish those measures "necessary against prevention and spread of infectious disease."[130] The Southern Pacific Railroad stopped issuing tickets to Chinese until a quarantine could be put in place. In light of these developments, Kinyoun asked Wyman what he should tell the inspectors stationed at California's borders.[131]

The following day, he sent Wyman another cable seeking directions on how he should handle freight shipments to and from the state. Furthermore, could he act under the 1890 statute?[132] Wyman replied that he would answer him the next day. Concerning the bigger question, as to the 1890 law, he instructed Kinyoun to operate on a temporary basis under its authority. More importantly, he ordered him to operate under the 1893 quarantine law, as well, if the border inspectors received any orders requiring immediate action.[133]

Within the mix off all this correspondence, Wyman sent a cable on June 3, to the Treasury Department, concerning questions about the mandatory use of Haffkine and apprehensions from Japan's chargé d'affaires about restricting the travel of Japanese residents leaving San Francisco. Wyman argued that he had not issued any order requiring vaccinations.[134] He admitted that, because of the plague's existence in Chinatown, "temporary"[135] restrictions had been imposed by the local board of health that had caused a few limitations on the "Asiatics"[136] living in the area. However, the measure had never been intended as a discriminatory act against Japanese and represented nothing more than a "misunderstanding."[137]

Confronted with a diplomatic issue, Wyman addressed any intentional action towards the Japanese. Many of them lived in Chinatown and had been caught in the quarantine's net. The plague had raised eyebrows in Washington and, as any astute public servant knows, one does not want to anger one's superiors, especially in the political world. Of great interest, though, and showing his diplomatic skills to some extent, he unequivocally denied the mandatory use of Haffkine. But in reality, he indirectly had required its use by not allowing people to leave Chinatown until they had a certificate from Kinyoun. The only way to secure this document was to be vaccinated. He seemed to shift any blame to the local board of health and the city supervisors as being the parties making these requirements. In fact, he had been instrumental in having these entities act on his directives.

For the Record: Kinyoun's Letter of June 11

After the court's order, Kinyoun sent a lengthy letter to Wyman outlining those events preceding the judge's ruling and explaining how the situation had gotten out of hand. The document articulated that every effort had been made by him and the Service to communicate the facts of the contagion's presence. It also described a joint understanding by representatives of the Chinese Six Companies, its attorney John Bennett, the Chinese consular general, the local board of health and members of the Merchants Association on how to prevent its spread. All parties acknowledged that the Chinese and Japanese should be inoculated with Haffkine. At the suggestion of

Mr. Bennett, a conference had been held the following day in hopes of persuading those affected to participate in the solution.[138]

Following the meeting, he thought everything to be in place, but on learning of this plan, a group of whites, including a few white doctors, began telling the Chinese the vaccine was dangerous, could cause death and had already claimed lives. The Chinese Six Companies had been approached by a large gathering of Chinese inquiring about these rumors and urged they be inoculated first to prove its safety. They refused, which almost led to a riot. Afterwards, gangs went to the houses of various Chinese Six Companies officers. Upwards of 700 protesters surrounded the consular office, and, had the police not arrived, there could have been a major incident. All the while, a paper circulated in Chinatown asking all its residents to boycott the immunization.[139]

On May 20, the Chinese consul, Mr. Ho Yow, officers of the Chinese Six Companies and others representing the Chinese invited Kinyoun to a meeting. They informed him that because of recent developments, along with the paper threatening anyone who received an inoculation, they could no longer encourage any of their fellow Chinese to have it. The group also questioned what authority he had to implement this procedure. He responded that it had been recommended—but not ordered—by Wyman, contrary to many people's opinion.[140]

If the disease could not be quickly controlled, then other measures could be expected by the state's health organizations. This could lead to neighboring states barring entry from those departing California. The gravity of the emerging crisis continued to boil over. During the group's meeting, 1,000 Chinese massed in front of the consulate and commenced stoning the building, until the police dispersed the crowd.[141]

At the same time, house inspections continued, along with offers of vaccination. Unfortunately, all the houses and businesses had been closed to avoid inspection.[142] It seemed a "Chinese highbinder element,"[143] had caused people to resist the inspections and had gone so far as to threaten violence to anyone who supported the inoculations or received one. A Chinese newspaper editor had received the vaccination in hopes of convincing others of its safety. A mob soon attacked him, resulting in his hiding inside his house for three days. Events were spiraling out of control.[144]

Everyone seemed to be denying the vaccine's benefits. White doctors continued to spread false rumors of its side effects, claiming that five people had died with others becoming very ill. But witnesses would see these same individuals walking the streets days later. Kinyoun pointed out that the press had gone to great lengths, publishing fabrications about the disease and the vaccine.[145]

Worse yet, Morrow had used Wyman's publication about the drug—in which he stated it should not be used on those individuals possibly exposed to the plague—to everyone's detriment.[146] In his ruling, he had denied its existence.[147] Kinyoun, though, wrote that the judge had indirectly admitted its existence, when he stated, "this method would be highly dangerous for people who had been exposed to plague, and therefore could not be safely taken."[148] In other words, if there was no plague, then how could anyone be exposed to it?

Towards the end of his letter he reported that, even with all the negative sentiment concerning Haffkine, 284 whites, 530 Japanese and 58 Chinese had been vaccinated out of the 25,000 residents in Chinatown and San Francisco.[149] The situation had literally turned to chaos through misunderstanding and the deception of numerous troublemakers.

New Troubles

After the quarantine was lifted, the local board of health asked the Service for help.[150] At the same time, the city's board of supervisors declared the plague's existence and issued a directive telling the local health board to establish a corridor encircling Chinatown.[151]

Those parties acknowledging the plague began setting up countermeasures to Morrow's ruling. Moreover, a distinction had been found in his ruling, whereby it applied to intrastate transportation, as opposed to interstate transportation, or travel between the states.[152] This distinction would eventually give rise to more litigation.[153] Regardless, Wyman and Kinyoun had embarked on a very problematic, if not precarious course in trying to navigate around the court's ruling.

Kinyoun told Wyman that the local health board requested the use of Angel Island for the detention of 7,000 people. The state board of health also asked for the Service's help in maintaining the inspections of ships and trains departing from San Francisco.[154] On the same day, he reported another possible plague victim.[155] Wyman directed him to operate under the interstate quarantine regulations already in place, pending the city supervisor's regulations.[156]

The state board informed him that it did not have any regulations concerning transportation inspections and that the local health board could not legally intercede because it was a state matter. Because of these factors, he had no authority to inspect the rail lines.[157] Wyman, though, instructed him not to stop the inspections, but to make sure no discrimination occurred in the process.[158] In the meantime, cases and deaths continued to increase during this period.[159]

Wyman had referred him to Section 3 of the act. It stated that if local and state board regulations proved ineffective, then seek their counsel as to what would be appropriate, especially where they will not or cannot make the necessary laws to contain the situation. He directed Kinyoun to let him know, so they can be included into those regulations being written by the city supervisors.[160] He had decided to take charge of the crisis. The situation had turned into a nightmare, and the judge had opened the floodgates. His ruling essentially allowed infected individuals to leave and potentially spread the contagion throughout the Western United States.

In the midst of all this maneuvering, Kinyoun informed Wyman that the state board of health had asked Governor Gage for assistance to help the local board of health with certain parts of the quarantine due to suspicions by the latter. The governor refused.[161] As an aside, Kinyoun wired Wyman, stating that the Secretary of War had approved the use of Angel Island as a quarantine camp at China Cove.[162]

On June 5, attorneys representing the Chinese filed a second injunction, *Jew Ho V. Williamson ET AL.*, against the local health board.[163] Kinyoun alerted Wyman that everything had come to a "standstill."[164] At least 1,000 Chinese and Japanese had left the city to other parts of the state.[165] He stated that there would be a mass "exodus of infected persons"[166] if the court granted the injunction. In earnest, he asked if the 1890 Quarantine Act could be wired to him in hopes of it overriding the possible decree.[167]

Morrow ruled in favor of this second injunction, staying any attempt to place the Chinese in the holding camp on Angel Island. But he delayed ruling on the newest cordon around Chinatown. Meanwhile, more bad news arrived during a meeting with the state health board. Gage had been doing all he could to smear the local health board and continued denying the plague. He stated all actions had come to a standstill.[168]

On a personal side, he informed the Service of an attempt to bribe him with a sizable sum on the morning of the filing of the first injunction. It would be paid if he used his position to quash the regulations imposed on the Chinese. Additionally, he had learned that physicians had been approached to deny the plague's presence in return for money in hopes of raising the quarantine. Worse yet, Chinese had been threatened with death by other Chinese if any of them went to the quarantine camp, the thinking being that it would constitute an admission of the contagion. Lastly, the Merchants Association had decided against providing the health board with any funding, except for providing food.[169]

Following these developments, the local health board voted to terminate the quarantine 20 days after the last reported case.[170] But on June 13, the worst of all fears surfaced after examinations determined that three Chinese reported to have died from heart failure and bronchitis had in fact died of plague. The third case appeared to have succumbed to pneumonic plague—the deadliest of all forms. More troubling, the victim had been discovered outside Chinatown, meaning it had spread beyond the containment zone, unless the decedent had been moved postmortem.[171] Either way, if the disease had entered this cycle, it would mean a greater state of acceleration and attendant death.

On June 14, the court lifted the barricade around Chinatown under a writ of habeas corpus. The quarantine had been ruled illegal because it discriminated on the basis of race. Kinyoun stated that the decision indirectly recognized plague when it stated that those afflicted or exposed could be detained within the area. Even with this ruling, he told the carriers to deny transportation to anyone leaving the state not possessing a health certificate. Now, he intended to contact the health boards of surrounding states about the situation in California, especially in light of the false statements being fed to the State Department by the governor's office.[172]

A state of limbo hung over everyone. The district attorney telephoned Kinyoun inquiring about his orders restricting travel to individuals not having a certificate. He told him these measures would result in his being held in contempt of court. Kinyoun replied that he only took orders from the surgeon general or the Secretary of the Treasury. In response, the district attorney pointed out that Morrow's earlier order stated the president's statement had been ruled too general and therefore not applicable to San Francisco.[173] Kinyoun, though, stated that the "public health reports"[174] do name the city, and, accordingly, the 1890 Quarantine Act applied.[175]

June 16 would prove to be a bellwether date for him and the Service. Earlier in the day, he notified Wyman that people departing the state only needed to certify that they had not been exposed and had not been in an infected area. By this measure, compliance with this requirement had been mitigated to merely an oral acknowledgment by the exiting party, absent any proof.[176]

Contempt Citation

As predicted by the district attorney, Frank L. Combs, a contempt of court citation for violating the judge's earlier order had been served on Kinyoun. He had been charged with obstructing the travel of Wong Wai from the city to Eureka, California. In his defense, he claimed the ruling only restricted passage within the state and not necessarily from state to state.[177] Wyman directed him to have Combs represent him at his hearing. He told him to review all matters concerning the quarantines with him.[178] In response, Kinyoun asked for any additional regulations concerning quarantines that might aid his case.[179] On receiving this telegram, Wyman told him that there were none.[180]

The next day, Wyman took things into his own hands. He issued Kinyoun two orders. The first directed him to cease all inspections, except those at the border.[181] The second told him to inform the inspectors to stand down.[182] At the same time, Gage sent a cable to McKinley about the situation. In turn, Acting Secretary of the Treasury Spaulding replied to Gage on behalf of the president, acknowledging the suspension of the quarantine for the time being.[183] But he also issued a statement in support of Kinyoun, stating:

> So far as known to the Department Surgeon Kinyoun has endeavored only to carry out the Department regulations.[184]

Wyman advised him that the Secretary of the Treasury had wired the attorney general asking him to direct Combs to represent him. He concluded the cable stating that the doctor had only been following instructions and did not intentionally violate the restraining order.[185] The importance of his wire lay in its reaffirmation of Spaulding's opinion about his conduct, stating, "convinced no intention on the part of Surgeon Kinyoun."[186] For now, the government stood behind him. Unfortunately, the Service had now come under the microscope as to its conduct. The two men had tried to put in place countermeasures based on their interpretation of the law. But the Chinese remained determined in their resistance.

On June 18, the district attorney appeared on Kinyoun's behalf in federal court. As expected, the judge had little sympathy for the Service's actions, but did grant a week postponement for the hearing. Combs argued that it had not been Kinyoun's intent to violate the order, he had since stopped the inspections, and all other restrictive measures would be approved by the court in advance.[187]

As a matter of legal maneuvering, he moved that the matter be placed on hold, but Morrow stated Kinyoun must account for his actions. He held that no one could interpret the court's ruling except the court. What's more, the federal court constituted the only body that could determine the merits of any interstate regulation, not even the president of the United States.[188]

In another flurry of "Confidential" exchanges, Wyman told Kinyoun to cease any further restraints upon the Chinese for those traveling to Eureka.[189] He directed him to forward all the proceedings for his examination.[190] Several days later, he advised Wyman that Combs had stated that only the court could place into effect state regulations promulgated under the 1890 and 1893 Quarantine Acts. Kinyoun stated he asked him to seek a review of this question, but Combs had refused his request. Because of this, he asked Wyman for another attorney.[191]

Apparently exasperated and alarmed with the unraveling situation, Wyman asked him to clarify whether the court now had unlimited sway over all matters of quarantine. He instructed him to consult with the district attorney for direction.[192] Kinyoun replied that ordinary operations of the Service were not affected by the order.[193]

Subsequently, he reported that Combs was acting contrary to the best interests of Wyman. Once more, he requested another attorney. He pointed out that this would be needed to protect the Service and himself.[194]

Kinyoun wired Wyman on June 23, again complaining about the district attorney's abilities. He wrote that there had been no plans to introduce any evidence about the plague, but merely to enter a denial on his behalf.[195] After meeting with the Acting Secretary of the Treasury and its solicitor, Wyman informed him that they were neither going to interfere with Combs's handling of the case nor appoint new counsel.[196] Within this array of dispatches, along with what could be considered adding insult to injury, he directed him to discharge the border inspectors.[197]

Legal Scrambles and Morrow's Ruling

By June 25, the petitioner's evidence had been submitted to the court,[198] with Morrow awaiting the Service's.[199] For Kinyoun, it looked bad. Telegrams continued to be shuffled back and forth between him and Wyman. But worst, the press had a field day with him.

During this exchange, another matter arose between him and the district attorney.[200] Apparently, after receiving Wyman's wire denying his request for a new attorney, Kinyoun sent Combs a letter, directing him how to handle the case. Coombs responded on July 2, stating he had received it an hour prior to Kinyoun's hearing.[201] He replied:

> I have to inform you that the course laid down in your letter to be hereafter pursued is so contrary to my own ideas of legal propriety, and in my opinion would be so fatal to your interest that I absolutely refuse to proceed in accordance with your view.[202]

Besides refusing to follow his demands, he defended his previous actions, stating:

> I have further to say that I have tried to conduct your case in the best possible manner and it seems to be conceded all around that I have, but I am unwilling needlessly to shoulder responsibilities upon others which are now in issue.[203]

The most interesting part of the letter centered on the last half of the sentence, beginning "but I am unwilling needlessly to shoulder responsibilities upon others."[204] By this statement, he appeared reluctant to widen the scope of the case. In a letter a year later, Kinyoun accused him of being in cahoots with the anti-plague factions.[205] Maybe Combs did not want to challenge the power brokers: the press, the leading industrialists and Governor Gage.

Regardless, Kinyoun had an uphill battle in proving his innocence. Fortunately, the case had been continued because the prosecution was searching for more witnesses to testify against him.[206] At the same time, Wyman informed him that the suit had been sent to United States attorney general for review by the Acting Secretary of the Treasury.[207]

Wyman wired the state health officer of Texas on June 27, telling him there had been 10 confirmed cases of plague with another 4–5 likely, pending a medical analysis.[208] From his end, he kept presenting the Service's findings to other potentially affected neighboring states.

The day before the hearing, Kinyoun informed Wyman the court had ignored evidence presented on his behalf. He implied in so many words that Combs held little regard for the case and therefore he expected an unfavorable ruling.[209] On the day of court's decision, the Acting Secretary of the Treasury and the acting attorney general exchanged telegrams expressing interest in the case's outcome.[210] This must have seemed either amusing or very agonizing to Kinyoun when, at the 11th hour, they did not show up to help him and acted only as observers to the outcome. It appeared his superiors had started to distance themselves from his troubles.

On July 3, Judge Morrow delivered a lengthy review of the findings. First, he weighed the evidence set forth by the complainant. His analysis went to great lengths assessing the accusations leveled at Kinyoun of whether he had contravened the injunction of May 28. Distinctions were made between the ruling and his supposed actions.[211]

Second, Morrow reviewed various affidavits in support or in opposition to the matter.[212] The most evidentiary of these documents came from Assistant Surgeon B.J. Lloyd attached to Kinyoun at San Francisco's port. He recalled witnessing a conversation on June 19 between him and Captain Miner Goodall in the Quarantine Office in the Ferry Building. The captain worked for the Pacific Coast Steamship Company.[213]

Goodall had asked Kinyoun to inspect the company's ships. He replied that all the inspections had been cancelled by the surgeon general. But in Lloyd's affidavit, he stated that the men referred to an earlier encounter on June 16. In that conversation, the doctor asked Goodall if he had not heard that travel within the state no longer required a health certificate. The captain stated he did know about this change.[214]

Lloyd proceeded to state that he had been on quarantine duty on June 16 and 17, inspecting vessels at the dock and on request would issue certificates in accordance with the recent injunction. But on one of these days he remembered seeing three Chinese talking with one of the ship's representatives. He asked Lloyd if he could secure a certificate for them. After answering his question, he related:

> Whereupon the Company's agent notwithstanding my assertion turned to the Chinamen and said: "We don't want you anyhow. We have orders from the Company not to take them." To the best of my knowledge and belief the said Company's agent was Captain Wallace.[215]

He concluded his statement by saying:

> I repeatedly stated to individuals applying for certificates and to employees of said Steamship Company that certificates were not required of those persons who were traveling only within State limits but were given to facilitate the movement of the Company's vessels.[216]

The contents of this affidavit served to benefit Kinyoun's position and appeared to show a possible conspiracy to set him up for contempt. The court's opinion described a similar story as presented in Lloyd's affidavit, although referring to a different name of the captain. In this case, four Chinese had approached him seeking permission to secure certificates so they could board the *Orizaba* and travel to Eureka.[217]

They claimed the steamship would not let them aboard because they did not have a certificate. It being alleged in an affidavit provided by the complainant that a Milton Bernard, an employee of the law firm representing Wong Wai, had been present with the Chinamen and heard Kinyoun deny them a certificate. However, in Kinyoun's affidavit, he denied ever meeting with the Chinese and Bernard.[218]

The opinion concluded that the injunction had not been violated by him. The injunction had only dealt with the quarantine in San Francisco allowing anyone to travel within the state. The restraints recommended after the ruling only addressed travel outside California to other states, which had not been in issue or addressed in Morrow's opinion.[219]

Moreover, as to Captain Goodall, his testimony corroborated Kinyoun's statement. He acknowledged there had been no requirement of health certificates, but merely a suggestion by the defendant.[220] It had never been a requirement, as purported by these three or four Chinese. If anything, he had merely made a helpful recommendation to Goodall so the ship might avoid being placed under quarantine.

At the end of the court's opinion, it ruled he had not intentionally violated the injunction, resulting in the case's dismissal.[221] With this ruling, the first of several acts in the plague had come to an end. Unfortunately for Kinyoun, the play had just begun and the next two acts would be ever more grueling, as the stage expanded with others jamming the theater for a front row seat.

The First Ending

As the crisis in San Francisco approached a lull in July 1900, one certainty could not be disputed anymore. Bubonic plague had arrived in America, whether anyone wanted to believe it or not. As officially noted by the Service in its Annual Report for 1900[222]:

> This disease during the period from July 1, 1899, to June 30, 1900, has been more widespread in its prevalence than at any other period of the world's history.[223]

The reality of the situation was that the plague had entered the country and every effort to abate its advancement ended up being counterpunched by the state's political and commercial interests. What these groups had overlooked consisted of the sheer weight of evidence supporting the contagion's existence and the precarious state of the nation's health.

All any person had to do was examine the official world death count of the plague from June 30, 1899, to June 30, 1900. During this period 421,141 people had died, as reported by 29 countries, with India accounting for the largest number.[224] In reality, the number represented an understatement of the actual number of deaths due to the lack of mass communication and public health services in comparison to today.

Even with all the evidence, those controlling California's government seemed oblivious to the facts. As previously noted, many believed the disease only affected people from Asia. Furthermore, the commercial interests of San Francisco outweighed the plague's existence. Nothing could be truer than these simple facts.

The real fallacy of the crisis lay in the three lawsuits brought against Kinyoun and the Service. Although he prevailed in the third suit, everyone had missed an opportunity to rectify the situation and avert a potential health disaster. The answer lay in using the Haffkine vaccine and the Yersin serum, which the court ruled had little if any value.

If the court had been more cognizant of the plague, it could have changed the situation dramatically. Plague represented a far bigger impediment to civil liberties and the rights of the state, the most important liberty being life and the pursuit of happiness with the implication of good health.

Kinyoun must have been in shock at how Morrow and the citizens of San Francisco reacted to the disease. It had only been a few years since he had been hailed a hero in many of the country's major newspapers for his diphtheria vaccine and other achievements. The world he had known suddenly turned upside down on him with more unimaginable hardships beckoning on the horizon.

XIV

Venomous Pens

The Scorpion's Shadow

With the first indication of plague in San Francisco in June 1899, Kinyoun came under the scorpion's shadow. The press began scrutinizing his every move and would pounce upon him like a pack of wild boars at every opportunity, hoping to rip his out jugular. Probably nobody in the annals of American History has received such a vilification as he. But his resilience against the constant onslaught of criticism and mockery remained firm. No matter what the headline or the story's content, he showed up to work with the same determination to contain its spread.

As previously noted, the period from the late 1890s into the early 20th century had become known as the era of Yellow Journalism, a style of reporting primarily devoid of facts, or twisted to a point of invisibility, preaching sensationalism with the intent to deceive or create antagonism and disbelief of the facts for gain. Unfortunately, at this point in the country's history, it had become a known journalistic practice, especially in California.

Politics and the well-being of commercial interests went hand in hand with this type of reporting. All these groups appeared as a well-oiled machine manipulating the public in order to satisfy their lust for greed, power and monetary advantage. It operated much like a shark's demeanor during a feeding frenzy.

Kinyoun had been no stranger to the press. Several years before, while studying in Europe, he had perfected how to replicate the diphtheria serum and other cures. With these achievements, he received many accolades from newspapers across the country. His stature as an expert in the science of bacteriology had become well-known within the many circles of medicine. At the time, one would have never thought his reputation would become the scorn of almost every newspaper in California.

The press has always been a peculiar but important institution in the American democratic experiment. It can sweep one into the limelight and national prominence. But at the same time it can be brutal and destructive in the blink of an eye. During this era of journalism, Kinyoun quickly became the eye of the needle, as if a large microscope was looking down at him and dissecting his every move. In his case, right or wrong did not matter, because the red demonic eyes of yellow journalism combined with the selfish interests of politics and commercial greed had become his editors.

Words of Denial

As news of the plague became known, the initial reaction could be best described as unsure. It had been less than a year since its first appearance in San Francisco. Although its arrival proved inconclusive, Kinyoun did receive some backlash from the newspapers and others in the community. The criticisms soon faded, along with the serpentine head of the media. But lines in the sand started to unfold in fear of the Black Death's next advent and its consequences.

Numerous publications comprised the local and regional newspaper entourage. These included *The Bulletin*, *The Chronicle*, *The San Francisco Call* (or *The Call*), *The Examiner*, the *Fresno-Morning-Republican*, the *News-Advertiser*, the *Record-Union*, *The Bee*, *The Evening Bee* and *The Saturday Bee*. There were other newspapers reporting on the plague, but these constituted the core. *The Bulletin*, *The Chronicle* and *The Call* of San Francisco represented the main anti-plague advocates, whereas *The Bee*, *The Evening Bee* and *The Saturday Bee* in Sacramento, the state's capital, recognized the plague's existence.

With the first reported case of the plague in March 1900, the papers began disputing its existence. Consequently, it did not take long for the anti-plague factions to voice their denial. Most of the reporting attacked Mayor Phelan and the local health board, questioning their knowledge against other medical authorities refuting its presence. From the outset, the media criticized anyone remotely suggesting the contagion resided in Chinatown. Kinyoun would initially escape the newspapers' ire and that of the political, commercial interests. This would soon change, and he would become the main focal point of the deniers' wrath.

Another non-believer would be Henry T. Gage, who had been elected governor in January 1899. He would become Kinyoun's chief opponent and supposed protector of the commercial interests. Gage envisioned San Francisco as the major port for the Asian markets after the Spanish-American War. In recent years, the city had been slipping in population to Seattle and Los Angeles, thereby making the presence of any highly infectious disease detrimental to his aspirations for the city as the largest Pacific port and city. He most probably well knew its presence could cause serious harm to the city's economy.

In time, the plague became an everyday headline. On May 30, one caption read, "The Farcical Side of It,"[1] printing, "the scare arranged by the Bubonic Board of Health is a fake and a fraud."[2] It called "Quarantine ... a silly farce."[3] On the same day, *The Call* ran a banner headline claiming:

> INVESTIGATING EXPERTS INSPECT CHINATOWN AND FAIL TO FIND A SINGLE CASE OF ANY ILLNESS[4]

On June 14, two days prior to Judge Morrow's ruling on the injunction brought by Wong Wai, *The Bulletin* ran an editorial titled "No Plague in San Francisco."[5] *The Chronicle* ran a similar story, theirs titled "Governor Officially Brands Bubonic Plague Scare a Fake."[6] These sensational commentaries were likely political salvos fired ahead of the judge's ruling. Although his decision was unknown, these publications wanted their opinions known, along with the governor's. The evolving viciousness of the attacks centered on telling the world it had been a hoax. The purpose behind the rhetoric was likely to calm the outside commercial interests so they would not stop trading with San Francisco.

The Chronicle's article reported that Governor Gage had sent a letter to Secretary of State John Hay decrying the whole matter as bogus.[7] Upfront, it identified and chastised those responsible for the "Fake,"[8] writing:

> It places the blame where it belongs—upon the Bubonic Health Board and upon the Federal Quarantine Officer, Dr. J.J. Kinyoun—and sets forth succinctly under fifteen heads the facts and the reasons for all the Governor's conclusions.[9]

Gage's letter "bore the names of several prominent San Francisco medical and business men"[10] supporting his anti-plague claims. It also contained the names of other well-known individuals.[11] They were:

Medical:
L. C. Lane, president Cooper Medical College
C. N. Ellinwood M. D., professor Cooper Medical College
Winslow Anderson M. D., M.R.C.P. London, M.R.C.S., England
Professor College of Physicians and Surgeons of San Francisco
Edwin S, Brayfogie, M. D.

Business:
Levi Strauss, president Levi Strauss & Co.
A.B. Spreckels
James H. Budd, former governor of California
William Alvord, president Bank of California
Robert J. Tobin, secretary Hibernia Savings and Loan Society
Adam Grant of Murphy Grant & Co.
Lewis Gerstle, president Alaska Commercial Company
Isaias W. Heitman, president Nevada National Bank
Henry F. Fortman, president Alaska Packer's Association[12]

The governor had secured some of the most important and influential men not only in San Francisco, but the state. They represented the titans of San Francisco society, but what was their true purpose in supporting Gage and others as to the non-existence of plague? The obvious answer would be the impairment to the city's future growth if the disease existed and put part of the community under quarantine, thereby cutting off trade.

In another part of the article, it attempted to portray itself as a crusader for the less fortunate. It reported that the "Chinese … have been reduced to the verge of starvation by the unwarranted action of the Health Board."[13] The Chinese undoubtedly felt suppressed, but were unlikely on the edge of starving to death. In fact, they had barricaded themselves in their houses, so inspections could not be conducted as to their health and living conditions. It had become well known that they possessed countless secret passages in and out of Chinatown granting them unlimited access to food.

This column would be just the beginning of many more articles aimed at the local health board and the doctor. One unidentified account printed a more unique and even humorous description of him: "Kinyoun seems to be on the toboggan. And it appears to be a case of 'slide Kinyoun slide.'"[14] But the worst had yet to be published against him, and in short order the press would have a field day trying to discredit him professionally and personally.

On June 15, he issued a directive to all the railroads, steamships and other carriers prohibiting the sale of tickets to all citizens wanting to leave California, regardless of race or ethnicity, without a health certificate.[15] The following day, *The Bulletin* headlined its story with "Kinyoun Quarantines State."[16] Although not totally true, his order did prevent people from going to another state, absent a certificate. Judge Morrow had previously ruled on May 28 that quarantining Chinatown amounted to an intrastate action that only California could impose and not the federal government or its agents. It could only act as to interstate matters. In this case, Kinyoun, Wyman and the Service had acted on this authority causing the press to become outranged over this new directive.

On June 16, the court cited Kinyoun for violating its earlier injunction.[17] Immediately, the city's newspapers became incensed and started printing more derogatory articles about him, as evidenced by *The Chronicle*'s headline on June 20:

His Recall Is Demanded
Angry Citizens Say That Kinyoun Must Leave
President Asked to Remove the Official[18]

The onslaught would continue for over two weeks, with daily tirades by most publications. *The Bulletin* wrote an editorial asking, "Will the Bubonic Board Resign?"[19] Kinyoun, along with Mayor Phelan, had been considered ex officio members of the group.

On the heels of this commentary, *The Chronicle* printed an editorial titled "The Abatement of a Nuisance,"[20] wherein it took direct aim at him. Its lead sentence served as the trier of fact: "it may be unnecessary to take further evidence.... Dr. Kinyoun is an unfit person to be intrusted [sic] with official duty here ... or elsewhere."[21] The editorial attacked—though not by name—*The Bee* and *The Evening Bee*,[22] referring to them as:

> Some fool papers of the interior whose editors do not know enough to understand that the press of this city have been fighting for the bread and butter of the entire State have intimate that the attacks on Dr. Kinyoun have been "political." That is the reply of all official rascals when caught in evil doing.[23]

It then turned its wrath upon the him:

> We know nothing whatever about the "politics" of this Dr. Kinyoun, if he has any, and never heard any one allude to the matter. But whatever his politics he is an unfaithful, foolish and vindictive man who cannot be got rid of too quickly.[24]

In the mix of the anti-Kinyoun propaganda, the daily Chinese newspaper *Chung Sai Yat Po* published an article on June 22 about his upcoming trial. The story's content could be readily understood by the cartoon preceding the story, centered squarely at the top of the page. The caricature was very political, if not quite

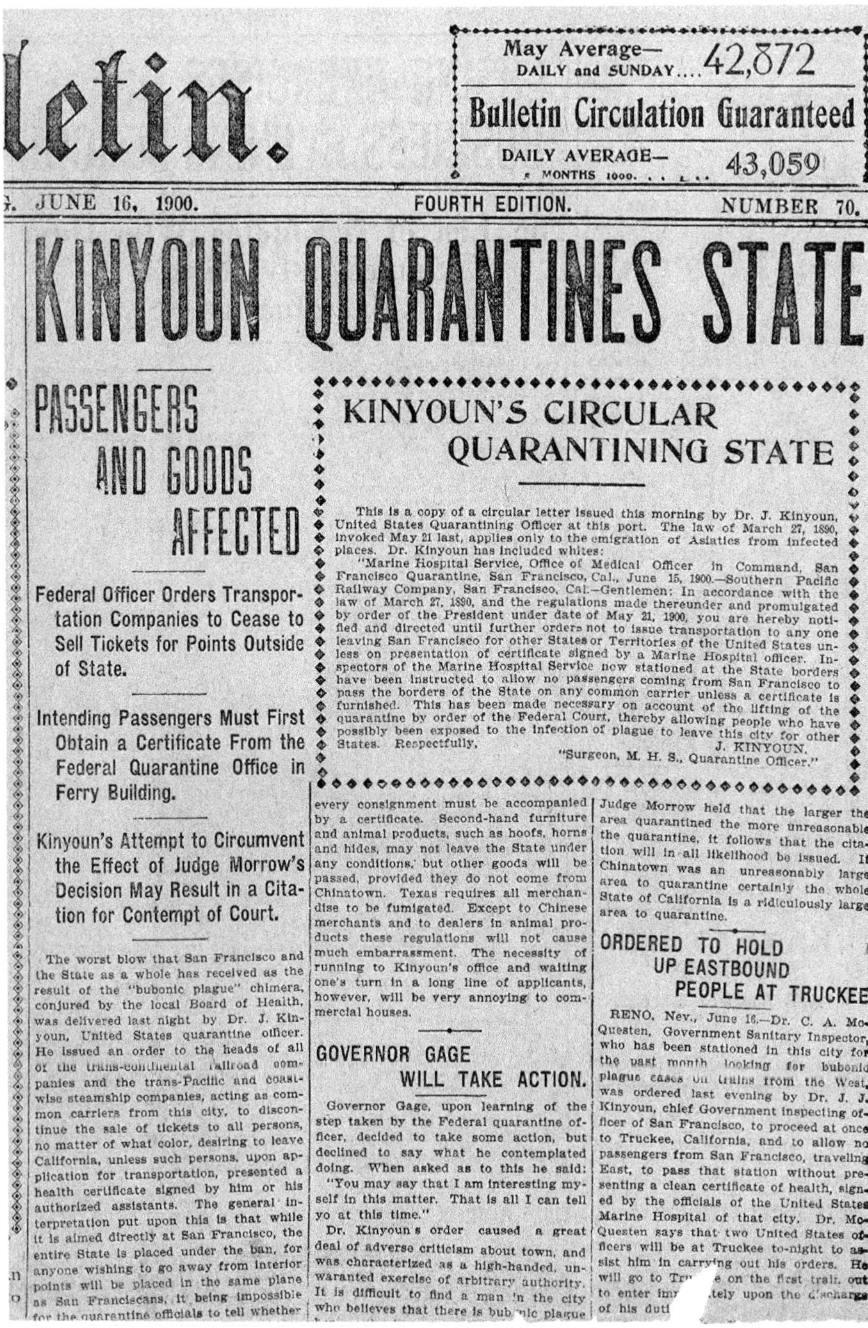

letin.

May Average—
DAILY and SUNDAY....42,872

Bulletin Circulation Guaranteed

DAILY AVERAGE—
MONTHS 1000. 43,059

JUNE 16, 1900. FOURTH EDITION. NUMBER 70.

KINYOUN QUARANTINES STATE

PASSENGERS AND GOODS AFFECTED

Federal Officer Orders Transportation Companies to Cease to Sell Tickets for Points Outside of State.

Intending Passengers Must First Obtain a Certificate From the Federal Quarantine Office in Ferry Building.

Kinyoun's Attempt to Circumvent the Effect of Judge Morrow's Decision May Result in a Citation for Contempt of Court.

The worst blow that San Francisco and the State as a whole has received as the result of the "bubonic plague" chimera, conjured by the local Board of Health, was delivered last night by Dr. J. Kinyoun, United States quarantine officer. He issued an order to the heads of all of the trans-continental railroad companies and the trans-Pacific and coastwise steamship companies, acting as common carriers from this city, to discontinue the sale of tickets to all persons, no matter of what color, desiring to leave California, unless such persons, upon application for transportation, presented a health certificate signed by him or his authorized assistants. The general interpretation put upon this is that while it is aimed directly at San Francisco, the entire State is placed under the ban, for anyone wishing to go away from interior points will be placed in the same plane as San Franciscans, it being impossible for the quarantine officials to tell whether

KINYOUN'S CIRCULAR QUARANTINING STATE

This is a copy of a circular letter issued this morning by Dr. J. Kinyoun, United States Quarantining Officer at this port. The law of March 27, 1890, invoked May 21 last, applies only to the emigration of Asiatics from infected places. Dr. Kinyoun has included whites:

"Marine Hospital Service, Office of Medical Officer in Command, San Francisco Quarantine, San Francisco, Cal., June 15, 1900.—Southern Pacific Railway Company, San Francisco, Cal.—Gentlemen: In accordance with the law of March 27, 1890, and the regulations made thereunder and promulgated by order of the President under date of May 21, 1900, you are hereby notified and directed until further orders not to issue transportation to any one leaving San Francisco for other States or Territories of the United States unless on presentation of certificate signed by a Marine Hospital officer. Inspectors of the Marine Hospital Service now stationed at the State borders have been instructed to allow no passengers coming from San Francisco to pass the borders of the State on any common carrier unless a certificate is furnished. This has been made necessary on account of the lifting of the quarantine by order of the Federal Court, thereby allowing people who have possibly been exposed to the infection of plague to leave this city for other States. Respectfully,

J. KINYOUN.

"Surgeon, M. H. S., Quarantine Officer."

every consignment must be accompanied by a certificate. Second-hand furniture and animal products, such as hoofs, horns and hides, may not leave the State under any conditions, but other goods will be passed, provided they do not come from Chinatown. Texas requires all merchandise to be fumigated. Except to Chinese merchants and to dealers in animal products these regulations will not cause much embarrassment. The necessity of running to Kinyoun's office and waiting one's turn in a long line of applicants, however, will be very annoying to commercial houses.

GOVERNOR GAGE WILL TAKE ACTION.

Governor Gage, upon learning of the step taken by the Federal quarantine officer, decided to take some action, but declined to say what he contemplated doing. When asked as to this he said:

"You may say that I am interesting myself in this matter. That is all I can tell yo at this time."

Dr. Kinyoun's order caused a great deal of adverse criticism about town, and was characterized as a high-handed, unwaranted exercise of arbitrary authority. It is difficult to find a man in the city who believes that there is bub nic plague

Judge Morrow held that the larger the area quarantined the more unreasonable the quarantine, it follows that the citation will in all likelihood be issued. If Chinatown was an unreasonably large area to quarantine certainly the whole State of California is a ridiculously large area to quarantine.

ORDERED TO HOLD UP EASTBOUND PEOPLE AT TRUCKEE

RENO, Nev., June 16.—Dr. C. A. McQuesten, Government Sanitary Inspector, who has been stationed in this city for the past month looking for bubonic plague cases on trains from the West, was ordered last evening by Dr. J. J. Kinyoun, chief Government inspecting officer of San Francisco, to proceed at once to Truckee, California, and to allow no passengers from San Francisco, traveling East, to pass that station without presenting a clean certificate of health, signed by the officials of the United States Marine Hospital of that city. Dr. McQuesten says that two United States officers will be at Truckee to-night to assist him in carrying out his orders. He will go to Tr[illegible]e on the first train out to enter im[illegible]tely upon the discharge of his duti[illegible]

KINYOUN QUARANTINES STATE, *The Bulletin*, June 16, 1900.

humorous. It showed Judge Morrow in the center standing over the bench pointing at Kinyoun tied to a chair tipped backwards with a noose around his neck.[25] Standing behind him, a Chinese man injected the back of his head with a hypodermic needle labeled "Common Sense Serum."[26] Obviously, it represented a vengeful mockery of the doctor's use of the Haffkine vaccine to inoculate people against the disease.

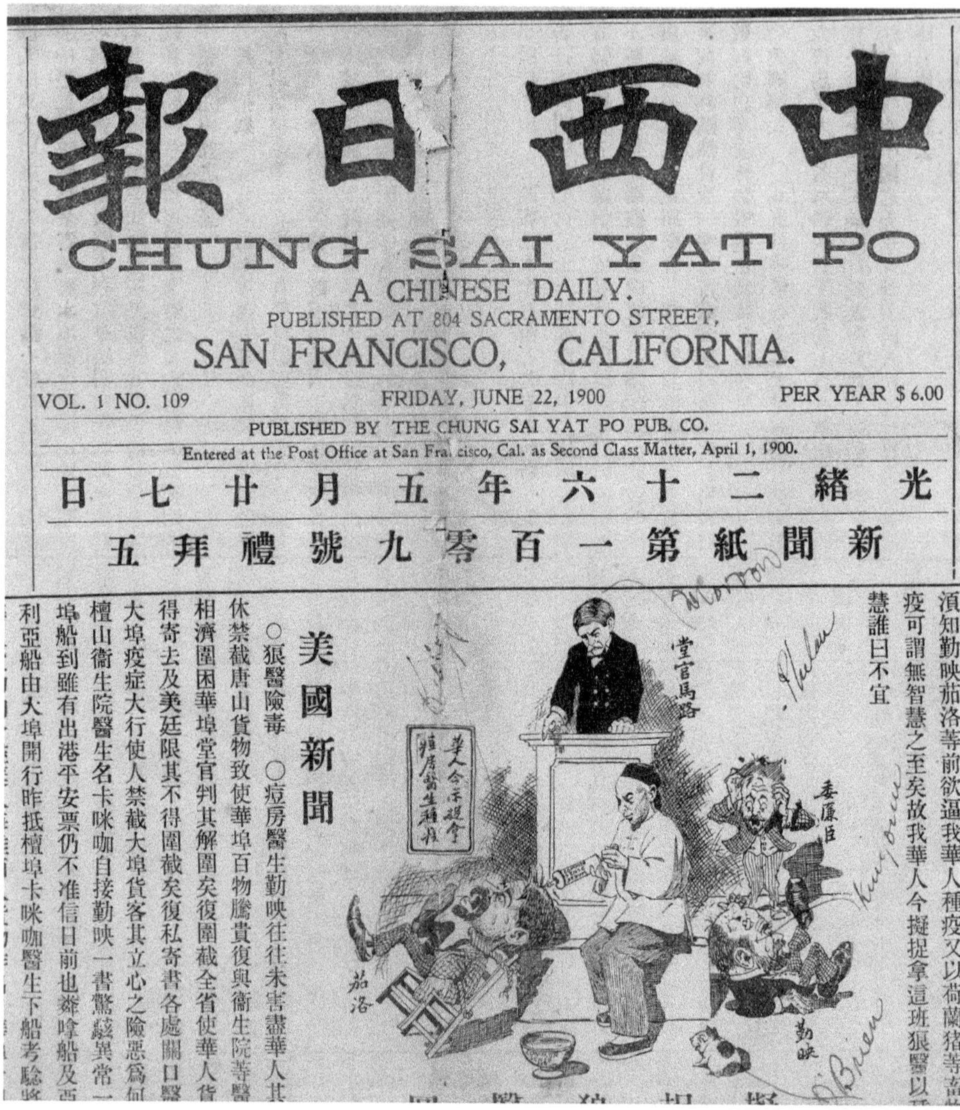

中西日報

CHUNG SAI YAT PO

A CHINESE DAILY.

PUBLISHED AT 804 SACRAMENTO STREET,

SAN FRANCISCO, CALIFORNIA.

VOL. 1 NO. 109 FRIDAY, JUNE 22, 1900 PER YEAR $ 6.00

PUBLISHED BY THE CHUNG SAI YAT PO PUB. CO.

Entered at the Post Office at San Francisco, Cal. as Second Class Matter, April 1, 1900.

光緒二十六年五月廿七日

新聞紙第一百零九號禮拜五

須知勤映茄洛等前欲逼我華人種疫又以荷蘭猪等畜
疫可謂無智慧之至矣故我華人今擬捉拿這班狠醫以
慧誰曰不宜

美國新聞

○狠醫險毒 ○痘房醫生勤映往往未害盡華人其
休禁截唐山貨物致使華埠百物騰貴復與衛生院等醫
相濟圍困華埠堂官判其解圍矣復圍截全省使華人貨
得寄去及美廷限其不得圍截矣復私寄書各處關口醫
大埠疫症大行使人禁截大埠貨客其立心之險惡爲何
檀山衛生院醫生名卡咪咖自接勤映一書驚蔌異常一
埠船到雖有出港平安票仍不准信日前也雅嗙船及西
利亞船由大埠開行昨抵檀埠卡咪咖醫生下船考驗

Political satire: Kinyoun et al., *Chung Sai Yat Po*, June 22, 1900.

On the other side of the judge's bench the picture portrayed Mayor Phelan with his hands on his head and a wide-eyed expression of alarm. Underneath him appeared another drawing of Kinyoun lying on his back with cuts and bandages on his head. Beneath him sat a guinea pig bearing a likeness of Dr. O'Brien. The guinea pig represented the animals used for testing and verifying plague. The article showed the extent of the press's attack on the doctor and others by making them appear as bungling, beaten-up buffoons. If anything, the cartoon showed how low and personal this newspaper had become in trying to discredit these men.[27]

Another article about him appeared on June 22. *The Call* published it under the headline "The Lesson of Kinyounism."[28] The story read like a primer on how the plague originated and could be prevented in the future, thereby avoiding the likes of Kinyoun, or as it was called, "Kinyounism."[29]

The story stated that with the quarantines removed, the doctor cited for contempt and the local board of health now hapless, these "irritations"[30] to the city were gone. *The Call* partly excused the activities of both parties but took great exception to the condition of Chinatown. It blamed the health board for ignoring its duties and creating the present mess. The paper stated that the quarter had long been known for its "indisputable foulness."[31] It proceeded to provide a lengthy description:

> It is known that the sanitary regulations enforced in other parts of the city are neglected in the Chinese quarter, that the buildings there are ill ventilated, ill provided with plumbing and sewer connections ... and are unhealthy, foul-smelling and filthy. It is known ... they are overcrowded ... undermined with dismal tunnels ... reeking with dirt and inhabited by people who swarm like rats in their burrows and have no regard for sanitation or cleanliness.[32]

The Call took aim at the health board and the wealthy landlords owning the tenements for not complying with the sanitation regulations and fixing up their properties so they could be habitable. The column stated that some of the landlords stood as the richest men in the city and should be held accountable for the condition of their properties.[33] It noted:

> It is a monstrous abuse of power to compel even the poorest property-owners in other localities to obey the health laws while these rich landlords are permitted to ignore them, defy them and mock at them.[34]

Two ironies can be found in *The Call*'s story. The first is its admission as to the unsanitary conditions of Chinatown and the haphazard enforcement of the health codes. By making these accusations, the paper in essence admitted the presence of plague based on the deplorable conditions in the quarter, which created a ripe environment for the disease. Nothing could be truer with plague. Garbage, trash and filth led to pests, rodents, or rats, which carry fleas bearing bubonic plague. The doctor knew this, as did the local health board, explaining the reason for the house inspections.

The second one constituted the lack of due process and equal protection in code enforcement, especially as to the wealthy landlords. Administration of the health regulations had been limited, if not non-existent, in Chinatown and other poorer sections of the city. The lack of supervision suggested favoritism towards the wealthy owners, as opposed to others of lesser financial and political means. This begged the issue of overt discrimination between the wealthy and the poor.

As ruled in the injunction, the violation of equal protection had been the primary legal complaint leading to Morrow's decision to remove the quarantine. The same complaint could be argued concerning the enforcement of the city's housing regulations, although involving a different set of circumstances. If the board and the economically endowed landlords had addressed these deplorable conditions earlier, then the plague might have been abated or have spread to a much lesser extent. These articles pointed out a severe lack of evenhandedness in administering the codes and a great deal of apparent favoritism to the elite, it being these individuals who had contested reports of the disease because of their other commercial interests and political dealings.

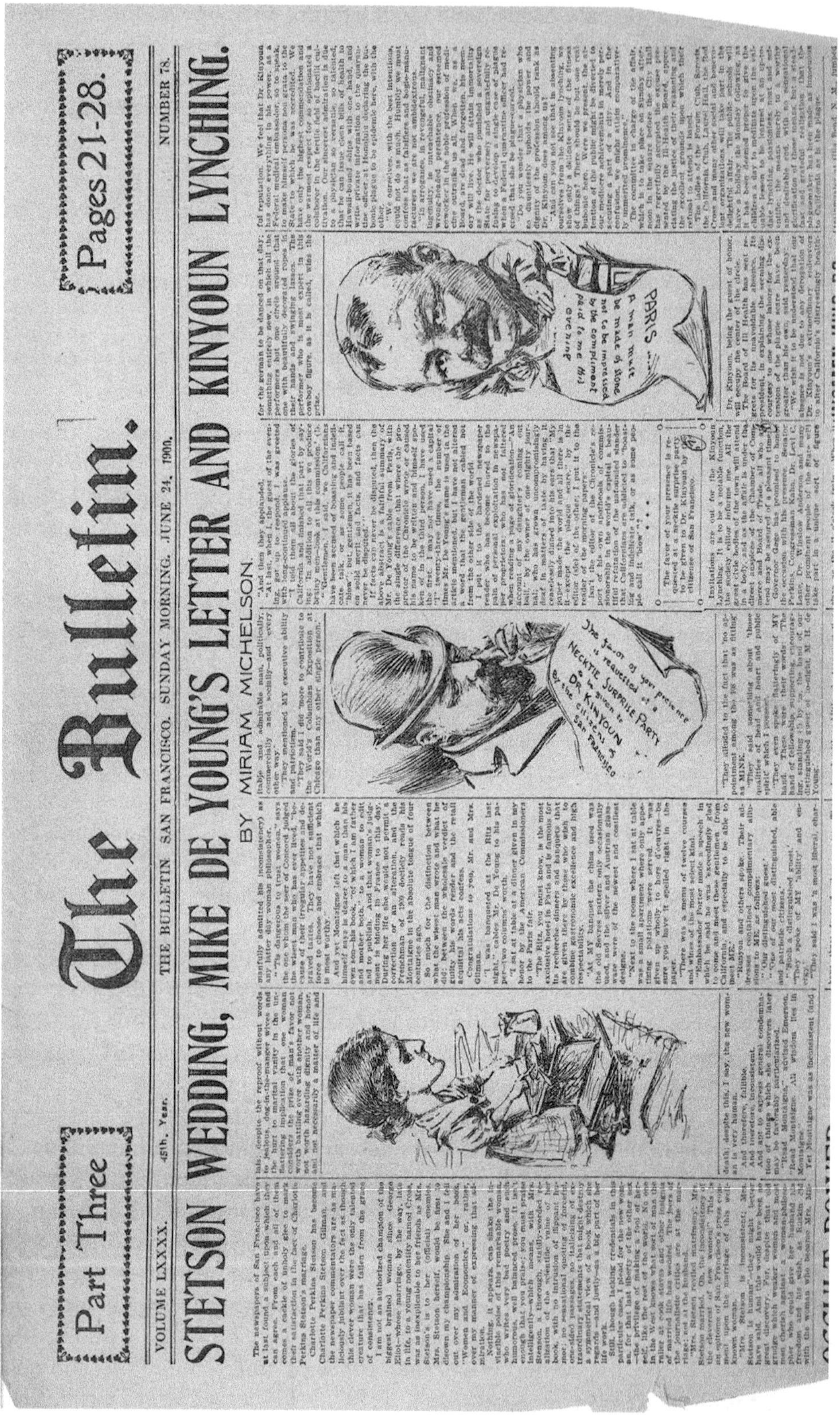

Part Three

The Bulletin.

Pages 21-28.

VOLUME LXXXX. 45th. Year. THE BULLETIN SAN FRANCISCO. SUNDAY MORNING. JUNE 24, 1900. NUMBER 78.

STETSON WEDDING, MIKE DE YOUNG'S LETTER AND KINYOUN LYNCHING.

BY MIRIAM MICHELSON.

Probably the most vindictive headline occurred on June 24, by *The Bulletin*. It read:

STETSON WEDDING, MIKE DEYOUNG'S LETTER AND KINYOUN LYNCHING.[35]

In the middle of the upper half of the page is a picture of him with his left finger touching his nose, as if mimicking Santa Claus, showing him reading an invitation with the following message:

> The favor of your presence is requested at a necktie surprise party to be given to Dr. Kinyoun by the citizens of San Francisco.[36]

The first paragraph trumpeted:

> Invitations are out for the Kinyoun Lynching. It is to be a notable function, the society editor informs me. All the great civic bodies of the town will attend in a body, and ... may be assured of a pleasant time.[37]

The article read as the social event of the year with attendees including Governor Gage, the Chamber of Commerce, the Red Cross, the Forum Club ladies, the California Club, the Board of Trade and other distinguished dignitaries. The story went to great lengths to ridicule and mock him, leaving little doubt to anyone that he had become the city's number one adversary.[38]

On June 25, *The Bulletin* ran another front-page story, titled

KINYOUN ENEMY OF THIS CITY, ON TRIAL FOR CONTEMPT OF UNITED STATES CIRCUIT COURT[39]

As part of the article, it printed a diminutive caricature of him standing somewhat slumped, looking rather short in stature and large in frame with an extended belly.[40] Another headline, published by *The Evening Post* on June 26, read

KINYOUN AND HIS WIRINGS
Evidence of Contumacy Are Read in Court[41]

And on July 3, *The Chronicle* published an article titled

KINYOUN ON THE GRILL[42]

And yet another headline read "Quarantine Kinyoun,"[43] with subheads "The Arrogant Doctor a Sorry Sight in Court"[44] and "Fresh Evidence of the Evil He Tried to Do the Community."[45] He had become the center of the press's bull's-eye and their ongoing malicious attacks. But he remained steadfast to the truth at great personal risk to his reputation and life.

He appeared in Judge Morrow's court on July 2 to plead his case. Evidence was presented by him and Captain Goodall. In his testimony, he explained that his order had not been issued barring travel within the state, but only between the states, contrary to the statements of other witnesses. Before the hearing, he had submitted letters and telegrams to Wyman and others in Washington as a transcript of his actions.[46] While on the witness stand he underwent, the paper reported, "an unmerciful

***Opposite:* STETSON WEDDING, MIKE DE YOUNG'S LETTER AND KINYOUN LYNCHING, *The Bulletin*, June 24, 1900.**

grilling"[47] from the opposing counsel. During the examination

> Kinyoun became confused and finally fired up and wanted to argue matters. He could not give straight answers to the pointed questions put to him and resorted to his usual policy of evasion to get over obstacles thrown in his way. While he admitted that he had stopped extra [sic] State traffic, he denied that he had quarantined the state; he denied also that he had stopped any one from leaving San Francisco.[48]

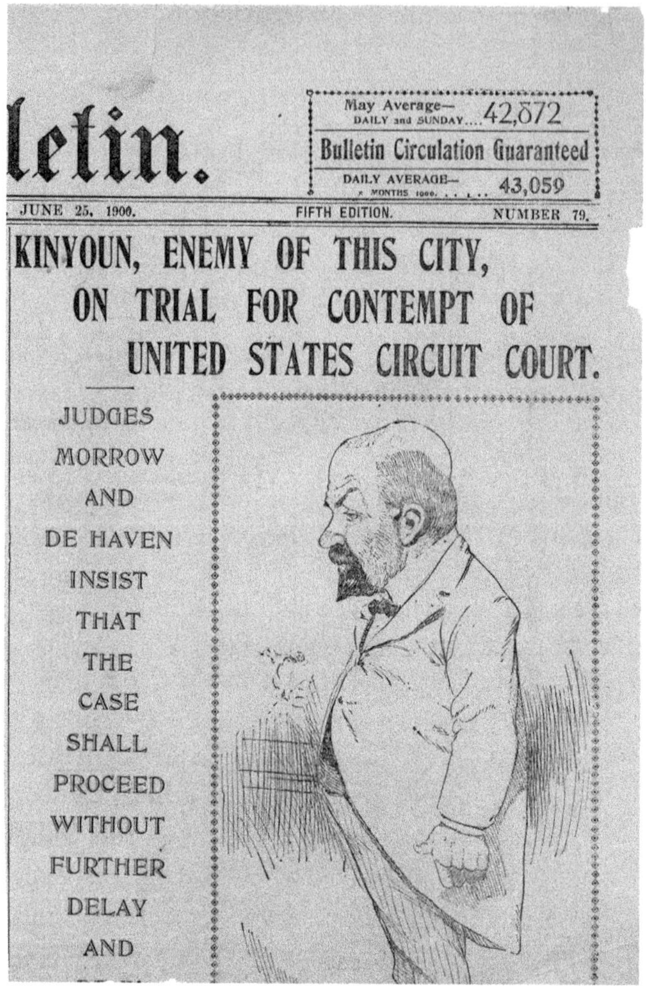

letin.

May Average— DAILY and SUNDAY.... 42,872

Bulletin Circulation Guaranteed

DAILY AVERAGE— ... 43,059

JUNE 25, 1900. FIFTH EDITION. NUMBER 79.

KINYOUN, ENEMY OF THIS CITY, ON TRIAL FOR CONTEMPT OF UNITED STATES CIRCUIT COURT.

JUDGES MORROW AND DE HAVEN INSIST THAT THE CASE SHALL PROCEED WITHOUT FURTHER DELAY AND

KINYOUN, ENEMY OF THIS CITY, ON TRIAL FOR CONTEMPT OF UNITED STATES CIRCUIT COURT, *The Bulletin*, June 25, 1900.

Any person on a witness stand would tend to become anxious, let alone in a trial of national significance. The object of the column had been to portray of him as weak, incompetent and evasive. However, one thing did come out of his testimony and from other witnesses not reported by this newspaper. He had not intended to quarantine the state, or interfere with intrastate travel. To his credit, on July 3 Morrow ruled in his favor and stated that he had not violated the injunction and therefore dismissed the charge.[49]

Even with this decision, the press would not admit the truth and would find other ways to discredit him. On July 4, *The Chronicle* wrote "Kinyoun Discharged."[50] Beneath the heading was the subheading "Petty Evasion and Hyprocrisy [sic] Save the Misfit from Contempt."[51] Although acknowledging his acquittal, the paper still expressed its discontent:

> The subterfuge and the rank and palpable evasion resorted to by Kinyoun during his defense were of avail, and the tremendous harm done to this State will go unpunished, save before the bar of public opinion. Before that tribunal Kinyoun has still to answer and evidence is not lacking that he will have to pay the penalty.[52]

The Chronicle and other newspapers were determined to deny and tarnish the facts and blame him for all the harm inflicted upon California. They would not believe anything he said about the plague. The crisis had become a tug-of-war between the federal government and the state, as evidenced by the article. The papers would on occasion capitalize the word "State," apparently as an expression of its sovereignty or their "states' rights," a sentiment strongly held by many of its politicians. Although California had been on the Union side in the Civil War, it experienced a large degree of independence from Washington, D.C., because of the distance from the country's seat of government, especially when it took a fair amount of time to travel between the coasts. This factor may have created a certain hands-off approach to interference by the federal government.

Another important consideration can be seen in the constant referral to the merchants and other business interests of the state, thereby showing the underlying reason for the ongoing denials. If in fact the presence of plague became true, the city and the state could lose a tremendous amount of businesses, jobs and revenue. Newspapers survived on advertising, and without large commercial companies to buy ads, the papers would struggle financially.

After Kinyoun's reprieve, the papers returned to their ongoing premise of denial. On July 31, *The Bulletin* published an extensive article titled "Dr. Silas Mouser, Whom State Employed, and Surgeon-General Sternberg Say Dread Disease Was Never Here."[53] Dr. Mouser, viewed as a highly regarded expert on bacteriology, had been hired by the State Health Board to make an evaluation as to the disease's presence. On completion of his analysis, he would not disclose his findings, stating that since the state board had engaged him, he was therefore not at liberty to release its contents. The article initially seethed with frustration about the release. Eventually, its tone took on a different demeanor, writing how others of stature discounted the plague's existence.[54]

Mouser's actions seemed erratic plus patronizing to the anti-plague factions. On the one hand, he would not release his findings, but on the other, he talked somewhat freely about his findings, hinting at its absence. He took the liberty to send a copy to Surgeon-General Sternberg,[55] who had become known as the "Father of American Bacteriology."[56] Sternberg had been visiting San Francisco as part of an army inspection. In an interview, he commented how important the city had become to the military, especially faced with developments in China and other places in the Far East.[57] For the record, Kinyoun and Sternberg knew each other.[58]

During the surgeon-general's visit, he met with Mouser and agreed with his findings that the plague did not exist.[59] The article took great advantage of their meeting and Sternberg's conclusion, reporting:

> He said so, adding his high authority to the opinion of the Health Board's expert.[60]

In reviewing this rather intricate piece of journalism, several hidden messages can be seen in the fine print. First, it jumped to the supposition that Mouser had determined the absence of plague by his loose comments, even though his report had not been released showing how he came to this conclusion. Second, it went through a trilogy of those in the know who had arrived at the same opinion, but did not supply any proof. Worst of all, it used Sternberg as the country's highest expert on all things bacteriologically, probably because of his rank and medical reputation.

More importantly, the article disqualified the surgeon-general in the same breath it taunted his credentials. This became evident when he referred to San Francisco as being militarily key to the nation's recent Asian acquisitions and future aspirations. And what parties stood the most to gain from the country's new territorial expansionism? The commercial and political interests of San Francisco as the country's leading western port.

Although not making direct reference to Kinyoun, *The Call* and *The Bulletin* on July 31, and *The Chronicle* on August 2, reported joint dismay with the lack of transparency by the state board of Health and the release of Mouser's report. He had been considered an expert on bacteriology, but by his flaunting the absence of plague, without providing proof, these newspapers began to question it.[61] *The Call* titled its article "Expert Says There Was No Plague Here,"[62] and *The Chronicle*'s headline read, "Suppressing the Truth."[63]

The papers reasoned that since he had been paid with public funds, his report belonged to the people and should be released forthwith.[64] As a result, *The Bee*, a pro-plague newspaper, filed a writ of mandamus against the board's suppression of the report. Several weeks later, Judge Hart rendered his opinion, stating that the board could not withhold Mouser's findings.[65]

This turn of events represented a strange twist to an already complicated situation and became even stranger at a time when the anti-plague and pro-plague newspapers appeared to be on the same side. In the end, Mouser's report stated that he had tested three guinea pigs with plague bacilli and all survived the experiment. Afterwards, he even gave his grandson one of the animals as a pet. His daughter assisted him with the experiment and later laughed at the question of whether the gift to her son could be considered dangerous.[66]

Clearly, the anti-plague papers wanted the findings made public to support their position. *The Bee*, on the other hand, wanted to see the report, too. However, the original story about Mouser stated the bacilli used in his examination had also been reviewed by other physicians, who had thought the victims had showed signs of the disease. Therefore, one had the same victims, but two different thoughts. The strangest question was why the state board did not want to release the report, when many of its members sided with Governor Gage and his anti-plague position.

Regardless of who wanted what and for what reasons, the plain truth of the matter became apparent. One newspaper sought the truth regardless of the consequences, whereas the others sought to falsify the truth in fear of the consequences with no concern for the public.

In early August, the last of the first round of anti–Kinyoun newspaper salvos asked, "Has Kinyoun Gone Mad?"[67] The article sensationalized his handling of the steamship *Coptic*'s passengers and how it had gone through an inspection apparently on Angel Island much to the dismay of all on board and now the community.[68] But the subheading revealed another reason for the paper's outrage. It read, "Action of Quarantine Officer Seems to Be Planned to Drive Traffic from This Port."[69]

The doctor had detained the ship for an inspection, as part of the regular quarantine procedures for incoming ships from the Far East. In this instance, the inconvenience of the process reached the newspapers. The article claimed the passengers had been outraged by the examination procedures; they had to disrobe as part of the process.[70] To the contrary, the *Town Talk* reported that other sources claimed these accounts to be "not well founded,"[71] with the only complaining parties being two missionaries who had not wanted to be inspected because of scars on their bodies.[72]

However, the overriding opinion of the press claimed his actions constituted "needless brutality and outrageous indelicacy."[73] As a result:

> ... Kinyoun's methods were having the effect, designedly or unintentionally as the case may be, of driving business away from the port of San Francisco.[74]

As before, the newspapers primary motive in discrediting him centered purely on the city's commercial interests and the consequences of his ongoing actions. Quarantine inspections now, and even today, can be intrusive. Nonetheless, he had to be thorough, and he knew all diseases could be very difficult to uncover. Still, the ships from Asia had become the primary carrier of the plague, just as the ships from Europe had been the primary carriers of cholera, diphtheria and other maladies years before.

The dominant reason for all the newspapers' animosity derived to some extent from competition from Seattle and Los Angeles. San Francisco had started seeing a slower growth in population based on the last federal census. With these other cities experiencing a population increase, it could mean a rise in their commercial growth. With the plague claiming lives, fortunes could change dramatically. Unfortunately, money and its attendant prosperity had now blinded the city to the facts, and the powers within were not going down without a fight.

A Solitary Friend

Even with all of the hatred and personal attacks on Kinyoun, at least one California newspaper stood by his side: *The Bee*, located in the state's capital. It had a different perspective on the plague. It weighed the evidence and concluded it did exit in Chinatown and therefore San Francisco. Throughout his remaining tenure in the port, *The Bee* defended his actions. One of its first articles supporting the plague's presence appeared on June 19, after he had been cited for contempt. In its evening edition, known as *The Evening Bee*, it ran a story titled "The Facts Are Not with the Governor."[75] The response had been written because of an attack it had received from another paper.[76]

The column's premise centered on Gage's letter to Washington on June 14, calling the plague scare a "Fake."[77] As will be recalled, the governor had listed various community leaders, including four doctors, who had aligned with his anti-plague stance.[78] In an article dated June 19, *The Bee* took exception to their authority, pointing out that none of them had examined the physical evidence and, accordingly, would be worth in a court of law about as much as "a farmer or a sheepherder."[79]

More importantly and of some humor, it reported that the only authority Gage had brought to San Francisco as an expert was Dr. George F. Shardy, a highly respected and distinguished physician from New York. Gage had summoned the doctor betting he would conclude the absence of plague. However, after conducting his examination, Shardy told the *San Francisco Call* and the *New York Herald* that the plague was present.[80] In summation, *The Bee* wrote:

> Facts are stubborn things, friend Record, and the facts are against Governor Gage.[81]

In mid–June, *The Bee* again expressed its support for Kinyoun in the article "Present Status of the Plague."[82] The article read:

> By political bulldozing at a time when political allegiance is of the highest importance to the Administration the Washington authorities have been induced to tie the hands of Dr. J.J. Kinyoun, the Federal Quarantine Officer who has been trying to the utmost of his ability and against the greatest possible odds to save the country from the dangers of bubonic plague[83]

In the following paragraph, the newspaper singled out the true culprit behind the denials, writing:

> The element which places present commercial interest above considerations of public health and is too deaf to hear beyond the jingle of the coin in its pocket has raised a hue and cry about the ears of Dr. Kinyoun at a time when the State should lend him every co-operation and extend expressions of gratitude for the courage and firmness he has shown.[84]

The Bee chastised the other San Francisco newspapers. It singled out *The Chronicle*, stating that it "and the other papers … must take the people of California for fools."[85] The article expressed consternation as to why such normally levelheaded newspapers would "act so foolishly."[86] In its conclusion, *The Bee* again made reference to Shardy being brought west to refute the plague after his examination concluded otherwise.[87]

Two days later, *The Bee* again took the other papers to task, when it wrote, "Every newspaperman in the California metropolis knows there has been (plague)."[88] It stated this position would cause "incalculable injury to the State."[89] And, "Why do they not tell the truth?"[90] In apparent frustration over the lingering state of affairs, it concluded the article noting:

> Falsification can do no good. On the contrary, the idiotic denial of a fact causes outside people to believe that something frightful is being concealed.[91]

On July 3, *The Bee* published a response to Judge Morrow's ruling. The headline read, "Vindication of Dr. Kinyoun."[92] Once again, it reported he had not violated the court's ruling restricting intrastate travel.[93]

One of the ongoing problems with the crisis centered on the victims, as to whether they died from the disease or from some other illness. Many had been secreted from the public, thereby covering up not only the actual number of afflicted, but those who had died. *The Bee* ran two articles about one case that demonstrated how the facts had been manipulated by others.

On July 3 the headline read, "Fresh Case of the Plague in San Francisco."[94] The victim's name was Lee Wing Tong, living at 767 Clay Street and described as a laborer. On July 4, he had been transferred to the City & County Hospital at the recommendation of Dr. Ernest Pillsbury. Coincidentally, he had been the expert witness for the

Chinese Six Companies in the *Wong Wai vs. Williamson, ET AL.* case. Pillsbury diagnosed Tong with typhoid. An examination followed upon his admittance revealing a tender, large bubo in the left groin, an enlarged stomach, and a 104-degree temperature. On July 6, he passed away. Dr. Orphlus from the Cooper Medical College performed a comprehensive autopsy, which included his organs. The impressive aspect about this medical procedure was the people in attendance.[95] They consisted of:

> ... Dr. Douglass Montgomery, bacteriologist of the University of California Medical College; Dr. J.J. Kinyoun, the Federal Quarantine Officer; Dr. Ryfkogel, bacteriologist of the State Board of Health; Dr. W.H. Kellogg, bacteriologist of San Francisco Board of Health; Dr. Krone, of Oakland; Dr. Jellinck; Dr. Shields, and Drs. D.A. Hodghead and H. D'Arcy Power, representing the Chinese Six Companies who came in later.[96]

Ironically, Pillsbury, the attending and admitting physician for Tong, had become sick and could not attend the procedure. *The Bee* reported that doctors representing the Chinese Six Companies did not offer an opinion on the case, although other doctors acknowledged San Francisco had the plague.[97]

The autopsy results showed the contagion's presence beyond a reasonable doubt. The bacterial analysis also revealed that Tong did not have typhoid fever, as diagnosed by Pillsbury. Prior to his death, pus had been extracted from the bubo and injected into a guinea pig. The important element of the test centered on the specimen having been taken prior to the victim's passing. Since the pus constituted live tissue, this ruled out the possibility of the guinea pig's death resulting from a non-live decomposing specimen taken after death. Until this victim, body samples had been taken from dead victims, casting doubt as to it being plague. *The Bee* ended its article stating that there had now been 13 cases and Mr. Tong had been a live case, negating those who denied its existence.[98]

During this period, Gage had been solidifying his political base with those individuals supporting the anti-plague stance. He rearranged the state board of health to support his position. As part of this process, he removed Dr. A.M. Henderson and replaced him with Dr. W.J. Hanna. Henderson had expressed his belief that the plague did exist, resulting in his replacement.[99] When interviewed about his thoughts on not being re-nominated, he said:

> This action of the Governor grows out of my attitude on the plague situation in San Francisco.... I still hold to my position that plague existed in San Francisco. This action is not a surprise to me.[100]

The Bee concentrated its reporting on the increasing number of victims. The *Occidental Medical Times* also acknowledged the disease's existence and reviewed the history of the initial 11 cases.[101] On July 14, *The Bee* allied with the *Times*' story. It explained that the process for determining plague had been recognized on well-founded scientific procedures providing definitive proof as to the correctness of the diagnosis through bacteriological analysis.[102]

It published two related articles, the first of which was titled "Governor Gage Should Apologize."[103] It applauded Kinyoun's efforts and the local board of health in remaining steadfast. The story reprimanded Gage for not accepting the scientific findings of numerous medical authorities who initially had gone along with

VINDICATION OF DR. KINYOUN.

Judge Morrow Purges Him of Alleged Contempt.

SAN FRANCISCO, July 3.—In the United States Circuit Court to-day Judge Morrow held that Dr. J. J. Kinyoun, local Federal Quarantine Officer, had not been guilty of contempt of Court in requiring persons leaving this city during the plague excitement to secure health certificates from the authorities.

The Judge found that travel within the borders of the State had not been

WANTED TO CALL IT BLOOD-POISONING.

Still Trying to Conceal True Character of Plague Cases.

The anti-plague bureau in San Francisco is still making every possible effort to prevent admission that there has been any plague in that city. In spite of the incontrovertible evidence with regard to the last case of plague, referred to in The Bee yesterday, Dr. Hirschfelder, in whose ward in the City and County Hospital the case occurred, desired to sign a certificate that death was caused by septicaemia or blood poisoning. Hirschfelder is in charge of what is knewn as the Cooper side of the hospital—referring to the ward in charge of physicians from the Cooper Medical College—and the autopsy was conducted by the physicians from the Cooper institution. Brady, who was in charge, is the assistant to Dr. Orphuls, the bacteriologist of the school, and he was very thorough in his work. Orphuls has been emphatic in his statements that the cases found were those of true plague, but the authorities of the school, including Drs. Laine and Ellingwood, have been the main supports of the Governor in his declaration that no plague has existed. They have been referred to by him as authority on the subject, and the fact of their connection with the Cooper school vaunted, when everyone who knows anything of the facts in the case knows that the one man in the school able to speak with authority on the subject, both because he has examined personally into the cases and because of his knowledge of the subject, is Dr. Orphuls. The Governor passed by Orphuls and took Laine and Ellingwood, who had not personally examined into the cases and had not made bacteriological examinations of tissues.

The influence of the school, therefore, has been used as against the statement that plague has existed, and Hirschfelder has attempted to carry out this plan. The autopsy, however, was too well attended to admit of any such evasion, and it is understood that the fact of the establishment of the existence of the disease in this instance has been duly reported to the Governor.

The one circumstance in connection with the case, however, calling for censure, is declared to be the act of Dr. Pillsbury, employed by the Six Companies, in sending the case to the City and County Hospital to endanger the lives of the inmates there, under a diagnosis of typhoid.

FRESH CASE OF THE PLAGUE IN SAN FRANCISCO.

San Francisco has got another case of bubonic plague, and the circumstances surrounding this are such as to leave no doubt of the character of the disease, in addition to confirming the necessity for the warning that has been given by the San Francisco Board of Health, by the State Board of Health, by Dr. J. J. Kinyoun, the Federal Quarantine Officer, and by The Bee, that it must not be taken for granted that an apparent immunity for thirty days is evidence that the danger from plague is over. The case in question is particularly interesting from the fact that it was under observation before death, and the authorities have a full history of the case. The autopsy was performed by physicians not connected with the Board of Health, many of whom have been somewhat suspicious of the existence of plague, and in the presence of two physicians representing the Chinese interests.

The case is that of Lee Wing Tong, a laborer found at 767 Clay Street and sent to the City and County Hospital July 4th by Dr. Ernest S. Pillsbury, who has been the expert physician of the Six Companies retained to combat the statements of Dr. W. H. Kellogg, the bacteriologist of the San Francisco Board of Health, and Dr. Kinyoun. The Chinese had been perfectly well up to a week before he was taken to the hospital, but did not go to bed until July 2d. He was then delirious, and was seen by a Chinese physician. Later Dr. Pillsbury saw him and had him sent to the hospital, with the statement that he probably had typhoid fever.

When he arrived at the hospital the man's temperature was 104 and he was found to have a large, tender bubo in the left groin, beside having a tender and distended abdomen. He was placed in Dr. Hirschfelder's ward, who, after an examination on the 5th, had the man isolated and placed under close observation. He died at 6:30 on the morning of the 6th, and a post mortem was held the same day, conducted by Dr. Brady, assistant to Dr. Ophuls of the Cooper Medical College, who made a very thorough job of it. Every organ was examined, including the brain. Among those present were Dr. Douglass Montgomery, bacteriologist of the University of California Medical College; Dr. J. J. Kinyoun, the Federal Quarantine Officer; Dr. Ryfkogel, bacteriologist of the State Board of Health; Dr. W. H. Kellogg, bacteriologist of the San Francisco Board of Health; Dr. Krone, of Oakland; Dr. Jellinck; Dr. Shiels, and Drs. D. A. Hodghead and H. D'Arcy Power, representing the Six Companies, who came in later. Dr. Pillsbury was invited to attend, but was ill.

The autopsy showed all the symptoms of the plague, and only plague symptoms. There was absolutely no evidence of typhoid. Bacteriological examination showed the presence of the plague organism beyond question. Before death a portion of the pus from the bubo in the groin was taken and injected into a guinea pig. This pig died of plague. The fact that the pus was taken before death avoids the criticism that the pig might have died from some substance injected which had been rendered of a deadly character through decomposition.

The physicians of the Six Companies have not expressed themselves on the subject, but the other physicians are pretty well convinced that San Francisco has the plague. The house in which the case was found has been quarantined and guarded by the police, and the ward in the hospital has also been thoroughly quarantined.

This is the thirteenth case of plague in San Francisco that has been verified. The first case was on March 6th, and the last previous to this on June 9th. The cases have, therefore, run over a period of four months and there has been nearly a full month between the last two. The opportunity for those who have alleged that no plague has existed at all to point to the fact that no live cases have been discovered is missing in this instance.

WANTED TO CALL IT BLOOD-POISONING., *The Bee*, July 10, 1900.

his position, only to reverse themselves after reviewing the evidence. It requested that he apologize to the doctor, the local board and all those who had come forward demanding the truth. It summed him up by stating, "His attitude has all along been silly in the extreme."[104]

The second article commenced with a large bold headline and subheading:

WANTED TO CALL IT BLOOD-POISONING
Still Trying to Conceal True
Character of Plague Cases.[105]

This article revealed Cooper Medical College's role in denying the plague and called out Drs. Ellingwood and Lane, who had supported the governor.[106] Although Orphlus had conducted a thorough examination of Tong, the Chinese Six Companies' physician, Dr. Pillsbury, should be subject to "censure"[107] for sending him to a hospital. By his act, others had been potentially exposed to the disease, either because of a misdiagnosis, or possibly because of political reasons. As to the college, *The Bee* noted it was used as a basis of authority between the differing parties, when the facts proved otherwise. Moreover, it knew, or should have known, the medical facts about the situation. And Lane and Ellingwood should have known better, too, but they were proponents of the governor's ongoing denial and had never attended the autopsy of the victims.[108]

Pause and Passion

By September, the crisis had reached a standstill. Both sides of the conflict stood firm in their respective positions. Each side championed the truth, but only one—consisting of Kinyoun, the Marine Hospital Service, the local board of health, *The Sacramento Bee* and others outside California—spoke the facts. During this interlude, the number of plague cases diminished to some degree. Yet just when 30 days had passed, signaling the area plague-free, another case appeared and again led to more denials by the newspapers. Other suspicious things occurred, leading the plague believers to claim an ongoing cover-up. Consequently, the plague flames remained stoked, and the factions continued to remain at odds.

Judge Morrow had ruled Kinyoun had not violated his earlier injunction because his action of establishing checkpoints at the state's border. His injunction had addressed intrastate travel, or travel within the state, a legal province belonging to California. Prior to the contempt hearing, Wyman had cancelled the checkpoints as part of the pre-trial maneuverings, and after the ruling he did not reinstate the border inspections or the requirement of health certificates. This omission created a void, resulting in no one doing anything to contain the disease.

As a result, Texas; Colorado; Mexico; Sydney, Australia; and Ecuador threatened quarantines against California.[109] Texas Governor Joseph O. Sayers wrote to Wyman stating he had lost confidence in those officials handling the situation in California and sought assurances the malady would not spread. Wyman asked Kinyoun the same question.[110] In response, he quoted a report received from Dr. O'Brien stating the health department to be "absolutely powerless"[111] in its ability to clean up Chinatown and rectify the situation.[112] As of October, there had been 19 plague cases, thereby causing these states and countries to impose quarantines.[113]

In October, the situation started to flare up again. *The Bee* headlined a story on October 17:

MORE PLAGUE IN SAN FRANCISCO.
Secret of the Most Recent Attack on Dr. J.J. Kinyoun.[114]

The paper reported that three Chinamen had died of the disease from October 5–14.[115] Kinyoun and the local health board and its bacteriologist confirmed the deaths as plague. He sent a detailed report to Wyman explaining the procedures performed on the three victims pre- and postmortem.[116] The victims had been living in close proximity to one another.[117] In addition, he reported the death of a young girl the month before: there had been no trace of the body, and a $100 bribe had transpired to cover up the cause of death. Towards the end of the article, *The Bee* revisited the matter of the *Coptic* and how Kinyoun had been blamed for violating the personal dignity of its passengers when they had been strip-searched for inspection. It confirmed that he had not been present at the ship's interment, nor the disrobing of its passengers, as claimed by *The Chronicle*. Instead, it had been proven he had been in Vancouver, British Columbia, when the purported incident had occurred.[118]

In early November, *The Call* reported in two articles that a hidden cemetery had been discovered on a hillside near Chinatown containing six graves. It claimed the Chinamen had been murdered because of gang wars involving the Highbinders. One of the victims appeared to be a Chinese baby, leading one to suspect otherwise.[119] The Chinese had been known to be uncooperative with health officials. To many, it had become common knowledge that the Chinese had been hiding their victims and their bodies in secret places to avoid discovery. On occasion, and based on leads, Kinyoun would go out in the shadows of the night and dig up dead Chinamen buried in unmarked graves, sometimes even digging underneath houses.[120]

On November 14, *The Bulletin* again took the doctor to task, reporting:

REPORTS SENT OUT INJURIOUS

Emanated from Marine Hospital Service.

Suspicion That Dr. Kinyoun Gave the Statement
That Plague Existed Here and Continues to Exist.

A Matter of Vast Importance to the People of California and San Francisco
in Particular as the Statements Are Spread Broadcast All Over the World.[121]

Kinyoun had sent reports to Wyman and others at the Service. It was his job to report the plague's ongoing presence and evolution.[122] However, the paper took a personal jab at the doctor when it called him "Dr. Kinyoun, who the people of San Francisco have wished to get rid of for many long days."[123] There had been several previous calls for his removal. But as time went on, the outcry for his departure by the anti-plague newspapers and other factions began to accelerate.

Another paper expressed its dislike for the doctor, running a very large picture of him with the caption, "FALSE STORIES OF PLAGUE CIRCULATED BY THE GOVERNMENT."[124] Depicting him with staring, almost sinister eyes and both ends of his mustache swirled into fine points,[125] the picture appeared to portray him as a villain.

The Evening Bee continued to press its point about the plague. On November 14, it ran a story updating the situation titled:

> THE BUBONIC PLAGUE
> AT SAN FRANCISCO
> The Truth Coming Out in a Half-Hearted Way Accompanied by the Usual Newspaper Denials.[126]

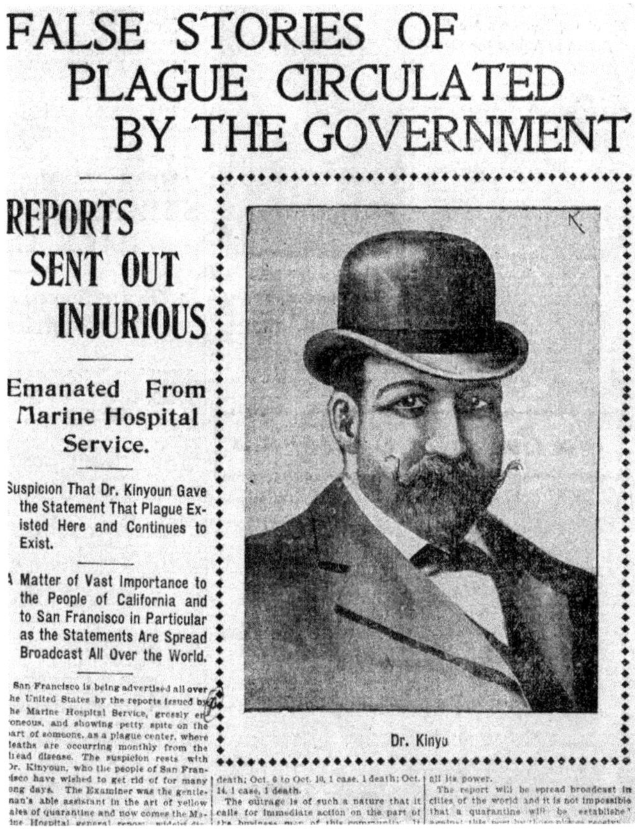

FALSE STORIES OF PLAGUE CIRCULATED BY THE GOVERNMENT

REPORTS SENT OUT INJURIOUS

Emanated From Marine Hospital Service.

Suspicion That Dr. Kinyoun Gave the Statement That Plague Existed Here and Continues to Exist.

A Matter of Vast Importance to the People of California and to San Francisco in Particular as the Statements Are Spread Broadcast All Over the World.

San Francisco is being advertised all over the United States by the reports issued by the Marine Hospital Service, grossly erroneous, and showing petty spite on the part of someone, as a plague center, where deaths are occurring monthly from the dread disease. The suspicion rests with Dr. Kinyoun, who the people of San Francisco have wished to get rid of for many long days. The Examiner was the gentleman's able assistant in the art of yellow tales of quarantine and now comes the Marine Hospital general report

death; Oct. 6 to Oct. 10, 1 case, 1 death; Oct. 14, 1 case, 1 death.

The outrage is of such a nature that it calls for immediate action on the part of the business men of this community.

all its power.

The report will be spread broadcast in cities of the world and it is not impossible that a quarantine will be established

FALSE STORIES OF PLAGUE CIRCULATED BY THE GOVERNMENT, *The Bulletin*, November 1900.

The article noted that *The Bulletin* had published a report of Kinyoun's plague tally to be 18, but in the same vein denied any confirmed cases. *The Bee* wrote that Dr. Williamson with the local board of health had reported 21 cases as of November 3.[127] Clearly, the anti-plague papers and *The Bee* wrestled in a tug-of-war over who was right. The tide started to change in November, with other groups beginning to acknowledge the contagion's presence.

On November 14, *The Evening Bee* ran a lengthy account of the change with a four-line bold type headline:

> The Medical Society of Northern California
> Unanimously Declares That the Bubonic Plague
> Exists in San Francisco, and Demands That
> Steps Be Taken for Protection.[128]

At the Society's autumn meeting, Dr. Wallace A. Briggs presented the following resolution:

> RESOLVED THAT IT IS THE PROFOUND CONVICTION OF THE CALIFORNIA NORTHERN DISTRICT MEDICAL SOCIETY THAT THE STATE BOARD OF HEALTH OF CALIFORNIA SHOULD IMMEDIATELY AND OFFICIALLY RECOGNIZE THE EXISTENCE OF BUBONIC PLAGUE IN THE CITY OF SAN FRANCISCO, AND SHOULD EXERT ITS

> UTMOST POWER TO LIMIT THE SPREAD OF THE DISEASE AND TO STAMP IT OUT AT THE EARLIEST POSSIBLE MOMENT.[129]

Dr. James H. Parkinson, the editor for the *Occidental Medical Times*, seconded the motion. As part of the accord, Dr. Briggs asked the Society to adopt it unanimously. Several members objected to the proposal and wanted more time to consider before voting. They reasoned that several of their learned colleagues had taken a contrary position about the plague and therefore should not be required to vote otherwise.[130]

In defense of the resolution, Dr. G.L. Simmons reminded the group about the arrival of cholera in San Francisco in the 1850s and its eventual spread to the Sacramento Valley, seriously impacting the region for years. He stated that the plague would pose the same danger if not dealt with soon.[131]

But several doctors stated that several of their members, particularly Dr. Silas M. Mouser and Dr. L.C. Lane, had already reviewed the plague evidence and concluded it not to be present. In response, Dr. A.M. Henderson advised the group that Mouser and Lane had derived their opinions from what they read from other sources and not from an actual medical observation. In the end, the resolution passed unanimously. Before adjourning, the Society praised *The Bee* for seeking the truth, unlike the other newspapers.[132]

The Evening Bee became relentless in trying to convince others about the seriousness of the situation and the ongoing denials. On November 15, it printed an article under the banner,

> "STATE BOARD ON RECORD CONFIRMING PLAGUE CASES."[133]

The story had a particular twist to it, where it went back to the beginning of the crisis when the organization had admitted its presence. In order to align the board to his stance, Governor Gage started stacking it with physicians in agreement with him. Dr. W.J. Hanna and Dr. Winslow Anderson were two such appointees. Since their appointment, they had been anti-plague supporters. Hanna reported that Surgeon General Sternberg and Dr. Mouser were non-plague believers. He touted Sternberg's opinion as proof positive of its absence. Later, Dr. G.L. Simmons stated that Mouser had offered Sternberg the opportunity to examine the slide samples from the victims.[134] But he replied that

> … he had not looked into a microscope for seven years and would not be competent to determine whether or not the specimens indicated plague.[135]

By this statement, Sternberg disqualified his earlier opinion in *The Bulletin* on July 31, where he stated agreement with Mouser that the plague did not exist in the city. His comment, although being truthful as to his competence, raised the question of why he even expressed an opinion. As the country's leading bacteriologist, he had not bothered to utilize the primary medical instrument of the day, the microscope, before agreeing with Mouser. Kinyoun, on the other hand, used it as one of his primary diagnostic tools, as did the leading European bacteriologists.

The Year Concludes

As one of the last salvos of the year, on December 20, *The Chronicle* published a story headlined "Kinyoun May Be Replaced."[136] It seemed that the Treasury Department had asked the collector at Fort Stratton to conduct an inquiry into his actions. The review had been initiated because of the *Coptic* incident. The column listed other examples of what it thought to be underhanded dealings. In particular, his notifying various Asian ports and Honolulu about plague being in San Francisco along with his advising merchant ships and sea travelers to avoid the port. The collector interviewed Kinyoun, and he acknowledged that officials in Washington might remove him.[137] In response to the collector's comments, *The Chronicle* stated:

> Dr. Kinyoun is of the opinion that his transfer is at hand. He believed that a change in location will cast no reflection on him and asserts that he is ready to go.[138]

There could be little doubt Kinyoun wanted to leave his post, especially since he never wanted to go to California. One must imagine that he would be elated to be transferred to another station or back to his Hygienic Laboratory. However, for the time being, he would remain on Angel Island.

At some point during this period, the local board of health passed a unanimous resolution thanking Governor Gage. On close reading, however, it appears to be a spoof. The motion, handwritten on official stationery, read, "DEPARTMENT OF PUBLIC HEALTH,"[139] with the address, "San Francisco, Cal.,"[140] written underneath. On the left side, layered in three lines, it stated, "OFFICE OF BOARD OF HEALTH CITY HALL."[141] The resolution read as follows:

> Dr. Buckley introduced the following resolution
>
> Resolved That it be the sense of the Board that Gov. Henry T. Gage in cooperating with the Federal and Municipal Authorities for the purpose of placing the Chinese District of this City in a Sanitary Condition and eradicating the germs of the plague practically conceded that the position of this Board was conformable to the truth, and that the accusation heretofore publicly made by the Governor against this Board was erroneous and unjust; and
>
> Be it further Resolved: that we appreciate this Co-operation in the interests of the public health, and that we Charitably accept this action as a sufficient retraction of the statements which he has heretofore published.
>
> Second Chief Sullivan
>
> Unanimously adopted.[142]

After 1900

The newspapers would wage war over the plague for years up to and even after the Great San Francisco Earthquake of 1906, when it reappeared. The problem with plague centered on its intrinsic, reclusive and secretive nature. Throughout history, the contagion would appear in a community resulting in several cases and then sequester itself underground, where it would fester. But within a year or so it would resurface with a vengeance, wiping out entire towns in a relatively short span of time. On its resurgence, the bacilli in many cases would transform into the worst phase of the disease, known as pneumonic. An infected person would pass it to another individual in the morning, only to be dead by noon, with the other one dead by midnight.

Kinyoun knew about the pneumonic phase and its severity, which had accounted for millions of deaths throughout Europe and Asia. One case of plague had been diagnosed as pneumonic outside the confines of Chinatown, thereby heightening the concern of its imminent danger. In some fairness to the anti-plague parties, many of them may have been unaware of this possible transformation of the disease, or only thought it would afflict the Asian population in Chinatown.

The white population may have felt a certain immunity from the malady because of their health, race and better sanitation practices, but their arrogance was totally unfounded. This position had been proven terribly wrong, as evidenced by the second and third great plagues in medieval Europe. The ultimate culprit would be the rat and flea combination, not yet connected by the scientific community, although the rat/plague connection had been suspected. Regardless, the plague had never discriminated based on one's race: it claimed all in its path.

Being a quarantine officer for many years, he knew pestilence and infestation usually went hand in hand with the entry and spread of disease. He had overseen the disinfection of countless ships, railroad cars, baggage and people over the last 15 years. But considering the times, when modern medicine, as seen through a microscope and other scientific techniques, had not been totally embraced let alone understood by the public and the medical community, it would be easy for opponents to mock not only the plague, but also the science behind it and Kinyoun as well.

As the year ended, the bickering between the plague and anti-plague factions persisted. Stories abounded with plenty of ammunition to sink the best of seafaring ships. One thing had become more prevalent: demands for his removal. Those on both sides of the argument remained in the dark as to where the situation would lead, or how long before it would end. As the standoff dragged on, Kinyoun's removal became an ongoing outcry, rallying others. At the close of 1900, one constant remained: people continued to die, and he would stay at the helm. All in all, the attempts to cover up the situation had failed, and the world knew full well that San Francisco had the plague.

XV

Darkening Clouds

The Home Front

Kinyoun wrote an 80-page letter on August 9, 1900, to Dr. Bailhache, purportedly either his uncle or Lizzie's. The letter went into great detail about the crisis and the state of his family.[1] He wrote that he very much felt like Davy Crockett at the Alamo,[2] but knew he was "right."[3] He remarked that as a result he would stand his ground against all the adversity. The whole affair had been mentally challenging to them, stating, "at the end of them all, if the end is reached, we are both alive and well, and ... we have come through fairly well."[4] As to himself, he commented:

> In fact, I believe I have grown just a few pounds stouter than I was in January; but as I expected to gain one pound each year, I do not know whether to attribute this to time or simply to having assimilated so much fat and "lies."[5]

Later in the correspondence, he wrote about the family's four children, who had the benefit of a governess for the first six months of the year.[6] He described a conversation with his sons, starting with Conrad, who, along with his siblings, had been receiving teachings in the Bible, centering on "biblical truths and orthodox beliefs."[7] One evening at dinner, Perry inquired about the presence of "false prophets."[8] After advising him that they do indeed exist, Conrad stated:

> ... there were lots of false prophets in California; the people follow false prophets; they don't believe in anything out here but, the dollar, and that is not right.[9]

The lad also had an opinion about Judge Morrow. He stated the judge didn't know his dad, but "he's the biggest man in the world ... he's mistaken, because he don't know papa like I do."[10]

The family, being pretty much confined to Angel Island, would on occasion make a few outings to the city, as the need arose for either personal business or small pleasures. Kinyoun complained that his health had not been the greatest; he had suffered four bouts of indigestion since arriving in California. He believed it to be his appendix. On one occasion, he considered a leave of absence.[11]

An Impasse

Towards the end of 1900, Wyman through a series of telegrams asked Kinyoun about the state of affairs in San Francisco. He wanted to know if the plague had been contained, what assistance the state and local board of health had taken, and the number of victims and their race. This correspondence occurred between October 20 and December 13, 1900, and set the stage for the coming year.[12]

Kinyoun sent several responses to his inquiries culminating in a lengthy report as to the overall situation. As to the actions of the health boards, he replied that nothing had been done by either party because they were waiting for the November 6 election to be over. No measures had been taken to contain it, provide a holding place or hospital, or establish disinfection procedures. The state board had previously hired inspectors for the cleanup process, but Governor Gage had dismissed them.[13] To the contrary, Dr. Ryfkogel, the state's bacteriologist, had been ordered to attend all postmortem investigations, serving as an "independent"[14] observer. The doctor advised, though, that the local health board could handle the situation for the time being without the state's help.[15]

He told Wyman that most of the victims had been Chinese. However, things would likely change soon, because the population in Chinatown would swell by 3,000 as Chinamen returned to the city seeking housing for the winter after working in Alaska over the summer picking fruit.[16] Kinyoun pointed out, "They live under the worst hygienic conditions imaginable."[17] By this statement, he put Wyman on notice that things could be expected to deteriorate, leading to a spike in cases.

Two days after Kinyoun's telegram, Wyman wrote to Governor Sayers in Texas. Sayers had visited Wyman in Washington and asked for an update. He told the governor that to his knowledge the state of affairs was not serious, in contrast to the doctor's previous wire.[18] The letter stated the contagion had "not manifested itself in the manner in which we feared ... and they have all been among the Chinese."[19] Wyman expressed the opinion that "the disease is more easily checked than yellow fever."[20] He commented that the local health board had been communicating with the state health board, and there was no need for a plague hospital since he did not view "the situation as critical."[21] Concerning commerce, except for items from Chinatown and those individuals showing signs of the illness, the status quo "would meet the present requirements."[22]

On November 2 and November 6, he sent additional cables to Wyman advising of more plague victims: two Chinese and one white. Neither death had occurred in Chinatown, nor did the victims have any connection to each other.[23] For some reason, Wyman had decided to downplay the truth of what had been happening. Most of the correspondence between them had been by telegrams, meaning that the receipt of communication was instantaneous. This did not mean that every wire had been read upon its arrival, but the implication would suggest otherwise, given the magnitude of the situation.

Considering this supposition, and assuming Wyman had read Kinyoun's telegrams before writing to Sayers, it would appear he had been less than forthright. But why would a person in his position not be straightforward with the facts as related by one of his officers? Perhaps he did not want to inflate the matter any further. Regardless, Wyman appeared less than candid, which could have a dire effect on the problem.

During this period, the local health board had been reporting plague cases to

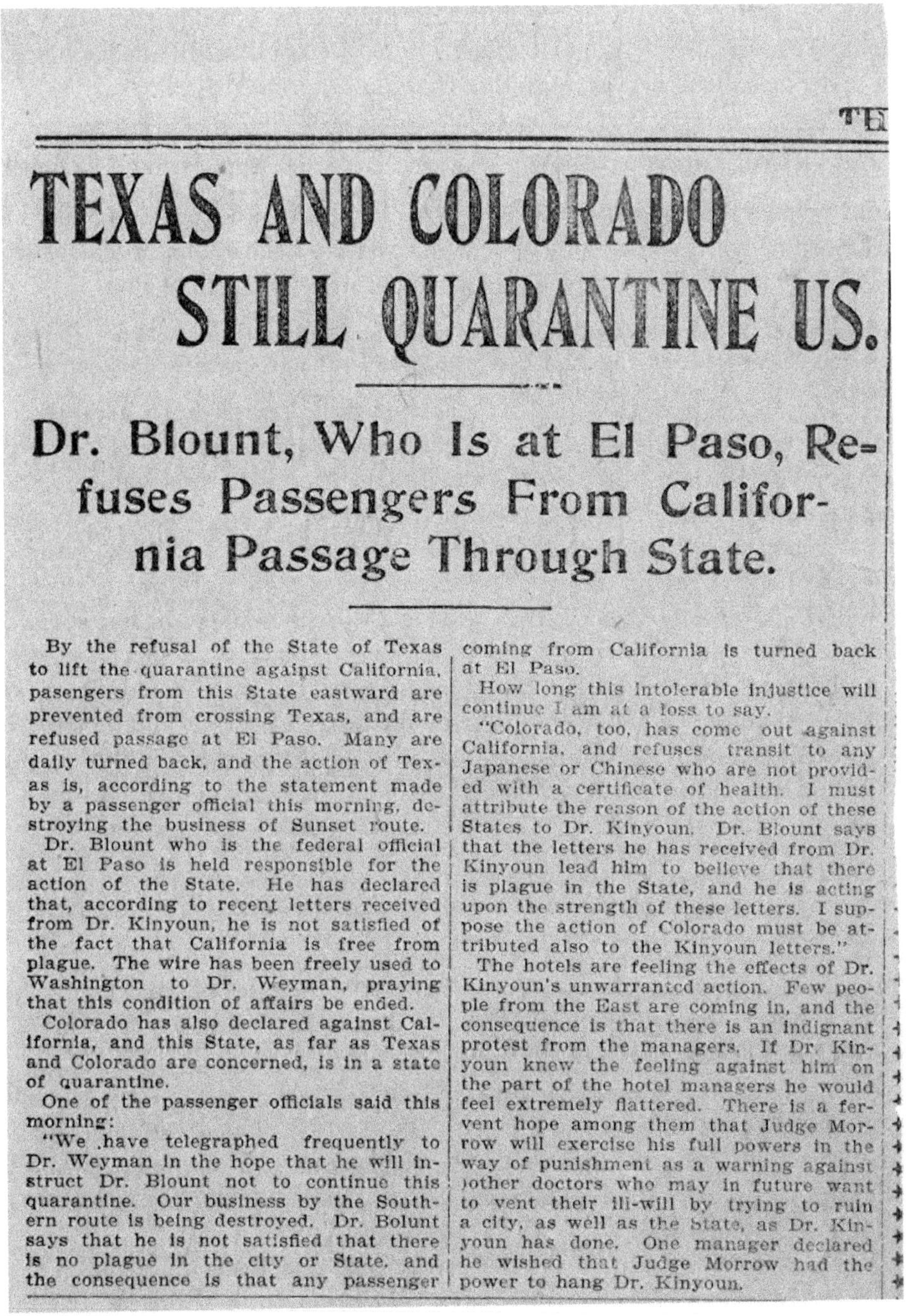

TEXAS AND COLORADO STILL QUARANTINE US.

Dr. Blount, Who Is at El Paso, Refuses Passengers From California Passage Through State.

By the refusal of the State of Texas to lift the quarantine against California, pasengers from this State eastward are prevented from crossing Texas, and are refused passage at El Paso. Many are daily turned back, and the action of Texas is, according to the statement made by a passenger official this morning, destroying the business of Sunset route.

Dr. Blount who is the federal official at El Paso is held responsible for the action of the State. He has declared that, according to recent letters received from Dr. Kinyoun, he is not satisfied of the fact that California is free from plague. The wire has been freely used to Washington to Dr. Weyman, praying that this condition of affairs be ended.

Colorado has also declared against California, and this State, as far as Texas and Colorado are concerned, is in a state of quarantine.

One of the passenger officials said this morning:

"We have telegraphed frequently to Dr. Weyman in the hope that he will instruct Dr. Blount not to continue this quarantine. Our business by the Southern route is being destroyed. Dr. Bolunt says that he is not satisfied that there is no plague in the city or State, and the consequence is that any passenger coming from California is turned back at El Paso.

How long this intolerable injustice will continue I am at a loss to say.

"Colorado, too, has come out against California, and refuses transit to any Japanese or Chinese who are not provided with a certificate of health. I must attribute the reason of the action of these States to Dr. Kinyoun. Dr. Blount says that the letters he has received from Dr. Kinyoun lead him to believe that there is plague in the State, and he is acting upon the strength of these letters. I suppose the action of Colorado must be attributed also to the Kinyoun letters."

The hotels are feeling the effects of Dr. Kinyoun's unwarranted action. Few people from the East are coming in, and the consequence is that there is an indignant protest from the managers. If Dr. Kinyoun knew the feeling against him on the part of the hotel managers he would feel extremely flattered. There is a fervent hope among them that Judge Morrow will exercise his full powers in the way of punishment as a warning against other doctors who may in future want to vent their ill-will by trying to ruin a city, as well as the State, as Dr. Kinyoun has done. One manager declared he wished that Judge Morrow had the power to hang Dr. Kinyoun.

"TEXAS AND COLORADO STILL QUARANTINE US." 1900.

the court.[24] Kinyoun wrote that its "attitude [is] now entirely changed; practically amounts to reversal of position assumed several months ago."[25] This represented not only a change, but a promising one. Wyman had asked him to meet with the judge concerning the issuance of health certificates for people traveling with the Southern Railway Company. Several attempts had failed, but while taking the ferry home one evening, he spotted Morrow sitting alone. The judge approached him and they had a 40-minute conversation.[26] Kinyoun asked why he had not directly ruled on the existence of the malady in the case, even though it did exit in the city and

> ... as an officer of the government to inform him of the fact and in confirmation of this information, I submitted to him proofs which I had obtained through my individual investigations.[27]

He told Wyman they had an extensive conversation over the rights of federal and state governments. This concept had been the primary issue in the earlier legal challenges.[28] The judge had firmly believed, like many others at the time, that

> ... the workings of the state's machinery ... was not within the province of the government to assume charge of the internal sanitation of a state unless it was abandoned by the state officials.[29]

He told Morrow that he held the same belief and had tried to operate and issue orders within the boundaries of the law. He noted that the constitution regulated "commerce between the states,"[30] but not within the states.[31] Such a statement would not necessarily appear compatible with a federal quarantine officer's duties. But in Kinyoun's case, his upbringing could have had some impact on his thinking. His father had been a Confederate officer and an attorney. More than likely, he had received a good dose of law and states' rights indoctrination growing up.

At the end their conversation, he commented that the judge "acted as a changed man."[32] He could tell he had been misled by the district attorney and the governor and believed the initial suit brought against him and others might have been different, if this conversation had occurred earlier.[33] As a summary of their encounter, he wrote:

> While I hold no animus toward the Judge in his course of action since I had the pleasure of stabbing him deep and turning the knife within the wound, I feel that I am in a position to play quits with him and am able to meet him on any question that might arise.[34]

Although not a flattering passage, it represented the thoughts of one who had been through a constant barrage of humiliation and disgrace by the plague adversaries. To his credit, he did not hold any ill will against the judge.

After their conversation, Morrow told him to feel free to approach him about any questions he might have as to the constitutionality of any regulation, or if he needed any counsel concerning the legality of a quarantine.[35] The judge went a step further and asked Kinyoun to contact him directly, "and he would give just as broad a latitude as the law allowed."[36]

As a prelude to problems facing the forthcoming year, Kinyoun cabled an extensive account of the matter to Wyman in early December. It was doubtful he knew about Wyman's correspondence with the Texas governor downplaying the crisis in California. One thing had become certain: the state of affairs continued to grow out of control. He wrote that reports stating that the local board of health had things under control were false. The press continued to lie about the plague, and there remained no funding, no inspection force, no inspections, no facilities, and no hospitals to care for the sick and dying.[37]

He stressed that the political interests had prevented any cleanup of Chinatown, deaths were being reported by victims' families as caused by other diseases, and at present there had been 160 Chinese deaths. Even the city physician, Dr. F.P. Wilson, who had been appointed by the local health board without pay, did not appear to be following the proper examination protocols set by the coroner. In some cases, he relied on the family's diagnosis and did not always conduct a postmortem analysis. And in other instances, he even identified the wrong cause of death: pneumonia when the true cause was probably plague.[38]

Mild cases of plague had been reported as diphtheria, phlegmonous erysipelas and typhoid pneumonia, although he believed there had been "no intent to mislead or deceive."[39] He reported that Dr. O'Brien and the health department had become "absolutely powerless"[40] in remedying the situation, although the court had been more cooperative. Concerning the white doctors treating the victims in Chinatown, he described them as less than impressive and said they could be considered as nothing more than "vampires."[41] In the end, Kinyoun believed the only solution to the problem would be the depopulation and destruction of Chinatown. As to the costs of eradicating the disease, he estimated that, based on the cleanups in Sydney and Glasgow, it would be $1,000,000, as opposed to an earlier projection of $7,500.[42]

A Second Opinion

In late December, Wyman took an approach to handling the crisis different from Kinyoun's. He ordered his chief of quarantine administration, Dr. White, to San Francisco. His orders included inspecting the quarantine station and its hospital, followed by a review of all matters concerning the Service. Wyman directed him to investigate quarantined food items that Kinyoun had embargoed because of plague-carrying pests. Lastly, he was to complete the assignment as expeditiously as possible.[43] On January 1, 1901, he cabled Wyman as to his arrival.[44]

In a week, he wired Wyman his first assessment, stating he had met with the Chamber of Commerce about the *Coptic* incident. He reported that Kinyoun's version was correct even in light of "some indelicacy."[45] Claims of the plague continued to be challenged, but he did observe one case on January 7. The media, the Chinese Six Companies, steamship lines and commercial groups remained steadfast as an anti-plague unit. They appeared cordial towards the Service, but detested Kinyoun. Concerning the food, he confirmed both the vegetable and the animal products to be dangerous.[46]

Wyman responded to White on January 9, and seemed indifferent to any impending epidemic. In his opinion, the climate in San Francisco differed from Calcutta and other plague-stricken cities. Concluding that such an outbreak would not occur for several years, he directed White not to create any excitement but be diligent in routine matters.[47] Wyman had decided to downplay the affair. Why the about-face? Lastly, Kinyoun and the local health board had been trying for over a year to conduct inspections, disinfections and inoculations. So why would he think White would have any greater success when previous efforts had been shunned by all the parties?

White wired Wyman on January 9, addressing a claim by the governor that

Kinyoun and others had been injecting corpses with the plague bacilli in order to prove its existence through postmortem examinations. He reported meeting with Drs. Kinyoun, Kellogg, Ryfkogel and Chambers at a suspected plague residence. They found a Chinese victim lying on a plank with one end supported by a box of food, or "chow,"[48] waiting to be eaten. After examining the man, he believed his death to be from plague. As to the question of manipulation of the bacilli in corpses, he found no evidence. He allowed that Kellogg and Ryfkogel were men of stellar reputations and knowledge.[49]

As a heads up, White cabled him on January 10 about a new development. *The Chronicle* ran an extensive article on January 9 outlining Governor Gage's annual address to the legislature denying the plague's existence and demanding Kinyoun's ouster. Gage claimed he lacked any experience with the plague, except through books, and had either mismanaged or intentionally altered postmortem examinations.[50] As a result, he asked for special "plenary power"[51] for a new "State quarantine officer"[52] and a "State Board of health."[53]

On the same day, Kinyoun sent Wyman a scathing wire about the governor, demanding his letter of December 6, 1900 be released to the press. He took exception to the accusation that he had placed bacilli in the dead. He argued that these new allegations reflected on the Service as well as himself.[54] There have even been accounts that he (Wyman):

> … has no longer any confidence in reports sent by me regarding plague here, as no further mention is made in Public Health Reports, I being disgraced and discredited.… Situation demands action be taken by you … allow me to defend myself. Rumors of Congressional investigation, which I hope are true.[55]

Replying the following day, Wyman stated there was no truth to recent press reports. Concerning the omission of plague accounts in the Service's annual report, he waived it off as a new procedure reducing the section on contagions as part of mid-year reporting. He advised him that he had heard nothing about a Congressional investigation, but thought one would be beneficial. As to releasing his letter of December 6, he would get back to him.[56]

Wyman next wired White and, trying to calm him down, stated that the situation seemed no worse than before.[57] White replied to Wyman and again stressed the need for a presidential commission to investigate the crisis. He defended the doctor: "Kinyoun exercises more self-restraint than I thought possible and much gratified by the Surgeon-General's wire yesterday."[58] He concluded by presenting the idea of holding a joint conference with local and state health boards, the mayor, shipping companies and the railroads.[59]

At this juncture, Wyman embarked on yet another course. He advised White that, going forward, the matter would be handled by the Secretary of Treasury and himself. There would be no need to contact the president at this time.[60] Being a bureaucrat, he would have known not to involve the nation's chief executive in such a political free-for-all. More importantly, that President McKinley and Governor Gage were Republicans made the matter rather delicate, especially having the president call for the commission as opposed to the Secretary of the Treasury. By having the

Treasury Secretary lead the investigation it would establish some separation between McKinley and Secretary Gage. This would leave the president room to maneuver if a commission's findings proved contrary to Governor Gage's claims.

Apparently, White had previously recommended Drs. Novy, Barker and Welch to be commissioners for a special plague investigation. These men, who were acknowledged experts in bacteriology, had been submitted for consideration in case a commission would be appointed. Wyman agreed to these individuals in the cable, but also wanted White to arrange a meeting with the local board of health and the mayor.[61]

Although this was a logical way to handle the crisis with everyone, including Kinyoun, in agreement, something did not seem right with Wyman. In Kinyoun's telegram dated January 10, he queried Wyman about rumors of a Congressional investigation. The surgeon general denied any such reports. However, two days later, he acknowledged White's request for a presidential commission.[62] A Congressional investigation and a presidential commission may seem like two different investigative measures. Wyman in turn denied one and recognized the other, when in fact both border on being one and the same.

In defense of the surgeon general, he obviously had tired of calamity. No doubt, he had been taking some heat from officials above him. The situation continued to show no sign of improvement; it was only getting worse. Even so, there remained some people who supported him. Mayor Phelan was one. In a letter to Dr. R.A. Forrest he wrote, "I believe Dr. Kinyoun to be an honest man, a rare quality in the quarantine service of this port."[63] The mayor had been involved in the outbreak since the beginning, and he too had received a great deal of criticism from the anti-plague group.

Broken Silence

The weight of the disparagement and the continuing stalemate in the crisis led Kinyoun to seek counsel from family friend Senator Cockrell. He had become frustrated and angry at the situation and felt abandoned by Wyman. He wrote to the senator about his role in the melee.[64]

His response indicated Kinyoun had complained about California Senator George Perkins and to some extent Wyman.[65] In his opening sentence, Cockrell stated, "They have been bombarding you pretty heavily and I believe without justifiable cause."[66] He qualified his comment, stating that the business community and press believed he had done "serious harm"[67] to the city. The senator told him that Perkins did not support his censure and said that he had done his job properly. On the other hand, Perkins thought it best he consider transferring to another port upon the conclusion of Dr. White's investigation.[68] In conversations with Wyman, he told him the surgeon general had said, "He stood by you squarely."[69]

He, too, recommended Kinyoun seek a transfer to another post, stating Wyman would probably send him to any available position. As a politician and seeing the complicated picture before all the parties, he advised him that a transfer would be best for everyone, especially the Secretary of the Treasury. He stated that such action would avert attacks upon the Secretary, implying this to be more important.[70] Cockrell, a longtime friend and an astute politician, could see that the situation would probably not improve until he left.

Kinyoun did not react well to the senator's response. As a result, he wrote him a 13-page letter articulating his opinion and laying much of the blame for the upheaval on the surgeon general. He told Cockrell that he suspected Wyman and Perkins had not given him the complete story. He bristled with antagonism at the anti-plague factions, the governor and Wyman.[71] He traced the beginnings of the controversy to four years earlier and the implementation of the National Quarantine Act. This legislation curtailed the state's quarantine authority and placed overall control with the federal government. Even with this change, states could remain participants, but to a much lesser extent.[72]

Kinyoun highlighted the major events, starting with the quarantine ordered by Wyman and the subsequent legal battles. He noted the ill will the governor held towards him, especially after the injunction. He quoted Gage saying that he "had effectively broken my back so that I would give no further trouble."[73] After the injunction Wyman ordered him to inspect the border traffic, which led to the contempt citation. Kinyoun stated that his actions had been ordered by Wyman and that after he was cleared of contempt, Wyman never offered an apology.[74]

Concerning the heightened state of affairs, he attributed it the *Coptic* incident, when several passengers had to disrobe as part of an inspection. Kinyoun stated he had been "charged with brutality and indecency towards passengers."[75] In fact, he had been 1,100 miles away in Victoria, British Columbia, and did not learn of the incident until a week after his return. The individual who documented the report knew full well the truth, but purposely sent false information.[76]

The letter turned to the governor's calling for his removal by what he termed as "Gage's Kindergarten Legislature."[77] In other passages, he referred to Gage and his followers as "political sycophants."[78] Furthermore, he criticized Wyman for not personally visiting California to assess the situation.[79]

The surgeon general had recently published an article titled "Bubonic Plague."[80] Kinyoun lashed out at him for disseminating his opinions about the disease, highlighting its ravages and saying that the vaccines were at odds with his orders and what was really happening. What's more, the anti-plague faction had used its contents to show that the plague did not exist. He stated it to be "unfortunate"[81] that Wyman had written it and made the distinction between one able to write an article about a disease and one who had actually studied it and experienced it firsthand, like he had.[82] In a sarcastic vent, he wrote that it

> … is a very good compliment to the Quarantine Regulations regarding plague, and rounds out the lack of knowledge in a way that could not be shown otherwise.[83]

The following four pages took direct aim at Wyman, detailing his faults along with Kinyoun's displeasure and frustration with him. He had become fed up with the whole matter and the surgeon general's handling of it, which he had cautioned against since the beginning, but to no avail.[84] By making these statements about his supervisor, although in a private correspondence, he was taking a great risk at losing his position, if it ever became public.

His greatest objection stemmed from the recent quarantine regulations. He stated that they were "antagonistic to all the local interests."[85] Kinyoun allowed that these rules "were conceived in ignorance, by persons who had no idea of the conditions to be met, or what was to be accomplished."[86] Changing the law led to increased anger among the political and business interests, leading to an uproar and consternation by a large portion of the public.[87]

He strongly disagreed with Wyman's directives on how to manage the problem, but as he explained to the senator in a highlighted passage, his job required him "to obey his orders,—and These orders are from Dr. Wyman's orders, who is solely responsible for the present conditions."[88] He had now pinned the blame on Wyman for creating the debacle. He reprimanded him, writing:

> My justification and my exoneration rests upon Dr. Wyman openly avowing his responsibility for my original actions. This he should, and will do if he possesses the courage of a man, and wishes to do what is honorable.[89]

The letter showed disdain for Wyman's management of the crisis. He thought he had been transferred to California to take over the laboratory on Angel Island.[90] The situation soon changed dramatically on the arrival of the *Nippon Maru* and the first suspected plague cases. From this point on, the whole affair worsened, eventually leading to his being the center of the controversy.

After 10 months from the first confirmed case, he had become exhausted by the whole affair. He had been a loyal servant of the Service, and now he felt cast adrift in an ever-turbulent sea of swirling sharks lunging at his sinking craft. Betrayal might best describe his feelings. Kinyoun had done everything he had been told to do by his superior and then found himself taking the fall for the latter's judgment errors. As a self-testament to his ability, he wrote that his 15 years at the lab established his ability. Besides, the national and state quarantine stations would not be what they were without him. And lastly, he had been the one who created the Hygienic Laboratory.[91]

He cautioned Cockrell against letting Gage re-establish a state quarantine service under the control of the state board of health, which he made part of his address to the legislature, in addition to asking for his removal. Such an act would become nothing more than a political plum tree for the governor filled by "political jobbers and railway and steamship interest."[92]

Towards the end of the letter, he expressed his true sentiment towards the surgeon general, writing:

> All these years, I have stood loyally by the side of Dr. Wyman, fought hard his battles, shielded him from mistakes, and propped up many of his weak-kneed policies, and on more than one occasion used my best efforts, and not without success, in keeping his political head from falling into the basket.[93]

He concluded the letter by making an analogy between his plight and the senator's while serving as a Confederate general at the battle of Vicksburg in 1863, where he had "so valiantly held [his] ground."[94] What would have been his feeling, Kinyoun wondered, if his Confederate commander, General Pemberton, had told him that the enemy hated his style of attack and that, as a result, he should be dismissed from the army, so as not to antagonize the foe? Kinyoun compared this hypothetical situation to his own.[95]

Whether Kinyoun actually sent the letter and Senator Cockrell responded to it has remained an unknown. He probably felt there was little recourse for Kinyoun but to accept his earlier recommendation and seek a new post elsewhere.

Desecrated

While Wyman and White were corresponding, Kinyoun came under another hailstorm from the press after the governor asked the Senate to remove him. With the 1900 presidential election over and Gage having secured a majority in the California legislature, the governor threw the entire weight of the government against him. The journalistic rampages now being hurled in his direction constituted nothing less than a full-blown witch hunt.

At its forefront, *The Chronicle* wrote on January 9:

> KINYOUN IS UNDER FIRE[96]

The subheadings alone told the story:

> Chamber of Commerce in Vigorous Protest Against His Methods
> Dr. White Asked to Have Him Removed.
> Indignities to the Passengers on the Coptic Told to the Investigator.
> Every Question of the Doctor Fully Met by Those Who Make Charges
> Against the Quarantine Service.[97]

On the same day, *The Bulletin* ran an editorial titled "The Message of Governor Gage."[98]

The article praised the governor for seeking Kinyoun's removal and thanked him for "his recommendations to the Legislature for the removal or restriction of the evil found to exist."[99] In no uncertain words, it went to great lengths expressing its opinion about him, as evidenced by the following:

> A point upon which the Governor dwells at some length is what may be termed the "case of Kinyoun." He shows how an incapable and arrogant public official, either through malice or through ignorance, inflicted great damage upon the business interests of the state.[100]

The editor also agreed with Gage's proposal to have a state health board that could control all local health boards. In its conclusion, it made a final reference to him, stating that his "professional opinion has little established value."[101] Unfortunately, he had become the specimen in the Petri dish under the microscope—still alive, but not for long. But one certainty about Kinyoun remained: his professional experience. Few others had the training and knowledge to understand the gravity of the plague, but nobody wanted to listen.

Other newspapers joined the chorus demanding his removal. On January 24, *The Call* in a "Special Dispatch"[102] ran a lengthy article under the headline:

> STATE SENATE DEMANDS DR. KINYOUN'S REMOVAL
> Health Officer Flayed by Members for the Irreparable Damage He Has Done.[103]

The story recounted the action of the Senate and how to appropriately word the resolution asking for his removal and present it to President McKinley and Treasury Secretary Gage. The deliberations became protracted with heated arguments by the proponents. Senator Wolfe addressed the assembly and said, "All we ask ... is that they remove him from the coast. He is an annoyance to us. Let them take him away."[104]

The resolution had been sponsored by Senator Cutter, who had become empathic about his discharge, stating that "in his baffled rage over the action of the United States Court in raising the quarantine on Chinatown in San Francisco, Kinyoun quarantined the whole state."[105] In summation, he proclaimed, "And he should have been hanged for it."[106] The debate ended with Cutter's remarks. A vote proceeded with a count of 26 to 9 in favor of the resolution.[107]

On January 25, *The Chronicle* ran an editorial with the headline "The Removal of Kinyoun."[108]

As part of the Senate deliberation, a secondary resolution had been considered, called a memorial, which still demanded his removal but included a statement that there should not be "any stain upon his professional reputation."[109] The paper pretty much stated that it could not care less whether the memorial version or the other one passed: "The prime object is to get rid of him."[110] All it desired was to "relieve us from the outrageous blight."[111] As a final stab, the editorial wrote:

> We were indebted to the Stuffed Prophet for the Phrase "innocuous desuetude," and now he has inflicted another on the country in the form of "head long national heedlessness." Great Grover![112]

Newspapers outside San Francisco printed articles about the governor's address. *The Los Angeles Times* ran a story titled "Dr. Kinyoun's Head Demanded...."[113] His removal had become a rallying call for those supporting Gage and his cover-up. Even the average citizen, who feared such a plague epidemic but did not grasp the science behind its existence, supported his banishment.

Other Voices

The Sacramento Bee came to his defense. Other publications supported him, too. On January 12, it initiated its campaign supporting Kinyoun and attacking Governor Gage.[114] The headline read:

> ANOTHER CASE OF PLAGUE FOUND IN SAN FRANCISCO
> Startling Answer to Governor's tirade Against Kinyounism and a Free Press[115]

The first sentence read, "Rare old Caesar used to remark, Whom the Gods wish to destroy they first make mad."[116] The next sentence noted that, just when Gage thought everything was all right, a new case of plague occurred in Chinatown. It referred to the ongoing denial and covering up of the facts by the political, commercial interests and press as "Kinyounism,"[117] a term previously used derogatorily against him.[118]

On January 15, it wrote a full-page article defying the governor under the headline:

TRUTH IS MIGHTIER EVEN THAN CALIFORNIA EXECUTIVE.
Facts Which Henry Theophilus Gage May as Well Try to Drown as to Stop the Rising of the Sun.[119]

The story gave a complete history of the crisis. It rebutted all contentions by the governor, including the five San Francisco newspapers and others like Drs. Mouser and Pillsbury, who had decided plague did not exist. The *Bee* slammed the newspapers, blaming them for the debacle and charging a conspiracy between them, the state board of health, the commercial sector and Gage, in order to protect the city's and state's prosperity.[120]

Concerning Kinyoun, it went to great lengths to clear his name and reputation, citing all the leading giants in the medical profession he had studied with, including Dr. Kitasato, who along with Dr. Yersin had discovered the menace. It set forth many of his contributions, including his work on diphtheria.[121]

The article took an intense swipe at Gage for conjuring up falsehoods. One example in particular was the claim that plague samples had been transported in someone's pocket to Kinyoun and therefore must have escaped en route. By this tale, it created an admission to the plague's presence by Gage and his cohorts. But no, it did not exist in their eyes, even though they as much as as admitted it by this contention.[122]

In conclusion, the paper wrote:

> The danger to the commercial interests is not the truth shall be reported and proper precautions taken, but that the idea shall prevail the truth is being suppressed for the sake of present sales and that Californians are willing to jeopardize the health of the Nation in the interests of commercialism.
>
> That idea is justified by the course of Governor Gage and the only result can be a lack of confidence on the part of the Eastern market that will cut down the sales of California fruits for years to come.[123]

And as to the doctor, it opined:

> Such attacks as have been made upon Dr. Kinyoun simply hold the State up to the contempt of the outside world and weaken its prestige. Attempts to suppress the truth result only in rumor that is far worse than the facts warrant and the sooner this principle is recognized the better it will be for the future of the State, commercially and otherwise.[124]

The *Honolulu Republican* also came to his defense with "Still Roaring About the Bubonic Plague."[125] The story reiterated fact after fact as to his credibility and the faith in his actions by the surgeon general and numerous highly regarded members of the medical profession. It noted that he had previously recommended that a committee of the most respected physicians be formed to review his findings.[126]

The paper took issue with Gage's claim that his actions had been vindictive with the sole design of damaging the state's reputation. What motive would he have had for such action, the paper asked, and how would he ever profit from such a deed, especially when all the commercial and political interests of the state were against him?[127]

Another paper ran a story titled "Bubonic Plague Conference."[128] It reported that at a conference of 19 state boards of health, all voted unanimously to censure the California State Board of Health, citing it "for a gross neglect of duty."[129] In recalling

Gage's address to the legislature, he proposed a reorganization of the state's health boards putting them under the control of the state board of health. If passed, the governor's proposal would censure these boards, since all communications to the public would henceforth go through the state health board, thereby potentially silencing them.

Other well-known publications supporting Kinyoun and the pro-plague factions included the *Occidental Medical Times* and the *Pacific Medical Journal*.[130] With all the ruckus something had to be done—and done quickly—to settle the matter. Otherwise, the present state of affairs would likely turn hostile.

The Commission

Dr. White wired Wyman on January 12, advising that various parties would support a presidential plague commission.[131] This hopefully would be respected by all sides of the controversy. On January 15, he cabled Wyman recommending Drs. Barker and Flexner as having the necessary "clinical knowledge"[132] to be commissioners. He also advised that another victim had died from the disease.[133] Wyman responded that Barker and Flexner had accepted the invitation, but that he was still waiting on Professor Novy's response.[134]

With these recommendations, Treasury Secretary Gage issued a "Letter of Appointment"[135] on January 19, creating a special commission to determine "the existence or non-existence of bubonic plague in.... San Francisco."[136] The appointees consisted of Professor Simon Flexner from the University of Pennsylvania, Professor F.G. Novy from the University of Michigan and Professor L.F. Barker from the University of Chicago, all eminent doctors and well versed in bacteriology.[137] They had been chosen for several important reasons. First, none of them had any connection to the government or the Marine Hospital Service. Next, none of them had had any association with the quandary in San Francisco. With these credentials, the hope was that the commission would be favorably received and viewed as impartial.

On January 23, Wyman informed the gentlemen of their appointment. He directed them to proceed to San Francisco forthwith, where accommodations awaited them at the Occidental Hotel. They were to conduct an unbiased, independent investigation as to the presence—or lack thereof—of plague. He recommended the University of California as a laboratory.[138]

They were to complete their mission in two or three weeks. Wyman instructed that, upon reaching a conclusion, they were to set forth their findings in a report written by the commission's recorder and signed by its chairman. Afterwards, the chairman would wire the finding to the Service and not divulge any of its contents until advised otherwise. Any expenses were to be paid out of pocket and submitted on vouchers for reimbursement.[139] Wyman further requested that they "pay their respects"[140] to the governor and mayor.[141]

Before commencing their work they selected officers, with Dr. Flexner as the commission's chair, Barker as the recorder and Novy as the bacteriologist. Flexner and Barber had received much of their training at Johns Hopkins Hospital.[142] Novy was an "organic"[143] chemist and, like Kinyoun, had studied abroad at the Pasteur Institute and with Dr. Koch.[144]

Two days later Senator Perkins informed Governor Gage that a special commission had been appointed by the Treasury Department to investigate and render an unbiased opinion regarding the situation. He stated that they were independent of any governmental agency and would not engage or converse with the public about their research and findings. Perkins informed him that they had researched the plague in India and China and knowledgeable about the malady from a microscopic and clinical standpoint. Upon the completion of their investigation, a report would be sent to Washington for review.[145]

Perkins revealed that the commission had been ordered at the request of states bordering California and not because of some impending harm. If the findings proved positive, then the need for corrective action would be necessitated to quell it before it became uncontrollable. The senator advised that the matter needed to be handled prudently and to date had been kept confidential with no mention to the area newspapers.[146]

It did not take long for Gage to express his indignation to the point that he sent McKinley a telegram voicing his disapproval along with a list of demands. He requested the state's participation and the inclusion of his choice of experts not only from within the country but internationally. And as before, he singled out Kinyoun as the central cause for all the ill will and damage caused to the state.[147] The following day, Treasury Secretary Gage responded on behalf of the president. The commission would proceed unimpeded by any additional members. All of them were regarded as authorities and would be acting independently of the doctor and other parties.[148] He stated that the members would be calling on him shortly and no "discourtesy"[149] had been intended by the commission's appointment. Its final report would be sent to him.[150]

Initially, White had been asked by Wyman to conclude his investigation within 2–3 weeks. However, this changed in light of the commission and Gage's letter to the president. As a result, Wyman asked White if he would remain in San Francisco.[151] White agreed.[152]

Gage tuned a deaf ear to the Treasury Secretary's response. He immediately leaned upon the University of California to cancel the commission's use of its laboratory. In another letter to McKinley, he proposed a commission comprised of three federal and three California appointees having the requisite scientific and medical background. The secretary replied that there would not be another commission. Faced with this rebuke, Gage took a different step and called on the legislature to abolish the commission.[153]

The Work Begins

By the end of January, all the commissioners had arrived in San Francisco and settled into the Occidental Hotel. They promptly began their investigation, and Flexner reported to Wyman that the members had met with the city's officials and approached the governor about meeting. Gage initially declined, but on February 16, he met with them. Flexner asked for a per diem allowance of $8.00 to purchase rats from areas alleged to be containing plague. The rodents would be examined for the disease as part of their investigation, which also included visits to those areas of Chinatown where people had been reported sick or had died.[154]

The commissioners set up a bureau in the hotel where individuals could meet with them and discuss the plague starting at 11:00 a.m. every morning. The press publicized their accessibility, which opened many doors for them with the various businesses and other private interests in the community. They also sent out letters to numerous doctors seeking an audience or their opinion about the disease's existence. Many responses were received, with varying opinions expressed. By this process, they learned how to approach the Chinese and earn their trust, so they would be allowed to examine victims.[155]

This approach led to the main commercial interests offering their welcome and working with them. These entities included the Chamber of Commerce, the Board of Trade, the Merchants Association, the Manufacturers and Producers Association, the Pacific Coast Jobbers and Manufacturers Association, the Southern Pacific Railway and the Pacific Mail Steamship Company. The city also assisted them by letting them use a room at City Hall as their laboratory.[156] It seemed that everyone wanted to cooperate so the crisis could come to a resolution.

More importantly, the Chinese Six Companies stepped forward and offered its assistance.[157] It issued a proclamation to all the Chinese advising them to report

> … all cases of sickness and death, no matter what the cause, to the offices of the Chinese Six Companies in order that daily inspections might be made.[158]

The Companies' secretary, Mr. Wong Chung, acting as interpreter, would accompany Dr. Barker on his daily inspections of reported victims and help in determining their "histories."[159] Later, the commissioners complimented the Companies for their assistance and stated that they "acted in good faith and that they made every attempt to give access to the sick."[160]

The task before them was not easy. Chinatown covered 14 blocks and they had only two or three weeks to conduct their investigation. As part of their findings, they provided an overview of the Chinese and their accommodations.[161] They gave special emphasis to the poorer Chinese; they found that within their dwellings the "rooms are small … shockingly unsanitary.… Devoid of light or means of ventilation … insufficiently lighted … filthy … situated in basements … damp and emit a foul stench."[162] They found most of the inhabitants to be well fed and clothed with many making good wages. To the contrary, though, they noticed a sizable number of prostitutes and many others smoking opium.[163]

By February 16, the commissioners had examined 13 cases. This concluded their investigation.[164] They wrote their report, containing a map pinpointing all the cases, and forwarded their findings to Wyman on February 26.[165] It contained an analysis of each case documenting the person's symptoms, length of illness, death, postmortem procedures and the victim's location. In some instances, postmortem examinations that required samples of blood and tissue were difficult to perform because the relatives did not want any desecration to the body. This had been a long-standing part of Chinese culture. But for the most part, they obtained enough samples to determine the cause of death.[166]

Upon receipt of the various tissues, they would be transported to the lab, where cultures were made on agar-agar. Following these procedures, the commissioners inoculated guinea pigs with the tissue samples. Any remaining tissues were put in alcohol and saved for future examination. After reviewing the evidence, they found six or possibly seven of the 13 cases to be bubonic plague.[167] The last sentence in their report read,

> The bacteriological examination of the foregoing 6 cases has, therefore, demonstrated the presence of the bacillus pestis in each.[168]

Finally, an independent group had established that the plague did exist in Chinatown. Kinyoun had finally been proven right.

XVI

The Price of Truth

The Papers Respond

While the commission began its fact-finding mission, the press continued to perpetrate its plague fabrications. At the same time, the governor, acting as the main anti-plague antagonist, continued his web of denials.

Several papers, however, took a different view. *The Bee* reported on January 31:

GOVERNOR GAGE UP TO HIS OLD TRICKS.[1]

It stated that after having insulted the president, he asked the legislature for:

> ... legislation as radical as that which was passed by the State of South Carolina and which initiated the Civil War.[2]

Gage had become desperate in trying to impede the truth, especially with the new commission starting its work. As a result, he proposed three bills to thwart not only the truth, but the commission as well. The first of these "Kinyoun Bills"[3] called for Kinyoun's removal, the second would create a revamped supreme state health board, and the third aimed to make it a felony to make false reports about the plague's presence.[4]

The Honolulu Republican, which had previously questioned Kinyoun's actions, ran a five-layer headline stating:

STILL ROARING ABOUT THE BUBONIC PLAGUE
Kinyoun Now Making an Effort for His Vindication.
SURGEON-GENERAL GIVES SUPPORT
Much Roasted Doctor Gets a Fair Share of Official Sympathy.
Meanwhile the San Francisco Press Lie Quiet and Patiently Wait the Raising of the Quarantine Officer's Head—All Kinds of Bluffs.[5]

While the headline was less than flattering, it did not represent the substance of the article. To the contrary, it inclined to admonish Kinyoun's distractors and offered an objective segment about the current state of the plague debacle. For once, a skeptical newspaper presented a balanced analysis of his role in this early 20th-century version of a Shakespearian tragedy.

It noted that Dr. White, who had been sent to survey the situation for Wyman, praised Kinyoun "in the highest possible terms,"[6] contrary to what the San Francisco newspapers thought about him. The story pointed out that rumors of his creating false plague reports to profit from the crisis proved untrue (what could he possibly gain monetarily?). Besides, no evidence existed to substantiate such a claim. As to the allegation that Wyman had lost faith in his abilities, it too proved false: Wyman acknowledged Kinyoun's plague count of 15 deaths.[7]

But other newspapers continued their attack. *The Bulletin* took aim on February 1, with the headline:

KINYOUN'S PLAGUE NOT UNDERSTOOD
Wild Stories Published in Sacramento Make Uniformed Legislators Doubtful.[8]

The Call on February 12 reported on the Kinyoun Bills' progress in the Senate:

COMMITTEE SIDES WITH GOVERNOR
Favorable Report on Health Bills to Senate.[9]

The article stated that the Judiciary Committee had approved the bills and sent them to the Senate for approval.[10]

On February 13, *The Bulletin* announced the group's findings under the headline:

"BUBONIC" BILLS ARE RECEIVED FAVORABLY
Partial Triumph Scored in Assembly by Friends
Of the Plague Measures.[11]

Although these headlines appeared to support these bills, they were debated at length with various amendments offered to secure their passage. The felony bill received a backlash from several House members, who, being journalists, felt that the proposed legislation trampled on press freedom.[12] Another bill sought $100,000 to clean up diseased areas.[13] The cleanup bill all but acknowledged the plague's existence, but was crafted cleverly to cover all contagions, for the probable purpose of avoiding its mentioning.

In support of Kinyoun, *The Evening Bee* continued to provide plague evidence. On February 15, the paper printed a large diagram with an accompanying headline on its front page, reading:

WHERE THE BUBONIC CASES WERE DISCOVERED.
Plan of Chinatown which Effectively Proves the Falsity of the
Assertion That the Cases Have Been Widely Separated.[14]

The map pinpointed the sites of 29 cases confirmed since March 6, 1900. It listed all the victims' names and addresses. The article stated that its drawing should establish once and for all that the cases had not been widely separated, but were instead closely connected by location. The victims were mainly in Chinatown, proving them not to be isolated cases.[15] It showed that the majority of them had occurred "in the block bounded by Stockton, Jackson, DuPont and Washington Streets, particularly east of Stout's Alley."[16] The landmark in the area was the Old Chinese Theater.[17]

Several days later, news surfaced that the commissioners had in fact found and examined several plague cases. On February 18, *The Evening Bee* ran a very large, top center, bold print headline reading:

FEDERAL PLAGUE COMMISSION HAS PRACTICALLY FINISHED.
Its Members Have Found Three Cases of Bubonic Plague
Themselves and Have Attended Autopsies on Six in
All—White Held Here to Await Results of Report.[18]

The story took issue with a recent report in *The Call*, where it maintained that the commissioners after three weeks had not uncovered any evidence of the disease. It also stated Gage had hired detectives and others to spy on them. The article revealed that, to the contrary, several cases of plague had been discovered during their examinations. Furthermore, Commissioner Barker had been feared to have contracted the contagion after investigating a case. To everyone's relief, it proved not to be plague, but a reaction he had to the Yersin vaccine. *The Bee* remained steadfast in chastising Gage over his denials and circumventing the commissioners. It noted that if he was not careful, the government could quarantine the state.[19]

On January 28, *The Evening Bee* in another center page column with abnormally large bold type print wrote:

GOVERNOR GAGE FEARS INVESTIGATION OF THE PLAGUE.
After Having Officially Stated That He Knows There
Never Was Any Bubonic Plague in San Francisco,
He Is Moving Heaven and Earth to Put Off
Any Inquiry Into Facts.[20]

The article praised the intrepidness of Kinyoun's efforts and scolded Gage for trying to cover it up. It described his stance as "pitiable"[21] for placing the state in such a position and called for his censorship.[22] Now confronted with a federal investigation by three of the country's leading medical scientists, he had boxed himself into a corner.

Early on, when the disease had become certain, Kinyoun had originally offered the governor a list of 12 to 20 "prominent scientists"[23] from which to select and conduct a separate investigation to verify his findings. He even offered to pay the expenses. Gage rejected his offer because he did not want to advertise even the possibility of its existence. But soon the matter had reached national attention.[24]

The Governor's Commission

Although the situation started turning in Kinyoun's favor, the governor had not finished trying to undermine the commission. At the 11th hour, on February 26, he established his own plague panel. Unlike the Treasury's quarantine commission, a question of impartiality could be asked, because three of its members were from of the anti-plague faction: Freemont Older from *The Bulletin*, T.T. Williams of *The Examiner*, and John P. Young with *The Chronicle*. In addition, it included H.T. Scott from the Union Iron Works and William F. Herrin of the Southern Pacific Railroad, plus Dr. S.M. Mouser from the state board of health as bacteriologist. Older, Williams and Young represented the three main newspapers denying the plague, while Scott and Herrin represented major commercial interests.[25]

Their first order of business was going to Washington and meet with Wyman. The group met on March 9 with Secretary Gage, Assistant Secretary Spaulding and Wyman. During their meeting, the parties reached an agreement on how to handle the crisis. On the same day, a flurry of correspondence occurred between the parties.[26]

Spaulding initiated the exchange by sending Chairman Young a letter from the surgeon general outlining the meeting's major points. The key elements included the state and local governments paying for the cleanup of Chinatown and any other areas.[27] He also stated that the intent of the government had been to cause minimum disruption to the commercial interests while at the same time keeping the matter from "the least possible excitement and alarm."[28] Lastly, Dr. White would be the Service's official supervisor.[29]

Wyman wired White stating that the situation in San Francisco did not compare to Glasgow, Santos, Oporto and Calcutta, where major outbreaks had occurred. He asked him to continue the assessments, disinfections and isolations as necessary, similar to those procedures conducted for smallpox.[30] As a result, Kinyoun had effectively been removed from any further duties, except those on Angel Island.

Following this development, Older apparently sent a telegram to Governor Gage reporting that "an agreement"[31] had been reached that would be to his satisfaction. The cable stated that White would represent the Service and no buildings would be destroyed as part of the deal. Of particular interest, he related that he had "spent an hour with President."[32] Previously, there had not been any traceable evidence of President McKinley's participation. To the contrary, in dispatches between White and Wyman, the latter had downplayed appointing a presidential commission, probably to keep him out of the matrix. However, by Older's reference, he had very much become involved in the matter.

A day before, the *Oroville Mercury* had released a story about the agreement under the headline:

SAN FRANCISCO HAS BUBONIC PLAHUE [sic].
Federal Commission Gives Result of Investigation.
GAGE TURNS TURTLE.
Confronted by a condition of Gravest Character,
The Governor Falls in Line.[33]

The article disclosed that its information had been received from a reporter with *The Bee* claiming the governor had finally admitted to the plague's presence. It stated he had agreed to partner with local and federal officials towards its eradication. The expense shared between the state and San Francisco approached $50,000.[34]

It exposed that the commissioners had told Mayor Phelan in a meeting ordered by Wyman the substance of their findings and the prevention measures needed for its containment. They stated that six victims and possibly a seventh had died from *Y. pestis*.[35] The panel said the situation was "a serious one and should be met with prompt action."[36] They recommended that the city

> ... depopulate Chinatown, form a detention hospital and that in the end it would probably be necessary to destroy the entire section. No half way measures would wipe out the disease.[37]

Stressing the gravity,

> one of the Commissioners stated that authorities could not afford to let a single Chinese body be buried without the most critical examination.[38]

The mysterious aspect about this article rested in its date: March 8, a day before Governor Gage's commissioners met with the government's representatives in

Washington. Somehow, *The Bee* had gotten a jump on the scoop and had released its findings to other newspapers. How could this have happened prior to their meeting on March 9, and the passing of official correspondence on the same date? It would appear as if the whole plan had been pre-determined prior to the arrival of Gage's representatives in the capital. Had Wyman and Secretary Gage been back peddling the plague since its arrival the year before? And had a conspiracy prior to the fact been created to deflate the seriousness of the malady in hopes of quieting the press and the special interest groups? One must entertain this possibility.

Other newspapers ran stories, including the *Fresno Evening Democrat*, which printed its opinion about Gage's meeting with the government's health hierarchy:

BUBONIC PLAGUE.
A REPORT MADE TO THE TREASURY DEPARTMENT.
San Franciscans in Washington, Conferring with the Federal Officials.[39]

The paper noted that the submission of the Treasury commission's report to the surgeon general resulted in Gage's commission arriving in Washington "almost simultaneously."[40] The rush in their arrival imparted their wanting to obstruct the report's contents.[41]

Afterwards, the newspaper printed a statement by the Gage commission acknowledging a difference in findings between the two boards. This account was preceded by a statement that Gage, Spaulding and Wyman indicated there had not been any new cases and all the other diseases had not been contagious with none being Caucasian.[42]

The final section of the statement represented quite a definitive change in the government's position as to past events in San Francisco. Substantiating this claim, Spaulding had issued a separate statement that "the existence of bubonic plague in San Francisco should excite no alarm there or in the country."[43] He stated it had not been epidemic, nor would it be, and he "would feel [as] safe living in San Francisco as in Washington."[44] In concluding, he remarked that there should not be any alarm as to the health of the city.[45]

This article shed several lights on the rapidly changing position of the government and the Service. With Spaulding's comments downplaying the plague, Kinyoun had become marginalized, meaning his tenure in California would shortly come to an end. It appeared that Gage's commission had achieved its goal of compromising not only the truth, but the government as well.

Betrayal, Cover-Up and Vindication

On March 15, Kinyoun received letter marked "Confidential" in the upper left corner from Wyman. It consisted of seven parts with the first section rebutting Kinyoun's earlier claim that the surgeon general had failed to give an update in the Service's annual report about the preceding year's number of plague victims. Wyman argued that was not true because they had been set forth in the Service's quarterly reports. Next, he acknowledged the number of plague cases between January 6, 1901 and March 2, 1901.[46]

The ensuing four paragraphs constitute the premise of the letter and set forth Wyman's suppression of the plague crisis going forward in alignment with the wants of Governor Gage's commission. He stated that

> The Bureau and Treasury Department are endeavoring to bring about harmonious action between the State and City Boards of Health, the Mayor of San Francisco and Governor of California.[47]

Because of the governor's denial of plague in his January address to the California legislature and his subsequent sending of a commission to Washington, Wyman wrote that the parties had agreed to work in harmony towards curtailing its presence under the supervision of Dr. White.[48] Furthermore, he is convinced "of the necessity of not giving out for publication all the facts in the case."[49] It was his hope that "by avoiding unnecessary publicity"[50] he would be able to rectify the plague situation in San Francisco,[51] but the agreement did not preclude him from "freely giving the facts when it seems necessary to do so."[52]

Wyman postulated that previous open communication had led to the present situation. It was now his hope and belief that eradication efforts would be undertaken with a positive outcome. He acknowledged that Kinyoun knew the everyday statistics about the plague as he did, but directed him not to release any of the information to the public.[53] In essence, the surgeon general had placed a gag order on him. At the end of his letter, he recommended Kinyoun review the public health reports issued of same date, covering a report by Mr. H. de. Brun of France and his dealing with the plague in Beirut.[54] Wyman noted it described his efforts

> … showing the distinction to be drawn with regard to danger, measures to be taken, etc., between the pneumonic and bubonic forms of the disease. So far as known at the present time, the disease in San Francisco is of the Bubonic form.[55]

Kinyoun responded to Wyman on May 28 with his letter marked "Personal."[56] It read:

> Dear Sir:—
>
> I return the enclosure to your letter of March 15th, marked "confidential."
> I cannot be interested in anything which compromises and humiliates the Service.
>
> J. J. Kinyoun[57]

Wyman's letter signaled the Service's capitulation to the truth and his surrender to the anti-plague factions, in particular Governor Gage. No longer would the facts be forthcoming, but only when politically expedient. Kinyoun had been sold out by his boss and in essence removed from his position by the appointment of Dr. White. Even worse, Wyman had muzzled him, so he could not interfere in the situation going forward. More significantly, it showed that he had caved in to the California anti-plague factions, right when he knew that the Treasury Department's plague commission had determined that the plague did exist.

It appeared that political cronyism had finally prevailed and the truth would be if not damned, at least curtailed at Wyman's discretion. Adding further insult to Kinyoun, he sent him a pamphlet making an apparent distinction between bubonic and pneumonic plague for his information. If anyone would have known the difference between them, it would have been Kinyoun more so than Wyman. For the most part it had remained as the bubonic type, but the doctor knew full well that it could and likely would convert to the pneumonic version in time. The world had now turned upside down as to the truth.

The day after Wyman's letter to Kinyoun, the truth finally succumbed to the deadly venom of yellow journalism, commercialism and back-room politics. *The Bee* acknowledged its passing with a fitting obituary:

INFAMOUS COMPACT SIGNED BY WYMAN.
Makes Agreement with Gage Not to Let Facts Become Known,
Contrary to Federal Law—Public Must Not Know Exactly How
The Situation Stands.[58]

The paper outlined the five elements of the agreement: First, "the report of the Federal Plague Commission ... shall not be made public."[59] Second, the Marine Hospital Service will report nothing about the plague in San Francisco, Washington, "or elsewhere"[60] and any and all reports from the Service concerning plague and its origins will be censored by the Service. Third, the newspapers in San Francisco have agreed not to publish anything about its existence or non-existence. Fourth, the newspapers and Governor Gage agreed not to further attack Dr. Kinyoun.[61] And fifth, Gage will aid in the cleaning of Chinatown and it will be conducted "as quietly and as free from publicity as possible."[62]

The Bee challenged the pact as unlawful. It cited Section 4 of the 1893 Federal Quarantine Act, which stated that the surgeon general "shall"[63] release all reports and findings of the nation's health. He does not have any discretion under the statute and therefore must comply with the law.[64] It stated that Wyman's stance was difficult to comprehend since he had "never handled an epidemic disease, either a single disease or a dozen."[65] Furthermore, the Service's standing as a reputable institution existed because of those officers and their knowledge under Wyman's command.[66] And "it would seem that the folly of his stand should be at once apparent."[67]

The paper noted that the Service had proven its ability countless times before by its staff. These individuals had guarded the country against epidemics of smallpox, yellow fever and cholera, proving their sense of duty and knowledge in handling these public health ills. Ironically, in the detection and control of all these maladies, Kinyoun had been the trailblazer. It reported that Wyman's actions represented "a complete stultification of his office and a blow at the Service itself."[68]

It stressed that the rest of the nation and countries like Mexico bordering California have an absolute right to know the truth for their protection. Finally, it maintained that Kinyoun possessed definitive documentation as to his findings that completely vindicated him. But the article labeled both Gage and the San Francisco newspapers as incompetent, vindictive towards him and falsifiers of his findings.[69]

Wyman's agreement with Gage's representatives would soon backfire. On March 23, *The Bee* reported under yet another banner headline:

GOVERNOR GAGE HAS BEEN FORCED TO ACT.
Texas Compels Him to Back Down from His Plague Position. Agrees to
Take Quarantine Measures in Chinatown.[70]

Several days before, the governor of Texas had threatened the federal government that he would impose the strictest quarantine possible against California. As a result, Gage jumped a train, gathered up his cohorts along with a few others and proceeded to San Francisco to address this new threat. A press release followed, stating that Gage had met with Mayor Phelan and other officials, and they had agreed that because of a lack funds in San Francisco, the state would pick up the tab for cleaning Chinatown and enforcing the state's health regulations.[71]

The article chided the governor, stating that his acts of suppression had done nothing but cause irreversible harm to the state and that, if he did not address the problem, other quarantines would be imposed against the state by the likes of Colorado, Texas and "one of the Dakotas."[72] In closing, it wrote:

> To-day [sic], in matters concerning the public health the real Governor of the State of California and the true friend of this State is the Governor of the State of Texas.[73]

Three days later, it ran another article, titled

> OTHER STATES DEMAND SUPPRESSED PLAGUE REPORT.
> Inform Surgeon-General Wyman That They Will Not Tolerate
> Violation of Their Rights—The Eastern Press Aroused.[74]

Although similar in its previous condemnation of Wyman's refusal to release the commission report, it pointed out several other important considerations in denying its release. It reported that every American state had requested a copy of it, citing the law requiring its release. As to the severity of the disease, it claimed it to be of the contagious type, with a 100 percent mortality rate, contrary to other accounts. Along with this revelation, the article took him to task for his failure to publish the findings.[75]

The Eastern press had also reacted in a negative way to the cover-up. It quoted the *New York Sun*, the *Seattle Post-Intelligencer* and the disapproval of other states. More importantly, it claimed the act to be a violation of the Vienna Convention, which required total openness about issues of sanitation, quarantines involving infectious diseases and epidemics. The standard practice had always been a complete disclosure of one nation's health to others.[76]

After much criticism, Wyman released the commission report in one of the Service's regular periodic publications. Apparently the delay had been attributed to allowing Governor Gage's commission enough time to meet with him, Secretary Gage and Spaulding.[77]

During this time, Kinyoun had reached out to Commissioner Lewellys Barker asking for the return of various papers he had given to him as part of the investigation. Barker stated that Wyman wanted to see them before their return and since Wyman had not seen them yet he would write the surgeon general asking that they be forwarded to him. The professor apologized for the postponement in releasing the commissioners' report, citing international reasons for the delay. He stated, though, that Wyman had promised that its release would be forthcoming.[78] As a testament to Kinyoun, he ended the letter with a tribute, writing:

> I do hope that the time will come when we shall have the opportunity to show how much we appreciate your work and how glad we should all be to see a lot of you.[79]

No.	Name.	Age.	Sex.	Color.	Place of death.	Date of death, 1900.
1	Wing Chut King	41	Male	Mongolian	1001 Dupont	March 6.
2	Chu Gan	22	....do	.....do	723 Sacramento	March 15.
3	Ng Ach Ging	37	....do	.....do	905 Dupont	March 17.
4	Lee Sun King	47	....do	.....do	Oneida place	March 18.
5	Law An	38	....do	.....do	St. Louis alley	April 24.
6	Lim Fa Muey	16	Female	.....do	739 Clay street	May 11.
7	Chu Sam	38	Male	.....do	717 Jackson	Do.
8	Chin Moon	16	Female	.....do	730½ Commercial	May 13.
9	Her Woon Jock	53	Male	.....do	740 Pacific	May 14.
10	Dang Hong	40	....do	.....do	706 Pacific	May 29.
11	Chen Kney Kim	49	....do	.....do	819 Clay	June 2.
12	Jay Man Tong	60	....do	.....do	759 Clay	June 9.
13	Lee Wing Tong	40	....do	.....do	767 Clay	July 6.
14	William Murphy	34	....do	White	427 Dupont	August 11.
15	Ham Tan	29	....do	Mongolian	900 Dupont	August 15.
16	Lea Do Hen	50	....do	.....do	710½ Dupont	October 5.
17	Chun Yen	37	....do	.....do	767 Clay	October 10.
18	Taik Dong Leong	39	....do	.....do	705 Clay	October 14.
19	Young Moon Li Chee	30	Female	.....do	802 Dupont	October 31.
20	Young Wah Noui	9	....do	.....do	802 Dupont	November 1.
21	Anne Roede	28	....do	White	Pacific Hospital	November 3.
22	Lee Ho	30	Male	Mongolian	844 Washington	December 7.
23	Chun Wey Lung	60	....do	.....do	780 Jackson	January 6, 1901.
24	Leam Wing Low	59	....do	.....do	633½ Clay	January 15.
25	Angela Colombo		....do	White	5 Lafayette place	Do.
26	Chun Ah Chou *a*	44	....do	Mongolian	814 Washington	February 5.
27	Lum Hong Yuen *a*	37	....do	.....do	28 Ross alley	February 6.
28	Wong Chi Lin *a*	50	....do	.....do	15½ Waverley	February 7.
29	Tom Shom *a*	51	....do	.....do	814 Washington	February 10.
30	Ng Ah Back *a*	45	....do	.....do	St. Louis alley	February 11.
31	Foong Ah Fong *a*	12	Female	.....do	747 Sacramento st	February 12.

Plague roster: commissioners' list and Kinyoun's.

In a postscript, two months later, Wyman wrote to Kinyoun asking whether he had received the papers from Dr. Baker; if not, he said, he would send them to him.[80]

On April 15, *The Bee* wrote a detailed article about the commission's findings under the headline

PLAGUE REPORT AT LAST SEES LIGHT OF DAY.
Surgeon-General Wyman Fails in His Attempt to Suppress Statements
of the Federal Commission—Vindication of Kinyoun.[81]

After a month cover-up, *The Bee* and the *Occidental Medical Times*, the main plague advocates, gained access to the commissioners' report. It confirmed once and for all the plague's existence. The article covered almost the entire front page of the paper and part of the second, leaving no detail untold. In many respects, it represented a microcosm of the account highlighting the more significant findings and a listing of all the cases examined during the investigation. The report, though, still had not been released to the public by Wyman. Somehow, these papers had received a copy.[82] *The Bee* stated that the findings represented an "absolute vindication"[83] of its reporting, the *Occidental Medical Times* and in particular Kinyoun,

> ... against whom a most outrageous and cowardly attack was made and continued by Governor Gage, the San Francisco newspapers and the San Francisco commercial interests.[84]

At last, the truth had won the day. He had now been vindicated, but at what cost to the citizens of Chinatown, San Francisco, California, the credibility of science, the Marine Hospital Service and his reputation? Many lives had been lost during the uproar, and the seeds of the plague had now become permanent on the continent. As to Kinyoun, it probably seemed like a hollow victory after all he had been through. His standing and career would at best be described as tarnished, if not destroyed. However, it had been his sense of duty because he knew the consequences, if the situation did not improve. The most disappointing thing about the entire matter had been Wyman's lack of loyalty to him. This had to have been especially painful after all their years of close professional affiliation.

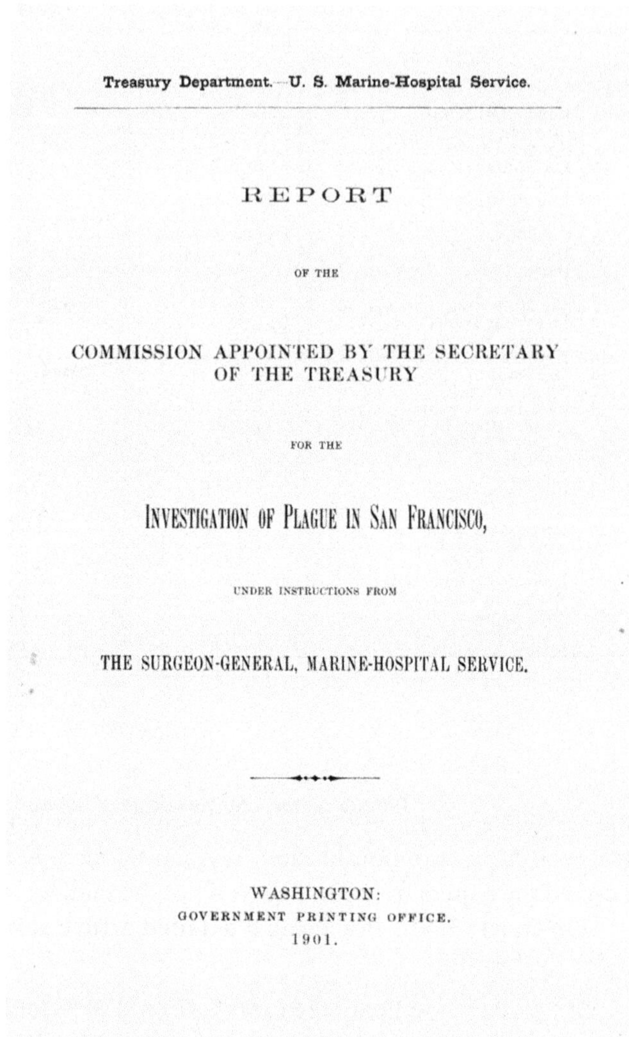
Treasury Department. U. S. Marine-Hospital Service.

REPORT

OF THE

COMMISSION APPOINTED BY THE SECRETARY OF THE TREASURY

FOR THE

INVESTIGATION OF PLAGUE IN SAN FRANCISCO,

UNDER INSTRUCTIONS FROM

THE SURGEON-GENERAL, MARINE-HOSPITAL SERVICE.

WASHINGTON:
GOVERNMENT PRINTING OFFICE.
1901.

Report of the Commission Appointed by the Secretary of the Treasury for the Investigation of Plague in San Francisco, Under Instructions from the Surgeon-General, Marine-Hospital Service. Washington, D.C.: Government Printing Office, 1901.

Political Reasoning and Aftermath

Governor Gage and President McKinley were Republicans. No direct evidence has been found of the two discussing the California plague. But did such a conversation occur, especially with the downplaying of the situation by Spaulding and Wyman after meeting with Gage's commission? In all probability, the answer is yes, especially in light of Commissioner Older from Gage's group having spent an hour with him. With so many parties involved in such a high-stakes dance of life and death, the president would have had to be part of the conversation.

After a year of bitter controversy and name calling, Wyman, Spaulding, Secretary Gage and McKinley may have decided to change the government's approach in trying to win over the anti-plague faction by taking a different route. Instead of arguing over the plague's existence, the focus changed to its cleanup. This would rectify the further spread of the contagion and at the same time omit any reference to it, allowing the naysayers to save some face, especially Governor Gage.

With this said, the opposing sides were left with a little pride and finally a symbolic resolution. A compromise had been reached with the underlying hope that life might return to a semblance of normal. Nonetheless, in any protracted controversy there usually has to be a loser. In this case, the casualty of this less than forthright comprise was Kinyoun. However, at this point no one really cared anymore because political cronyism and cynicism had won.

Moving On

As part of the compromise, Kinyoun would be expatriated from San Francisco and transferred to Detroit.[85] From there, his future remained uncertain. Fortunately, he had his own plans. During the waning days of the diabolical plague play, he had not been sitting idly by waiting for the proverbial last shoe to fall. He had been job searching, as evidenced by a letter in March from Milton Campbell, president of the H.K. Mulford Company.[86] The organization had become well known as a pharmaceutical company for its manufacture of serums and anti-toxins.[87]

It seemed he had inquired about employment opportunities. Campbell responded with an offer of $4,500 for the first year and $5,000 a year for the next four, conditioned on each party's satisfaction.[88] He wrote, "We believe that you would be of inestimable value to us in carrying out this high grade work."[89] The only caveat rested on his early acceptance of the position because the company had been considering the hiring of a prominent bacteriologist from Germany.[90]

Also during this period, on April 25, he had wired Wyman requesting a four-month leave of absence to accept an invitation to visit the Orient. He had been asked to study tropical illnesses.[91] In his opinion, it represented a onetime opportunity, and he felt it his duty, "both officially and professionally,"[92] to accept the offer.

Over the course of the next eight months, numerous letters would be exchanged between Kinyoun and Campbell. On May 1, Campbell congratulated him for his leave of absence to study in the Far East. He wanted to know when the doctor could start upon his return and wrote that he would raise his starting salary by $500 to $5,000. Campbell summarized his understanding of the terms for Kinyoun's trip to Asia, noting that if the Service denied this request, he could resign his commission and the Mulford Company would pay his expenses to Asia.[93] Upon his return, he would take over the company's "bacteriological laboratory."[94]

During the first week of May, when making arrangements to leave San Francisco, he was charged with attempted murder. As luck would have it, a deaf-mute fisherman accused him of having had several men fire their rifles at him while fishing offshore. Ironically, he had previously vaccinated the man. He hid in an army compound for several days before finally giving himself up to the authorities.[95] In this escapade, he received a letter from Wyman stating that he could not believe "so absurd a charge should have been made."[96] Wyman offered any necessary legal assistance and hoped the matter would be quickly resolved.[97]

He could not believe it either, but for once, luck appeared to be on his side. The police soon released him because they learned that an escapee being hunted by the military had fired several shots in the direction of the fisherman. There had been some suspicion that the deaf-mute was an accomplice of the fleeing prisoner. Under testimony, the fisherman failed to identify the doctor. In fact, Kinyoun had actually tried to protect the man from the shooting.[98] With his name cleared, he headed to Detroit for a short stint before heading overseas.[99] At last, he had been freed from the ever-tormenting shackles of San Francisco and its unscrupulous blindness to the for brooding shadow of death hovering above its hordes.

Amidst this transition, he had been asked to address the California Medical Society in Sacramento. He gave a lengthy dissertation about his experiences in San Francisco, even quoting verses from Kipling. He reviewed many of the cases he had examined and discussed some of the difficulties in diagnosing the contagion. As part of the speech, he went through the preliminary stages of the contagion and addressed the problems with suppressing it. He referred to a similar situation in Holland, where in 1664 the commercial interests had suppressed its existence, only to have it break out "violently."[100] The *Occidental Medical Times* published his presentation in its August 1901 periodical.[101]

Before leaving, but still in the throws of the plague debacle, Kinyoun had been working the sidelines of Congress to establish a national health department. In the process, he had angered a long-standing friend, Dr. Young, by sharing a confidential letter of his concerning the department's creation. Young worked for the Treasury Department. He accused him of being part of an effort led by a Dr. MacCormac and other individuals prejudicing several of his friends through misrepresentations set forth in the letter. As a result, he demanded to know why its contents had been shared with MacCormac, Dr. Woodward and a Major Owen.[102]

Kinyoun responded bluntly to the accusation, stating that the release of its contents stemmed from Wyman's opposition to the creation of a "Department of Public Health."[103] He alluded to the surgeon general's stalling on Senate Bill 1968. Moreover, he explained that Wyman's and his support of another bill, which he called the "Dead Bill,"[104] had been presented at the House of Delegates meeting in Atlantic City, as opposed to SB 1968. This other bill had caused him to share its contents. He stated that he had been able to stop the proposal, known as the "Marre Bill."[105] He pointed out that

> ... Wyman would stop at nothing to prevent the AMA (American Medical Association) from taking action for a Department of Health.—& would use every device known to have the Marre Bill passed in order that he might stop any further legislation. Your letter shows this to be true.[106]

As shown by this exchange, Kinyoun continued to pursue the establishment of a public health department, separate from the Service and the United States Army. Up to this point, the Service and the Army had for the most part administered the nation's health. The former primarily addressed the entrance and control of infectious diseases, whereas the latter dealt with the well-being of the country's military.

Both governmental bodies had proven effective in their areas of responsibility.

But Kinyoun had always argued for an independent agency, solely responsible for the nation's health. While serving as the lab's director, he had advocated for such an entity several times in his annual reports. Wyman's reaction to the proposition had been neutral up until this time, but as evidenced by the exchanges between Kinyoun and Young, his opposition had become apparent.

On the surface, this correspondence would appear to have little value, except for the creation of a national health agency. Underneath, the exchange had a more important meaning because it showed him again challenging the system and his superior, regardless of personal risk. One thing about him remained constant: his unwavering convictions about the nation's best interests.

When he knew plague to be present, he firmly stood by his findings, and during his days at the lab, he knew that the best course for the nation's medical future rested in a separate omnipresent body overseeing the nation's health. This letter, although speaking to one issue, clearly demonstrated his stature because it revealed his real personality. He was not afraid to make his opinion known for what he thought best. Wyman likely opposed the proposition for several reasons. First, he may have felt someone else might supersede him. Second, the new agency might have eliminated his position. Probably, the real reason rested on his wanting to keep the Service as the nation's chief health bureau and retain, if not possibly increase, his level of authority.

Kinyoun and his detractors, including Wyman, had their own reasons for rising up against him. And in many respects, they were right in their opinions because the science of bacteriology represented a complicated subject to not only the public, but also his scientific and medical peers. It would take until the early 1920s, after the Great Influenza Pandemic of 1918, before these communities finally understood and embraced it.[107]

For him, it could be said he literally knew too much about the subject, and therefore it operated as his Achilles' heel in the end. Regardless, though, he had been proved right, and soon his efforts to create a national health agency would start to become a reality: in 1902, Congress changed the name of the Marine Hospital Service to the Public Health and Marine Hospital Service.[108] This would be followed in 1912 by Congress renaming it the Public Health Service.[109]

With all the whirlwind still surrounding him, some good news arrived on May 10, from the Association of American Physicians office in Washington, D.C. He received a letter from the organization's secretary, Henry Hurr, informing him that he had been voted a member of the group.[110] Also, on May 26, he received a letter marked "Personal"[111] from Wyman. The letter said that since the murder charge against him had been resolved favorably, permission could now be secured for his departure to Asia.[112] Ironically, this letter, dated 11 days after his March 15 letter advising Kinyoun about his taking control of press releases, also shows that Wyman was possibly assisting his leaving his position. The question arises: Was this coincidental or happenstance?

As a farewell, Dr. W.W. McFay with the San Diego quarantine station sent Kinyoun a note of appreciation. McFay congratulated him on his vindication and thanked him for his kindness and help. He related that he had sent numerous copies of the commissioners' report to other people and in particular to Major Cole, the commander of the San Diego post. As an aside, he wrote of the humor he found in the deaf-mute man accusing him of murder, saying he was happy that the charges had been dropped.[113] In closing, he wrote that his leaving Angel Island must be "a great relief."[114]

To the East

On June 28, Wyman ordered Kinyoun to Yokohama, Japan and Hong Kong. He instructed him to visit Tokyo, Kobe, Kioto and Nagasaki. After completing his tour, he would be granted a four-month leave.[115]

The dispatch outlined his duties. On arriving at each port, he would make an assessment of the facility's operations and report whether it functioned in accordance with the Service's standards. Upon leaving each facility, he would send an analysis concerning its state of affairs. Weekly, he would send a letter of any significant health or operational developments and inform the Service of any change of address.[116]

Of special note, Wyman directed him to forward any information about:

> ... plague and other epidemic diseases as may be of use in the efforts of the Service to prevent the conveyance of these diseases to the United States. Special attention should be given to the methods which have been adopted in these foreign countries for the eradication of plague and to general sanitary conditions, which now, or in the future, may affect the health interests of the United States.[117]

These passages raise the question of where Wyman had been the last two years in light of what had transpired in San Francisco. To direct him to learn how to prevent the plague when in fact it had already made its arrival leads one to question why he never visited the city during Kinyoun's efforts to control the contagion. He had even studied it while in Europe. This must have been a surreal moment for him. Even the special plague commission had confirmed the plague's presence and had outlined what sanitation measures would be required to abate it. In fairness to Wyman, though, there was more to be learned about the menace, but in many respects Kinyoun already knew how to handle it.

In late July, he departed for the East aboard the *Nippon Maru*, the ship that in all probability had brought the plague to America in the summer of 1899. This must have been ironic for him, if not even a little eerie. Regardless, it would be his last trip as an officer with the Service.

Throughout his travels, he wrote many letters home, most of them to Lizzie, several official, and one sent to his father. Each of them was quite long and represented more of a diary, documenting daily routines, acquaintances and observations of Asian culture. His first letter, dated July 26, consisted of 24 pages and covered his departure from Honolulu to his arrival in Yokohama on August 4.[118]

On arriving in Honolulu and knowing that the passengers had to wait for a quarantine inspection, he proceeded to conduct it himself. When the inspector arrived and saw that Kinyoun had completed it, he allowed everyone to disembark.[119] After leaving the ship, he met with Dr. Cofer, the port's quarantine officer, who asked him to make an inspection of his quarantine procedures. Kinyoun wrote:

> He could now witness, the transformation, of the former quarantine officer of San Francisco, who was the personification of quarantine, into a prosaic doctor whose sole desire was to study disease—For Behold! Had I not kept my vow, and dispersed with the hirsute ornamentation, the badge of quarantine!![120]

By this passage, he was through with serving in this capacity. Instead, he wanted to examine the disease's recent presence in the city, which he later admitted amounted to an examination of the quarantine station. But, to his surprise, he wrote that he had learned a great deal from his assessments, more so than he had previously gleaned from reading firsthand accounts by other doctors.[121]

An interesting encounter occurred on his boarding the vessel for Yokohama: He learned it had been delayed because a "Japanese Steerage passenger"[122] appeared ill. Kinyoun was asked to examine the man and afterwards stated that "he was a fit subject for the Board of Health,"[123] meaning he had the plague. Once again, he and the *Nippon Maru* crossed paths with the Black Death.

Other than this initial experience, the passage to Japan appeared peaceful and without interruption with the passengers comprising various levels of society ranging from diplomats to a movie actress. One evening, he saw the *Peking*, the *Coptic* and a man-of-war appear in the distance. The *Nippon Maru* steered toward them and passed the ships at a close distance. All the passengers on the ships went to the decks and cheered the others as they passed by. And again he had encountered another former dark shadow—the *Coptic*—that had caused him considerable trouble towards the end of his San Francisco assignment.[124]

Part way through his letter, he described how he managed to board the *Nippon Maru* unnoticed by the press. He knew many of the reporters and realized they would be looking for him. So he disguised himself and wrote that though they searched and searched, they could not find him. He declared it to be very entertaining to see them pacing back and forth when in fact he had been right in front of them.[125]

After the ship landed in Yokohama, he conducted his research and examination of the city. He found it very clean, with one-story houses connected to one another. The people kept their houses neat and swept the street in front of their residences, which helped prevent the spread of disease, in particular plague.[126]

While stationed in Yokohama, he journeyed to Tokyo several times to meet with Dr. Kitasato. They had become friends over the years since meeting in 1891 while in Europe.[127] As part of the international courtesies to visiting prominent officials, the general manager of the steamship line Toyo Kisen Kaisha sent two letters of introduction asking that every effort be made to accommodate Kinyoun and his desire to study the plague and tropical diseases. The first letter was addressed to Professor H. Hozomi, the director of the College of Law at the Tokyo Imperial University, where he asked that he be introduced to Drs. Aoyama and Kitasato.[128] The second letter was addressed to S. Asano, Esq., president of Toyo Kisen Kaisha asking he be extended every courtesy.[129]

His observations of Tokyo, the country's largest city with a population of 1,200,000, differed in comparison to Yokohama. It appeared more modern, different from the usual Japanese quaintness. Kinyoun wrote that the modernization occurred after 1867, with the monarchy's restoration that led to increased construction, broader streets and grander buildings. He commented that the Japanese seemed in earnest to adopt Western culture. The architecture had a beautiful French flavor, especially the Naval, War and State Departments,[130] representing an iconic sign of what was yet to occur 40 years later.

Another letter offered further insight into Japanese society. One noticeable cultural difference occurred in Tokyo, where a feast had been held in his honor by the Kitasato Institute. He explained in great detail the experience as they entered the Maples restaurant. After passing through the front door, he and the other guests were greeted by six Japanese girls, who kneeled and touched the floor with their heads before saying words of welcome. They proceeded to remove everyone's shoes and took them to the second floor, where the banquet awaited them. Kinyoun stated that although embarrassed by walking in his stocking feet, he at least had been told about the custom the night before and therefore had prepared himself.[131]

The banquet's menu consisted of the following delicacies:

1. Tea
2. Cake
3. Fish soup
4. Sake and Lobster
5. Omelet of Fish & Stuff
6. Raw Clams, and raw fish on a Soya
7. Fried fish, green ginger root, & pickles
8. Fish Soup—(Principally Lobster)
9. Sliced Pear with grated horseradish
10. Sake and Tea
11. Beer-Cigarettes, Confections[132]

As he dined on each course, he expressed with great openness his appreciation for the qualities of each delectable round. The presence of geisha girls, who throughout the feast assisted everyone in many ways, added a special charm to the evening. At one point, he asked permission to remove his jacket due to the evening's heat. To his surprise, one of the geisha girls returned with a rather large kimono for him. After changing into the new attire, he described it as quite comfortable.[133]

The letter delved into the purpose of his visit: visiting Japanese cities that had experienced plague and sharing notes with many doctors and others. One of his primary focuses had been to learn as much as possible about it from Kitasato, who, alongside Dr. Yersin, had been credited with its discovery in 1894. He wrote that following the banquet, he finished collecting all of Kitasato's material on the bacterium and its presence in Osaka and Kiolee. As a bonus, on his return from Tokyo, he had the opportunity to visit a hospital for leprosy patients.[134]

Apart from his inspections, he remarked that he had gathered enough plague information to impress even Wyman and his "fastidiousness."[135] It should further compensate him and the Service for agreeing to the trip. And as a sign of his continual dismay with his superior, he wrote:

> But whether he thinks I have been able to render a "quid pro quo," matters but little to me, I am benefitted, if he is not.[136]

As part of his itinerary, he had been scheduled to meet Professors Ogata and Aoyama at the university (likely the Tokyo Imperial University), but it was closed due to vacation. He had met Ogata, who served as the professor of hygiene at the university, years ago, while studying in Berlin.[137] Professor Aoyama served as the professor of medicine.[138] Several weeks later, he headed to China, but before leaving Japan, Dr. Ogata presented him a letter written in Japanese on one side and Chinese on the other introducing Kinyoun as a liaison from the Service.[139]

The night after his return from Tokyo, he had dinner with Mr. Tuskahara, who had included Mr. Ito and one other member of the company. Other guests included Professor Kitasato; Mr. Hiashi, superintendent of quarantine; Dr. Hoshimo, the medical director of quarantine and apparently the director of the university's law department; Dr. Arnold of the Navy; Dr. Eldridge, U.S. sanitary inspector; and Mr. Howard, an agent of the P.M.S.S. Company. The affair was held at the Oriental Hotel, and afterwards the group retired to the plaza, where they continued their conversations, but in many different languages.[140]

At the evening's conclusion, Professor Kitasato made a short speech in German and presented Kinyoun with his cane

> ... as a mark of friendship & good will. This appeared all that was necessary to establish my standing.[141]

Several days later, he again had the opportunity to see Dr. Koch, who happened to be in the vicinity as well. Kinyoun had studied under him in his early years at the Service on a special visit to his laboratory in Berlin. He and Koch had a long conversation, where they "talked shop"[142] for over an hour. At this time, Koch headed the German Naval Hospital.[143]

Nearing the end of his inspections, Dr. Murata, the chief sanitary inspector for Kobe, arranged for him to meet with Ukegami, the chief of police for Osaka. The purpose of this visit, as of many others, consisted of reviewing the quarantine measures in place at various cities and ports. Although he had tired of being a quarantine officer, he still knew it was important to make sure other countries maintained rigid controls. The purpose was to assure that proper containment procedures had been put in place in the less sanitary areas of the world, thereby preventing the spread of unwanted contagions to the United States.[144]

He reflected back to other experiences in Japan. One interesting comment occurred while doing an assessment of the Nagasaki Naval Station. During his investigations, he would routinely take pictures of the facilities as part of his reports. In this case, he could not bring his camera because of Japanese security. This matter coincided with another image of Japan's transforming military on a trip back to Hong Kong, when he observed four Japanese torpedo destroyers sailing side by side in the distance.[145]

Kinyoun had wanted to visit the Royal Palace in Kyoto, but at the time no foreigners were allowed entry. Kitasato, though, had made a special appeal on his behalf.[146] After he had arrived in Hong Kong a letter arrived from him expressing his regrets that the government had denied his request.[147] The palace contained the treasurers of the shoguns, the all-powerful military rulers of Japan for nearly 700 years.[148]

October 4 represented an important day for the doctor and his father. It was his dad's birthday, and he had been accepted into the Service 15 years before on the same date. He wrote from the Hotel de Oriente in Manila, where he had been staying while working in the city's hospital. Kinyoun described how much he had learned about the plague and tropical diseases.[149]

In describing his experiences, he wrote that Canton had been his best source of medical information. To him, the city represented the typical Chinese city in southern China. Concerning the medical side of his journeys, he related how helpful all the personnel and hospitals had been in providing information. In Manila, he had the opportunity to examine plague victims, stating that the procedures used to detect it were the same as those utilized in San Francisco.[150]

Regarding plague, he stated it had become conclusive that rats spread the contagion. There had been more than 400 cases of the disease and, if proper measures could not be improved shortly, then a major epidemic would likely occur within the year. He told his father that he had a couple more weeks to spend in Manila, Hong Kong and Shanghai before returning home.[151]

Back Home

Sometime in December, he returned home and assumed his former position with the Service in Detroit. In his absence, the family had been sick: Alice and John had had diphtheria, but were doing better.[152] He remarked about rumors reporting Secretary Gage and General Spaulding had resigned:

> General Spaulding's retirement will almost break somebody's heart and I hope it will. If it does I will not be the chief mourner at the funeral.[153]

It had been Secretary Gage and Spaulding who had hatched the plan with Governor Gage's commissioners and Wyman to remove Kinyoun from San Francisco and temporarily suppress the federal commissioners' report.

Two days after Christmas, Kinyoun wrote a letter addressed, cryptically, to "My dear twins (No. 1)."[154] It probably had been sent to his friends on Angel Island (Lloyd, Lumsden, Walker and Ransom). He had used code names before, dubbing himself "Abutment."[155] Various names had been used during the plague in hopes of keeping his correspondence secret, especially from the newspapers.

The letter represented an outpouring of frustrations about his job and the future of the Service. Kinyoun revered the organization, but at the same time he had an unquestionable disdain for Wyman. Regarding his employ, he recognized that his former days of rank and respect had come to an end. He told the twins that he had a personal "grievance"[156] with the Service, and that although people had been sympathetic about his plight, he knew no one could stand by him without risking their career.[157]

His greatest fear involved a bill reorganizing the Service that in his opinion would make it subject to politics and the retention of its present leader. He went so far as to blame President Roosevelt and Wyman for its drafting, but no one would ever know because of its anonymity. He stated his objection to government matters being anonymous, but did not mind when it came from "zoophile cranks."[158] He argued:

> The bill as now proposed has nothing more nor less its object than the perpetuation of our present head and granting him a salary of $7,200 a year. There is a threat and practically a bribe in nearly every line of this wonderful epistle.[159]

He had become angry and felt betrayed by Wyman, along with worrying about the bill's effect on the Service. His greatest objection resided in it possibly undermining other officers:

> What has been meted out to me in San Francisco is the lot which may fall to all these men. I cannot therefore stand idly by and see not only the cherished ideals swept away by one fell swoop of the politician, but to have my friends and associates subjected to ignominy and insult without protest, is more than I have been brought up to stand.[160]

In the final paragraph, he wrote:

> I am unalterably opposed to any scheme which has for its sole object the aggrandizement of one man at the expense of all the rest and will maintain this attitude notwithstanding the threats, bribes, even cajolery, that is now sent out from Washington to bring everyone into line to pass a bill to perpetuate one man in office.[161]

As to the bill's title, he thought of a more fitting caption:

> "To Increase the Efficiency of the Marine Hospital" it should be "To Decrease to Deficiencies of the Corps" for the purpose of the King living forever.[162]

Kinyoun had decided to leave the organization. In this letter, he showed profound disgust with his employer. Furthermore, he had become thoroughly disenchanted with the future of the agency. He even lashed out at President Theodore Roosevelt.[163] By the tone of the letter, one can tell he did not care anymore what his superiors thought about his comments. Simply, he had had enough, and rightfully so.

He had been short-sheeted in the end by Wyman and many others. Who wouldn't be angry after being sued, ridiculed daily by newspapers, threatened, bribed, accused of murder with a bounty on his head? Not many individuals would have stayed the course, but to his credit he remained steadfast in his convictions about the plague and the well-being of the Service. He knew the greater risk: it becoming pneumonic and epidemic, with the possibility of killing thousands of people.

When he went to California, he had ascended to the height of his profession. He had been the young upstart who set up a lab so others could see and understand the importance of bacteriology. He had become a leader in the country's evolution to modern medicine. But all of this came to a very quick end the minute he stepped off the train in San Francisco. From there, he became embroiled in an ever-enlarging vortex of quicksand created by the state's naysayers. Those in positions of power did not want the walls of their precious fiefdoms to come tumbling down, even if it meant the sacrifice of countless innocent lives. Unfortunately for them, Kinyoun became their biggest obstacle, but tragically in the end, he too had succumbed to the plague.

XVII

Farewells

Resignation

After returning to Detroit, Kinyoun decided to leave the Service. He advised Wyman that he had written the president tendering his resignation effective May 1, 1902.[1] While awaiting a response, he received several letters of interest. The first one arrived in January, addressed to Senator Cockrell from Army Surgeon General Sternberg. He had sought the senator's influence for a position in the War Department and access to its medical index.[2]

Sternberg turned down the idea of letting other doctors access the directory because it was for public libraries. He knew "Dr. Kinyoun very well and would be glad to comply with his request, but under the circumstances [he was] not able to do so."[3]

The other correspondence came from longtime friend Dr. (Henry R.) Carter, who sent a rather pleading letter to him.[4] It opened with:

> What on earth do you mean by saying as soon as you settle in your new home.... You aren't going to leave us are you? Don't do it old man, don't do it ... don't do anything of the sort....[5]

Followed by:

> "Old man you are one of the men who helped make the service."[6]

Regardless of his deteriorated relationship with Wyman, many of his colleagues thought highly of him, as expressed by Carter. Those in the Service knew how much he had contributed to the organization, not only because of the Hygienic Laboratory but also his overall professionalism.

One of his supporters had been Major Walter Reed. Between June and July, he received two letters from him.[7] Reed had always looked up to Kinyoun as a mentor, and they had become friends.[8] During this period, Sternberg had decided to retire, thereby opening up the position. The first letter covered several topics and in particular dinners given in Sternberg's honor apparently as farewell ceremonies.[9] Reed reported that one of his friends had asked General Wood who his likely replacement would be and his reply was, "Why shouldn't Major Reed be?"[10] A month later, he wrote Kinyoun and stated that, to his dismay, Colonel O'Riley received the position.[11]

Kinyoun eventually received a response to his request. On February 14, Secretary of the Treasury Department Leslie M. Shaw reported that the president had

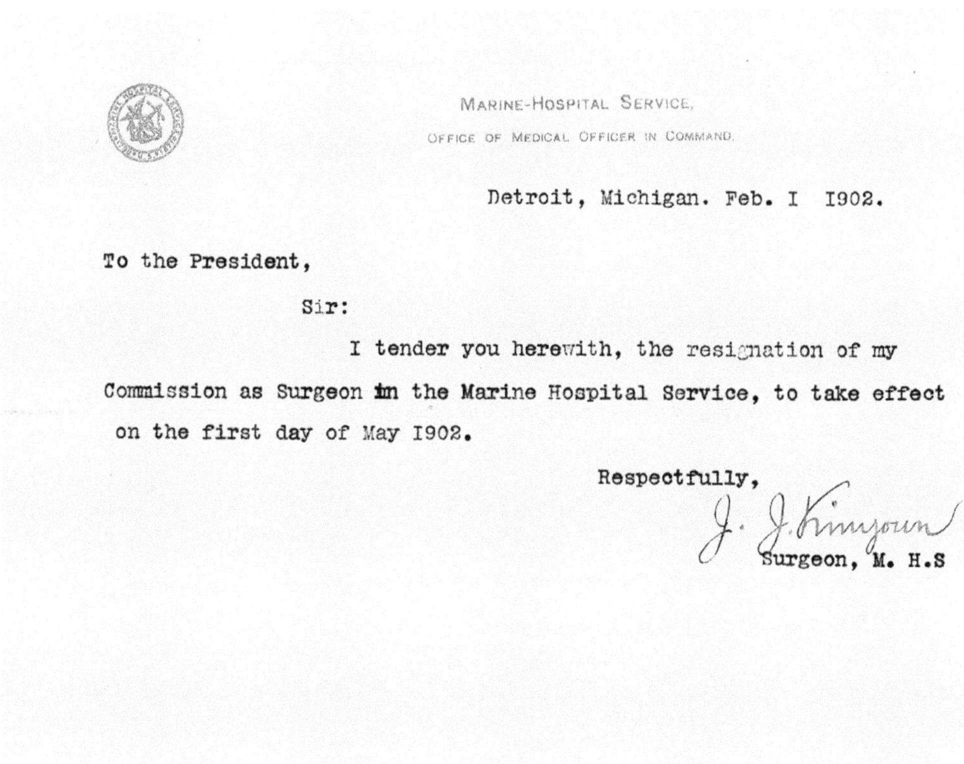
MARINE-HOSPITAL SERVICE,
OFFICE OF MEDICAL OFFICER IN COMMAND.

Detroit, Michigan. Feb. I I902.

To the President,

Sir:

I tender you herewith, the resignation of my Commission as Surgeon in the Marine Hospital Service, to take effect on the first day of May I902.

Respectfully,

J. J. Kinyoun

Surgeon, M. H.S

Kinyoun's resignation letter to the president, February 1, 1902 (effective first day of May).

accepted his resignation to be effective on April 19, 1902.[12] After 15 years of dedicated service, he would now become a private citizen. One can only speculate as to whether his career with the Service would have ended absent the plague crisis in San Francisco.

Before his departure, Dr. White had been sent by Wyman to replace him as the federal quarantine officer for San Francisco, although he remained at his post in a different capacity. White would soon face the same barriers and confrontations with the politicians and the press. Governor Gage proved to be guarded and withheld much of the $100,000 he had agreed to allocate for the cleanup of Chinatown; he parted with only $25,000.[13]

Other changes would occur. Dr. Rupert L. Blue soon arrived as the new quarantine officer, relieving White. Over the course of a few years, he proved successful in working together with the opposing parties in California and altered the public's antagonistic sentiments towards the plague. Eventually, his efforts paid off in bringing it under control and the crisis to a closure, of sorts.[14] Nonetheless, and without warning, the menace reoccurred after the 1906 San Francisco earthquake. This time, the public's reaction and response proved more resolute in its abatement.[15]

Wyman would remain the surgeon general until his death on November 21, 1911.[16] Blue would succeed him on January 13, 1912, and remain in the position until March 9, 1920.

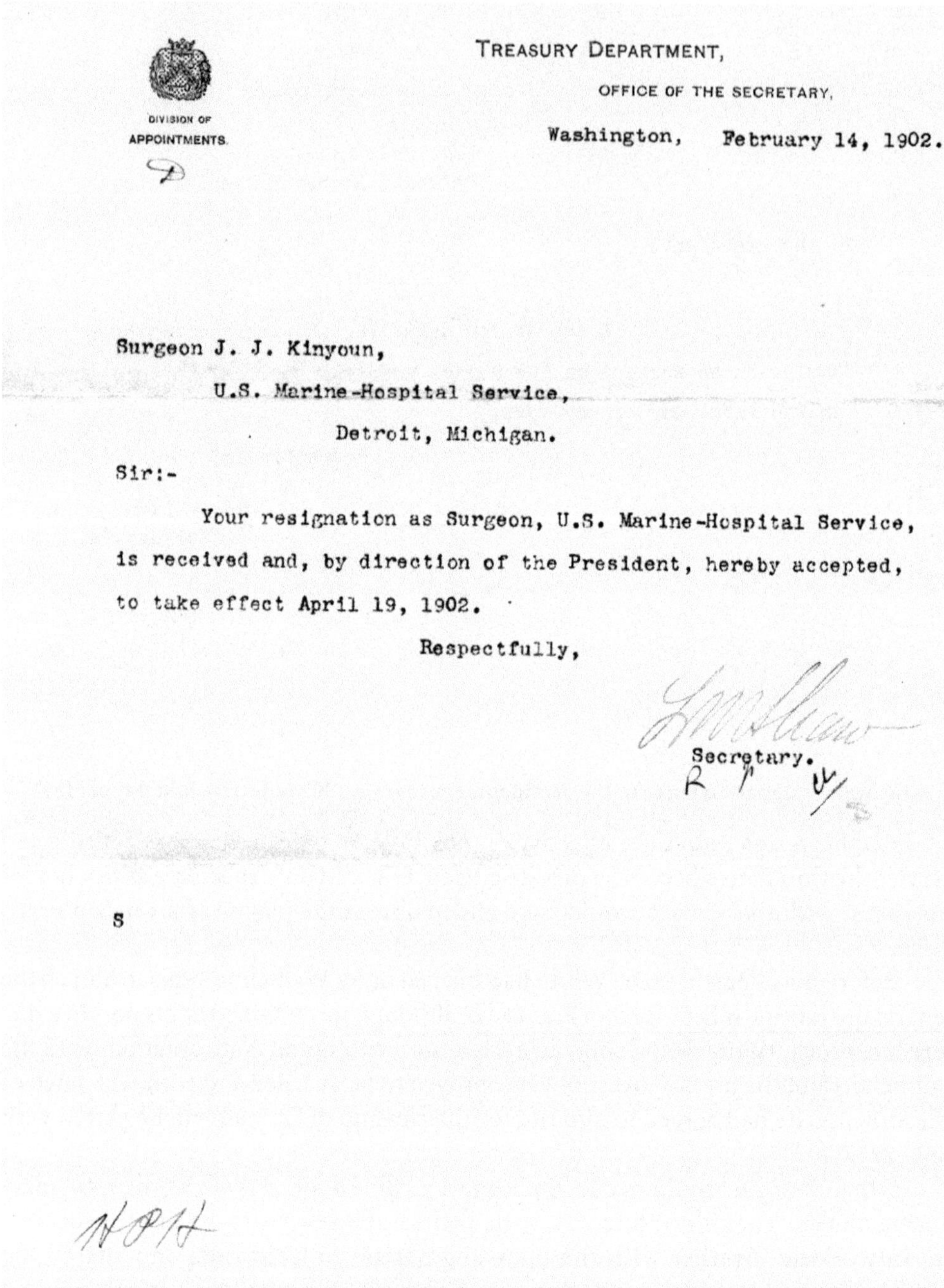

TREASURY DEPARTMENT,

OFFICE OF THE SECRETARY,

DIVISION OF APPOINTMENTS.

Washington, February 14, 1902.

Surgeon J. J. Kinyoun,

U.S. Marine-Hospital Service,

Detroit, Michigan.

Sir:-

Your resignation as Surgeon, U.S. Marine-Hospital Service, is received and, by direction of the President, hereby accepted, to take effect April 19, 1902.

Respectfully,

Secretary.

S

Kinyoun's resignation letter is accepted, February 14, 1902 (effective April 19).

Political Goings-On

On the heels of Kinyoun's departure political changes transpired that did not help the ongoing plague situation. The most notable occurred with the 1902 mayoral election and the entry of Mayor Eugene E. Schmitz.[17] He replaced Mayor James

Phelan, a Democrat, who had decided not to run for re-election. Schmitz, a violinist and orchestra conductor, had been tapped by attorney and political boss Abraham (Abe) Ruef to run for mayor on the Union Labor Party ticket.[18] Although not a Republican, like Governor Gage, he too denied the plague.[19]

In the June 30 "Annual Report of the President of the San Francisco Board of Health,"[20] Board President John M. Williamson wrote a scathing admonishment of Schmitz for his cronyism and failure to recognize the plague's seriousness. He pointed out that his department had gotten along with all the other municipal branches in the city "except the mayor's office."[21] Williamson called out Schmitz for replacing those board members appointed by Phelan and then seizing the department's office and installing his new health board without informing the former members. Concerning the plague, he stated that the mayor had never approached the board about its presence, except once asking for a recent plague victim's report.[22] Afterwards, he quoted a remark by Schmitz attacking the board for its stance and how it caused:

> … irreparable injury to the people, whose protectors you are supposed to be; it is against the welfare of the city, and is, in my opinion … justification for your removal.[23]

He recited a passage from the mayor, where he expressed regret in their removal. But Williamson refuted this attempt at an apology by citing Schmitz's executive order,[24] which lay out the real reason for their dismissal:

> Following is the cause for you are removed: to wit Continued injury and injustice to…. San Francisco…. California, and to their commercial and financial interest, in declaring … without proper foundation or justification in fact, that bubonic plague … has existed therein since March 6, 1900.[25]

Williamson expounded by stating their termination ought to be considered congratulatory of "all true exponents of municipal imperialism."[26] Because of their termination, the health board filed an injunction against the mayor for his interference in its operations and seizing its offices. After an initial hearing before Judge M.C. Sloss, the defendants moved to transfer the case to Presiding Judge Cook for a ruling. As of the date of Williamson's report no ruling had been rendered.[27]

He went to great lengths documenting government reports and sources about the contagion, chastising the mayor for not mentioning the federal commissioners' report confirming its existence. Next, he attacked the state board of health's pamphlet about the governor's special plague commission's report, referring to it as "palpably one of deception"[28] and writing:

> Its contents add nothing whatsoever to scientific information, and its conclusions contribute less to veracity. A superficial narrative … detailing the progress of the inspection and cleansing of the Chinese quarter carried out by the state.[29]

Williamson quoted a passage from Schmitz's dismissal letter, where it stated that the press and the state board of health and city officials, combined with the report of the governor's commission, were gospel, that plague did not exist. He noted that the report added nothing scientifically to support the position of the commissioners and lacked any scientific or medical background. Next, he turned his commentary towards Williamson, along with *The Examiner*, noting how his newspaper had been an anti-plague advocate.[30]

He addressed another material inconsistency regarding the cleanup effort being conducted by the state as part of the deal struck with the governor's commissioners and Wyman. The state board of health claimed it had cleaned 30,000,000 cubic feet of living space, but with only 300 pounds of sulfur. Williamson implied that these numbers did not add up and that the Marine Hospital Service had gauged the amount at 30 tons.[31]

On top of this factor, he revealed how three girls had died from the plague living at the same address as determined by the Service. But the state health board had claimed the deaths were caused by hemorrhagic septicemia. However, a fourth girl at the residence had been treated by the board with Yersin serum.[32]

He concluded his report by returning to the matter of the former board member's removal.[33] He wrote:

> ... it may not be amiss to state that, taking into consideration the attitude of the press in San Francisco, as well as that assumed by your Honor, it is difficult to determine whether membership on the Board of Health of this city and county is to be looked upon as a crime or as a joke.[34]

Williamson would remain defiant that the plague had and still existed in the city. He wrote about a new conspiracy between Schmitz and Gage, along with their associates, to thwart the cleanup process brokered with Wyman and others.[35] As to Eugene Schmitz and his political power broker Abe Ruef, both would end up in prison.[36]

Although the San Francisco mayor had become an anti-plague advocate, Californians elected a new chief executive on November 6, 1902: Dr. George C. Pardee, the mayor of Oakland and a regent at the University of California.[37] Gage did not appear on the November ballot because the California Republican Party did not approve his re-nomination.[38]

Pardee not only acknowledged the plague's presence, but immediately took steps to curtail its spread. New measures were instituted and in a public statement he agreed to work with the Service. At the same time, businesses started cooperating that helped prevent a quarantine of California by other states. Along with the cleanup efforts of Quarantine Officer Dr. Rupert Blue, the crisis lessened with fewer cases appearing.[39]

Starting Over: 1903–1907

In 1903, Kinyoun and his family moved to Glenolden, Pennsylvania, where he would work at the H.K. Mulford Pharmaceutical Company as the director of its new laboratory. Before he left the Service, he had been approached by the organization several times about running its lab. He had always had a passion for research, so the job appealed to him. He would leave the company in 1907.[40]

During his tenure at Mulford, he started writing numerous pamphlets on various medical topics about disease. These articles were written as either part of his job or because he had more time to document his numerous scientific findings. Many of these papers would be read at different medical association meetings or published in journals. These included *The Journal of the American Medical Association* and the

Journal of Experimental Medicine. His papers included the following: "The Prophylaxis of Plague" (1903); "Dysentery, With Special Reference to Its Bacillary Form" (1904); "The Action of Glycerin on Bacteria in the Presence of Cell Exudates" (1905); "The Prevention of the Spread of Infectious Disease" (1906); "Dried Tetanus Antitoxin as A Dressing for Wound" (1906); "Uncinariasis in Florida" (undated); and one on diphtheria.[41]

In December, the American Public Health Association consisting of the United States, the Dominion of Canada and the Republic of Mexico elected him into membership at its annual gathering in New Orleans.[42] Following this award, he became a fellow in the American Association for the Advancement of Science.[43] On a personal level, he received an invitation from the family of Senator Francis M. Cockrell to attend their daughter Marion's wedding to Edson Fessenden Gallaudet on February 14, followed by a breakfast on February 15 at Rauschers.[44]

On a personal note, he received a telegram on July 27, 1903, informing him of his father's death. The elder Kinyoun would be buried between his two wives in the Centerview Cemetery. John Kinyoun had played a major role in his son's development as a doctor and assuredly had been proud of his many achievements.[45]

Within this period, he worked on improving many maladies and created a more reliable administration of the smallpox vaccine that became known as the "Kinyoun Method."[46] This process required applying "the needle parallel to the skin surface."[47] The measure received approval from the Public Health Service and remained in use until the introduction of the bifurcated needle sometime in the 1960s. Among other illnesses, he worked on dysentery, hookworms and water sanitation. At one point, he assisted with the polio epidemic in New York City[48]

The following year, on January 11, 1904, Kinyoun received a letter from Dr. Rosenau, who had replaced him as head of the Hygienic Laboratory in 1899. Rosenau reported that the Service would soon move into its new laboratory. In light of this occasion, he asked the doctor if he could place his picture in the reception area honoring him as the founder and first director of the lab.[49] Kinyoun must have agreed because his portrait adorns the lobby of the administrative building at the National Institutes of Health.

He assumed numerous leadership positions in various medical associations. He served in 1904 as vice president of the American Society of Tropical Medicine[50] and in 1906 as the first vice president of the American Public Health Association.[51] Other affiliations included the Association of American Physicians and the American Association for the Advancement of Science.[52] In September 1904, the International Congress of Arts and Science extended him a membership invitation and asked him to attend and participate in its Universal Exposition being held September 19–25 in St. Louis.[53]

Of one occasion, Kinyoun revisited the Hygienic Laboratory in 1906, as an advisor on a special project. At this time, the laboratory had been working on the development of a "standard unit"[54] to measure the effectiveness of tetanus anti-toxin. He went as a representative of the Society of American Bacteriologists.[55] His return to the lab must have been a bittersweet moment.

Career, Awards and War 1907–1919

Over the next 12 years, he would be involved in numerous tasks and different areas of employment. During this period changes would occur reflecting his continued stature as a medical researcher. His reputation preceded him, as evidenced by his invitation to attend the "Semi-centennial of the Founding of the Pathological Society of Philadelphia,"[56] in early May 1907. The emblematic symbol of the organization was a portrait of Dr. Virchow, regarded by many as the father of modern pathology due to his concept that cells constituted the building blocks of all forms of life: plants, humans and even disease.[57] Kinyoun had studied with him while in Europe.

In October, President Charles W. Needham of George Washington University offered him a professorship of pathology and bacteriology in the university's medical department with a salary of $1,800. He accepted the position within a week.[58]

In June 1908, he also received appointment as the bacteriologist for the District of Columbia. He would be responsible for such "duties devolving upon him,"[59] with his primary focus being the prevention of diphtheria, scarlet fever, tuberculosis and other infectious maladies. His work schedule was not to exceed three hours per day, and he would be paid $3.00 per hour. All told, his maximum salary would be $468 per year.[60] This amount combined with his salary at George Washington University amounted to $2,264, less than half his starting salary at Mulford Pharmaceutical Company in 1902, but comparable to what he made at the Service six years before.

The Kinyouns by having lived in the capital for many years had risen not only in the medical community, but also socially within the highest levels of the government. It would not be uncommon for them to be invited to social gatherings at the White House, as in 1899 to attend a reception by President and Mrs. William McKinley[61] and in 1916 by President and Mrs. Woodrow Wilson.[62] After the doctor's death, Lizzie would attend numerous events at the White House, especially those held by Mrs. Franklin Delano Roosevelt.[63]

On March 9, 1909, he received an invitation to become a member the Cosmo Club, the most prestigious gentlemen's social organization in the capital.[64] The club was founded in 1878, by legendary American explorer John Wesley Powell with the purpose of advancing those engaged in literature, art and science. Over the years, its members have included 36 Nobel Prize laureates, Presidents William H. Taft and Woodrow Wilson, two vice presidents, 61 Pulitzer Prize winners, 55 recipients of the Presidential Medal of Freedom, 12 Supreme Court justices, and Alexander Graham Bell. After meeting in several places, the organization purchased the Dolly Madison House in 1886.[65] He joined the club and enjoyed it for many years.

Kinyoun and Wyman's paths crossed once more in 1911, even though the surgeon general had made it known he would never utter his name.[66] In September, Wyman sent a letter to the municipal and state health officer, transportation companies and other parties notifying them that Anacleto Palabay, afflicted with leprosy, had been placed in custody. In due order, he would be transported from Washington, D.C., to Seattle for deportation to the Philippines. He advised that the District of Columbia health officer (Kinyoun) had arranged for a special vehicle for him accompanied by a doctor to ensure ample protections for the discarding of any refuse.[67] True to his word, he did not mention Kinyoun by name, only by his title, indicative of his perpetual snub.

As part of the 1913 presidential inauguration for President-Elect Woodrow Wilson, he received appointment as an additional private on the capital's Metropolitan Police Force by the District's commissioners for a ten-day term, from February 28 to March 8. His services would be without compensation.[68] In all probability, this extraordinary position would allow him to attend the inauguration and related festivities.

In 1917, an ironic twist occurred that demonstrated how circumstances in life do not always follow a set track, as in his case. Kinyoun had been a member of the American Medical Association for several years. Memberships usually required the payment of an annual fee. After paying his dues, he received a certificate acknowledging its receipt for the forthcoming year. Ironically, it was signed by Rupert Blue, as president, who succeeded Walter Wyman on his death in 1912, as surgeon general and Kinyoun as the quarantine officer in San Francisco.[69] It must have seemed odd to Kinyoun that, absent the plague, he might have been or would have had the opportunity to be the surgeon general.

With America's entry into World War I in the spring of 1917, the Army's Reserve Officers Corps presented Kinyoun with a major's commission on March 22, 1918. The surgeon general of the Army wanted to use his expertise for "epidemiological"[70] containment for the military. Accordingly, he requested an indefinite leave of absence as the bacteriologist from the District of Columbia commissioners.[71] Over the next several days a flurry of letters transpired between the commissioners, Kinyoun and the surgeon general.

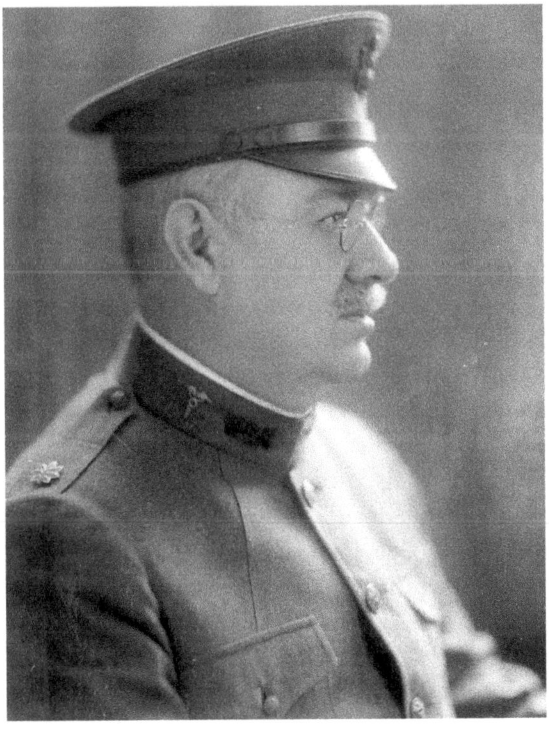

Dr. Joseph J. Kinyoun, World War I major, 1917.

The commissioners became upset over his appointment because it left them without a bacteriologist. They wrote to Kinyoun and the Army's surgeon general about their displeasure and required that the doctor provide a succession plan,[72] which he submitted on March 25 naming three persons who collectively could handle the job.[73] They accepted it,[74] and on March 26 he accepted the commission.[75]

Before he could legally accept the army's appointment, he needed to resign from the "Medical Reserve Corps"[76] of the Navy, in which he had been enlisted as part of the Marine Hospital Service. It approved his resignation on March 28.[77] After much finagling between Kinyoun and governmental branches, he received orders on April 2 to proceed to Raleigh, North Carolina.[78]

Final Journey

Unfortunately, his position in the Army would be short-lived. Within two months of his enlistment, the grim reaper would knock on his door with other plans for his future. On July 2, 1918, he received a prescription for morphine sulfate for one year.[79] Kinyoun had developed a cancerous growth. Knowing his fate, he sent two letters of instruction concerning his impending death. The first one dictated his burial instructions[80]; the second was his last will and testament.[81]

After years of overseeing the disinfection of ships, railroad cars, buildings, people, baggage and cargo, the exposure to formaldehyde and other dangerous chemical compounds had taken their toll on him. He discovered a knot in his neck, which proved to be lymphosarcoma, a fatal diagnosis.[82] By December, he had been relieved from his post and ordered to Washington, D.C., reporting to the Army's surgeon general.[83] Kinyoun's condition continued to worsen, and on February 14, 1919, at 4:45 p.m. he died in his home at 1423 Clifton St. N.W., Washington, D.C., with his wife Lizzie at his bedside accompanied by Army Captain Dr. George C. Smith. It was Valentine's Day, and he died at the age of 59.[84]

His body would be buried in the Centerview, Missouri, cemetery next to his daughter Elizabeth and near his parents. Lizzie would live for many more years, dying on May 21, 1948. She would be buried beside her husband and daughter in the cemetery.[85]

Postscript

Kinyoun had a determined personality. He knew the subject matter of plague better than most medical minds of the time. His education and studies abroad exceeded many of his peers, affording him an advantage over other medical scientists, let alone the average citizen and politician. With this background, he had studied not only the dangerous wanderings of contagions, but also how to perfect their cure and prevent their spread. Understandably, not all cures and preventions had the desired results.

The complexity of the situation in San Francisco centered on numerous fabrications. Most people of the time knew about the deadly ravages of the disease and its decimation of millions. But with this knowledge, instead of turning it into a way to protect life, it pivoted towards how to protect the city's and the state's commercial interests from being known as a plague harbor. As a result, his methodology came under unrelenting scrutiny and attack.

With every backlash, he became more resilient in trying to prove his findings as fact and not fantasy. But his resolve was incessantly condemned by the major San Francisco newspapers, to the point that they personally mocked him. Only the

Sacramento Bee stood by him. He had employed all known scientific know-how to prove his point and at the same time avert an epidemic. In the midst of this drama, even his supervisor, Dr. Walter Wyman, began to distance himself from the matter.

Since the plague debacle, others have examined his methods of discovery and prevention with conflicting viewpoints. Most scholars have accepted the veracity of his findings. The plague did happen and eventually showed up in surrounding areas. One of the main criticisms has been that the plague in San Francisco did not become an epidemic; compared to other regions of the world, the city was an unlikely place for an epidemic to occur. Although true to some degree, the conditions existed for such an outbreak in Chinatown, where living conditions and sanitation could be described as inadequate and poised as a perfect incubator for an epidemic. As in ages past, the plague would make a brief appearance only to subside and reemerge with a vengeance several years later. Kinyoun had pointed this fact out in his letter to Senator Cockrell.

What the Old World knew but the New World failed to comprehend was the effectiveness of the scientific identification of germs, the use of the microscope, vaccines and containment procedures. Microorganisms proved invisible to the naked eye. However, they have been as real as humans and just as mobile. Therefore, the movement of contagions needed to be stopped first, followed by sanitation efforts to clean the infected region, along with treating the afflicted with serums and vaccinations. Only then would the situation stabilize and lead to the contagion's eradication.

Within this mix existed several major stumbling blocks. One rested on cultural beliefs. This boiled down to trust in the facts in harmony with the cultural beliefs of populations. In the case of San Francisco, it came down to not wanting to believe the facts because the stigma of plague could irreparably damage the city's commercial prominence, livability and standing as an international port. The white population further complicated the matter by believing the disease to be only an Asiatic illness not affecting them. The only part even faintly true about this belief would be that white neighborhoods did in many cases have better sanitation than the Chinese in Chinatown. In truth, such a mindset amounted to nothing more than an enormous or elaborate misconception, because in the end the plague has never discriminated in its choice of victims.

The Chinese population had entrenched customs and was leery of outside interference in their everyday lives, especially regarding privacy, medical treatment and death. It must be remembered that they had long been forced into their own living district, exiled into Chinatown. The whites had discriminated against them for decades, which led to their deportation and being provided inadequate living facilities and public services. This became apparent in their housing and sanitation that could turn their environs into breeding grounds for disease. So upon being quarantined, even though it was plague, they reacted with impertinence and rioting. In their eyes, they had been imprisoned by the white population for the whites' protection and not theirs.

In all probability, they viewed it as having to rough it out behind a locked barricade with the potential of imminent death. Kinyoun and the local health department had tried to make house-to-house inspections, clean up Chinatown and aid the afflicted, but because of prior intrusions upon their liberties this did not come to pass. Possibly, if the Chinese had been treated differently and included socially and economically in San Francisco society from the beginning, the plague crisis could have been lessened with a better result.

Kinyoun's Legacy

Growing up, he would have experienced many sentiments from his parents, friends and surroundings after the Civil War, especially in his new home of Missouri. This factor may have had a strong bearing on his thoughts and opinions, but maybe not. In retrospect, a considerable number of individuals held deep-seated animosities towards others. Nonetheless, this does not make it right.

On arriving in San Francisco, he inherited an already tense situation with the exclusion of the Chinese and in many respects the Japanese from society and probably in other regions of California. He had stepped into a powder keg that ignited upon his discovery of the plague. With this eruption, he stood his ground, and although it could be viewed as aimed at the Chinese, his main concern centered on avoiding its spread. The sweeping ravages of death from the disease, as experienced in China and India, lay heavily on his mind and shoulders. Someone had to stand up to big business and the political machines to avert a potential health disaster that could have had national implications if the disease became epidemic.

Grandmother Allie always defended her father. She stated on many occasions that Wyman had done her father wrong. Her loyalty to his legacy remained resolute throughout her life. On occasion, she would speak harshly of those who had caused him so much grief, especially the newspapers, and grumble about how the Chinese had placed a $50,000 price on his head, according to her.[86]

The legacy of Kinyoun can be measured in many ways and on many levels. First and foremost, after joining the Service, he became its chief bacteriologist and within a short period started demonstrating his skills. Both of his supervisors, Hamilton and Wyman, recognized early on his unique abilities and accordingly sent him to Europe to study with the medical titans of the time. These men included Louis Pasteur, Robert Koch, Rudolf Virchow, Paul Ehrlich, Élie Metchnikoff, Émile Roux, Emil Behring, Friedrich Loeffler,[87] and Shibasaburō Kitasato.[88]

He visited Europe three times and on each occasion brought back formulas for the newest vaccines and serums being created by the learned. Other items included improved ways to handle sanitation and how to enhance municipal water quality. In many respects, he became a microcosm of these groundbreaking scientists. Two of his most significant contributions were Pasteur's revised rabies and the diphtheria vaccine. These represented only a few of the important medical breakthroughs. Even while studying abroad and running the Hygienic Laboratory, his thirst for learning remained steadfast, as evidenced by his receiving a degree in philosophy.

Another of his great attributes can be seen in his advocacy as a visionary. He remained steadfast in trying to improve the overall medical structure. In repeated requests to Wyman, he would outline the need for a larger laboratory, a separate building, and an agency to monitor the development, manufacturing and distribution of drugs for the safety of the public. His persistence eventually paid off with the passage of the Biologics Act in 1902.[89] The agency would evolve into the Food and Drug Administration, commonly known today as the FDA.[90] Some have claimed that he even had the foresight for what would become the Centers for Disease Control (CDC).[91]

As for the Hygienic Laboratory, it continued to evolve after his departure. In 1926,[92] Senator Joseph E. Ransdell, from Louisiana, introduced legislation making the lab a separate entity from the U.S. Public Health Service. Upon the bill's passage in 1930, the lab became known as the National Institute of Health (NIH), consisting of several sub-agencies, or institutes, each to research various maladies and health issues.[93] The NIH continued to expand by adding more institutes, thereby leading to its name being changed in 1948 to the National Institutes of Health, representing the inclusion of all the institutes.[94]

As a special aside, during World War II, a Liberty ship bore his name, the *Joseph James Kinyoun*. These ships were rapidly built and employed as supply and armaments conveyors to the war fronts. In 1968, the ship was scrapped in Hong Kong.[95]

In the end, he had studied and learned the new ways of the Old World and transported this knowledge to America. His far-sightedness unlocked the many doors of the germ theory. It became a fascinating journey for him and led to progressive results in health care and improved sanitation techniques, two important elements in the fight against disease.

In all probability, he would have been more than happy to remain as the director of the Hygienic Laboratory. Kinyoun had had a skyrocketing career until his transfer to San Francisco. Nonetheless, with this move, his soaring career at the Service would soon close. In the end, his greatest legacy would be as the founder of the world's largest medical research center: the National Institutes of Health. And as with the fate of all humanity, although a giant of early modern American medicine, he faded into the obscurity of time.

Chapter Notes

Introduction

1. Kinyoun Genealogical Papers.

2. Letter, Walter Wyman, Surgeon-General, Marine Hospital Service, to Passed assistant Surgeon J.J. Kinyoun, Director Hygienic Laboratory, U.S. Marine Hospital Service, Washington, D.C., 27 April 1899; Letter, Lyman J. Gage, Secretary, Treasury Department to Passed assistant Surgeon J.J. Kinyoun, U.S. Marine Hospital Service, Angel Island, California, 12 June 1899.

3. William H. McNeill, *Plagues and Peoples* (New York: Random House), 164–165, 168–169, 199.

4. *Occidental Medical Times*, Kinyoun, *Bubonic Plague*, 4–5, 8–9, 11.

5. *Occidental Medical Times*, Kinyoun, *Bubonic Plague*, 5; R.A. Forrest M.D., *Echoes of the Plague Scare in San Francisco* (San Francisco: N.p., 17 November 1900), 1; Ralph Chester Williams, *The United States Public Health Service 1798–1950* (Washington, D.C.: The Commissioned Officers Association of the United States Public Health Service, 1951), 97.

6. J.J. Kinyoun, M.D., *Bubonic Plague* (San Francisco: *Occidental Medical Times*, reprint, August 1901), 4–5, 7; Brent Hoff and Carter Smith III, *Mapping Epidemics: A Historical Atlas of Disease* (New York: Grolier Publishing, 2000), 71; William H. McNeill, *Plagues and People* (New York: Random House, 1976), 164–165; Sarah R. Riedman, *Shots Without Guns* (Chicago: Rand McNally, 1960), 116, 126–131, 137–139; CDC, *Natural History*, www.cdc.gov/ncidod/dvbid/plague/history.htm, accessed 5 August 2008, 1–2; Johannes Nohl, *The Black Death* (Yardley, PA: Westholme Publishing, 2006), 72–73, 83.

7. CDC, *Natural History*, www.cdc.gov/ncidod/dvbid/plague/history.htm, 1–2.

8. Hoff and Smith III, *Mapping Epidemics: A Historical Atlas of Disease*, 8; Webster's *Collegiate Dictionary Fifth Edition* (Springfield, MA: Webster's, 1947), 78.

9. Charlton T. Lewis, *Elementary Latin Dictionary* (Oxford: Oxford University Press, 1966), 612.

10. *The American Heritage Dictionary, Fourth Edition*, 535–536.

11. *Ibid.*, 613, 718.

12. *Ibid.*, 412.

13. *Ibid.*

14. J.J. Kinyoun, M.D., *Bubonic Plague*, 4–5; Bubonic Plague, accessed July 11, 2006, *Infection/Transportation*, http://en.wikipedia.org/wiki/Bubonic_plague, 2.

15. National Park Service, U.S. Department of the Interior, Public Health Program, accessed 16 July 2006. www.nps.gov/public_health/inter/info/factsheets/fs_plague.htm, 1.

16. CDC, *Information on Plague*, accessed 16 July 2006. www.cdc.gov/ncidod/dvbid/Plague/info.htm, 1–2.

17. McNeill, *Plagues and Peoples*, 138–140, 147.

18. *The American Heritage Dictionary, Fourth Edition*, 285; Hoff and Smith III, *Mapping Epidemics: A Historical Atlas of Disease*, 9.

19. McNeill, *Plagues and Peoples*, 138; CDC, *Information on Plague*, accessed 16 July 2006. www.cdc.gov/ncidod/dvbid/plague/info.htm, 1–2; *Questions and Answers About Plague*, 1–2.

20. *The American Heritage Dictionary, Fourth Edition*, 289; Hoff and Smith III, *Mapping Epidemics: A Historical Atlas of Disease*, 9.

21. *Ibid.*

22. McNeill, *Plagues and Peoples*, 179.

23. CDC, *Information on Plague*, accessed 16 July 2006. www.cdc.gov/ncidod/dvbid/plague/info.htm. 4–6, *Natural History*, 1–3; *Prevention and Control*, 1–3.

24. Discovery Channel, *Tracking the attack of the plague*, accessed 12 July 2006. www.exn.ca/Stories/2000/09/12/52.asp, 1.

25. Centers for Disease Control and Prevention. *Prevention of Plague: Recommendations of the Advisory Committee on Immunization Practices* MMWR 1996; 45 (No. RR-14): 2; CDC, *Clinical Features*, accessed 16 July 2006. www.cdc/ncidod/dvbib/plague/facts.htm, 1; CDC, *Diagnosis*, accessed 16 July 2006. www.cdc.ncidod/dvbid/plague/diagnosis.htm.

26. Centers for Disease Control and Prevention. *Prevention of Plague: Recommendations of the Advisory Committee on Immunization Practices* MMWR 1996; 45 (No. RR-14): 2; CDC, *Clinical Features*, accessed 16 July 2006. www.cdc/ncidod/dvbib/plague/facts.htm, 1; CDC, *Diagnosis*, accessed 16 July 2006. www.cdc.ncidod/dvbid/plague/diagnosis.htm.

27. Centers for Disease Control and Prevention. *Prevention of Plague: Recommendations of the Advisory Committee on Immunization Practices* MMWR 1996; 45 (No. RR-14): 2; CDC, *Clinical Features*, accessed 16 July 2006. www.cdc/ncidod/dvbib/plague/facts.htm, 1; CDC, *Diagnosis*, accessed 16 July 2006. www.cdc.ncidod/dvbid/plague/diagnosis.htm.

28. Bubonic Plague. *Types*, accessed 11 July 2006. en.wikipedia.org/wiki/Bubonic_plague. 3.

29. CDC, *Questions and Answers About Plague*, accessed 16 July 2006. www.cdc.gov/ncidod/dvbid/plague/qa.htm, 2–3; Centers for Disease Control and Prevention. *Prevention of Plague: Recommendations of the Advisory Committee on Immunization Practices*, 5.

30. CDC, *Information on Plague*, accessed 16 July 2006. www.cdc.gov/nicdod/dvbid/plague/info.htm, 2.

31. *The American Heritage Dictionary, Fourth Edition*, 285; Hoff and Smith III, *Mapping Epidemics: A Historical Atlas of Disease*, 9.

32. McNeill, *Plagues and Peoples*, 137–142.

33. *Ibid.*, 139, 170.

34. *Ibid.*

35. *Ibid.*

36. *Ibid.*, 137, 156, 171–177, 199.

37. Frederick F. Cartwright, *Disease and History* (New York: Thomas Y. Crowell, 1972), 8; Charles F. Mullett, *The Bubonic Plague and England* (Lexington: University of Kentucky Press, 1956), 366; McNeill, *Plagues and Peoples*, 122, 130–132.

38. Exodus, 9:1–12; McNeill, *Plagues and Peoples*, 96–97.

39. Exodus, 12:1–32.

40. 1 Samuel 5: 1–12, 6: 1–21; McNeill, *Plagues and Peoples*, 140.

41. 1 Samuel 6:3–5.

42. Exodus, 9: 1–12, 12:1–32, Samuel 5: 1–12, 6:1–21; McNeill, *Plagues and Peoples*, 96–97, 140; Cartwright, *Disease and History*, 5–7.

43. Cartwright, *Disease and History*, 8.

44. *Ibid.*, 30–31.

45. Cartwright, *Disease and History*, 16–17; McNeill, *Plagues and Peoples*, 137–138, 141.

46. Cartwright, *Disease and History*, 17–18; William Rosen, *Justinian's Flea* (New York: Penguin, 2007), 209–210.

47. McNeill, *Plagues and Peoples*, 137–138.

48. McNeill, *Plagues and Peoples*, 138; Rosen, *Justinian's Flea*, 209–211.

49. Rosen, *Justinian's Flea*, 210; Mullett, *The Bubonic Plague and England*, 261, 264.

50. McNeill, *Plagues and Peoples*, 141.

51. McNeill, *Plagues and Peoples*, 170, 175–179; Hoff and Smith III, *Mapping Epidemics: A Historical Atlas of Disease*, 69–71.

52. Hoff and Smith III, *Mapping Epidemics: A Historical Atlas of Disease*, 68, 70.

53. *Ibid.*, 69–70; McNeill, *Plagues and Peoples*, 175, 177–179.

54. Laurie Garnett, *The Coming Plague* (New York: Penguin Books, 1994), 237–238.

55. Garnett, *The Coming Plague*, 238; Mullett, *The Bubonic Plague of England*, 195.

56. Mullett, *The Bubonic Plague and England*, 261, 264.

57. McNeill, *Plagues and Peoples*, 199.

58. Bubonic Plague, *History*, accessed 11 July 2006. http://en.wikipedia.org/wiki/Bubonic_plague, 5–6.

59. *Ibid.*

60. McNeill, *Plagues and Peoples*, 164–165, 169; Kinyoun, *Bubonic Plague*, 4–6, 8.

61. *Ibid.*, 164–170.

62. Kinyoun, *Bubonic Plague*, 4–5, 7; Hoff and Smith III, *Mapping Epidemics: A Historical Atlas of Disease*, 71; McNeill, *Plagues and* Peoples, 164–165; Reidman, *Shots Without* Guns, 116, 126–131, 137–139; CDC, *Natural History*, accessed 5 August 2008. www.cdc.gov/ncidod/dvbid/plague/history.htm; Nohl, *The Black Death*, 72–73, 83.

63. McNeill, *Plagues and Peoples*, 164.

Chapter I

1. Mrs. Hale Houts, "Yadkin Boys," *Journal of North Carolina Genealogy* Vol. IX No. 2 (Raleigh: North Carolina State Library, 1963), 1131–1135.

2. Kinyoun Genealogical Papers; Letter, from J.H. Kinyoun to Elizabeth Conrad Kinyoun, 2 April 1862 (Durham, NC: Duke University Rare Book, Manuscript, and Special Collections Library); David S. Heidler and James Jeanne T. Heidler, *Encyclopedia of the American Civil War* (New York, London: W.W. Norton & Company, 2000), 1481–1484.

3. Walter Clark, *Histories of the Several Regiments and Battalions from North Carolina in the Great War 1861–1865*, Vol. 3 (Raleigh: Published by the State), 685.

4. Heidler and Heidler, *Encyclopedia of the American Civil War*, 1712–1713.

5. Joseph Kinyoun Houts, Jr. *A Darkness Ablaze* (St. Joseph, MO: Platte Purchase Publishers, 2005), 35–38.

6. Alice Eceles Kinyoun Houts, *The Mears Genealogical Questionnaire* (Kinyoun Genealogical Papers), John Hendricks Kinyoun, 1.

7. Frances H. Casstevens, *The Civil War and Yadkin County, North Carolina* (Jefferson, NC: McFarland, 1997), 110–111.

8. *Ibid.*, 106–107.

9. *Ibid.*, 115.

10. Houts, *A Darkness Ablaze*, 43–44.

11. *Ibid.*, 26–27.

12. Irving A. Watson, *Physicians and Surgeons of America* (Concord, NH: Republican Press Association, 1896), 378–379; "Death of Dr. J.H. Kinyoun," *The Centerview Record*, July 31, 1903; "In Memory of Dr. Kinyoun," *Journal Democrat*, August 7, 1903; Joseph James Kinyoun, *Memorandum, 1874–1896*, 1–4; Kinyoun, Joseph James, *Who's Who in America 1910–1911*, 1.

13. Petition and Letter, to Hon. Grover Cleveland, 26 January 1893.

14. "Death of Dr. J.H. Kinyoun," *The Centerview Record*, July 31, 1903; "In Memory of Dr. Kinyoun," *Journal Democrat*, August 7, 1903; Certificate of Membership The Home Library Association No. 171152, R.S. Peale, President, Chicago, October 29, 1888; Watson, *Physicians and Surgeons of America*, 378–379; Kinyoun Genealogical Papers.
15. Houts, *The Mears Genealogical Questionnaire*, John Hendricks Kinyoun, 1.
16. Watson, *Physicians and Surgeons of America*, 378–379; "Centerview Woman Found Dead," *Journal Democrat*, February14, 1923.
17. Watson, *Physicians and Surgeons of America*, 378–379; "Centerview Woman Found Dead," *Journal Democrat*, February14, 1923.
18. "Centerview Woman Found Dead," *Journal Democrat*, February 14. 1923.
19. H.H. Cunningham, *Doctors in Gray* (Baton Rouge: Louisiana State University Press, 1993), 3–6.
20. Joseph Kinyoun Houts, Jr., *A Darkness Ablaze* (St. Joseph, MO: Platte Purchase Publishers, 2005), 19–20.
21. *Ibid.*, 6.
22. Dr. Claude Heaton, *History of the Bellevue Hospital Medical College* (New York: Courtesy of Ehrman Medical Library, 1941), 20.
23. Irving Robbin and Samuel Nisenson, *Giants of Medicine* (New York: Grosset & Dunlap, 1962), 64–71, 72–77, 82–85.
24. Heaton, *History of the Bellevue Hospital Medical College*, 14.
25. Diploma: Bellevue Hospital New York to Joseph J. Kinyoun, M.D. in Gynaecology [*sic*] March 1882.
26. Certificate of Private Instruction in Operative Surgery and Surgical Dressing by Joseph D. Bryant, M.D. to Joseph J. Kinyoun of the State of Missouri. New York, January 12, 1882.
27. Diploma: Chemical Laboratory of the Bellevue Hospital Medical College, New York, to Joseph J. Kinyoun in Medical and Toxicological Chemistry 15 March 1882.
28. Diploma: Bellevue Hospital New York to Joseph J. Kinyoun, M.D. in Gynaecology [*sic*] March 1882.
29. Bellevue Hospital Medical School, City of New York, Lectures on Special Subjects. 1881–1882.
30. Joseph J. Kinyoun, *Biographical Sketch* (Undated), 1–2; St. Louis Medical College, Lectures. 1880–1881.
31. Hospital of the City of St. Louis, Mo. Mr. J.J. Kinyoun is admitted to the Practice of this Institution for one year. Dean: Geo T.H., October 1, 1880–1881.
32. Hospital of the Sisters of Charity St. Louis, MO. Mr. J.J. Kinyoun is admitted to the Practice of this Institution for one year. Dean: Geo T.H. October 1, 1880–1881.
33. Letter, J.J. Kinyoun to Lizzie Perry, 9 May 1881.
34. Alice Kinyoun Houts, Contents Booklet, 11.
35. Letter, J.J. Kinyoun to Lizzie Perry, 9 May 1881.
36. Jean Carter Dabney collected stories and Ann Bennett Houx, compiled and edited, *Book of Houx Stories* (Warrensburg, MO: 1995), 32–34.
37. Sequoyah A. Perry, Children of Silas Perry, 19 August 1978.
38. Dabney and Houx, *Book of Houx Stories*, 32–34.
39. Joseph K. Houts, Jr., *Quantrill's Thieves* (Kansas City, MO: Truman Publishing, 2002), 31.
40. *Ibid.*, 31–31, 131–139.
41. *Ibid.*, 131–139.
42. Letter, W.E. Ward to Miss Lizzie Perry, 14 August 1877.
43. W.E. Ward's Seminary for Young Ladies, *Announcement* (Nashville, TN: 1881), 1.
44. *Ibid.*, 2.
45. W.E. Ward, Principal, *Monthly Report Miss Perry*, April 1878.
46. W.E. Ward's Seminary for Young Ladies, *Announcement*, 1.
47. Letter, Joe Kinyoun to Lizzie Perry, 19 February 1882.
48. *Ibid.*
49. *Ibid.*
50. Letter, Joe Kinyoun to Lizzie Perry, 21 December 1882.
51. *Ibid.*
52. *Ibid.*
53. *Ibid.*
54. *Ibid.*
55. Houts, *The Mears Genealogical Questionnaire*, 1.
56. *Ibid.*
57. Quit Claim Deed, Johnson County, Missouri, R.W. Houx to S. Elizabeth Kinyoun, wife of Joseph J. Kinyoun, 7 April 1885.
58. Joseph J. Kinyoun, *Biographical Sketch*, 1–2; Joseph James Kinyoun, *Memorandum*, 1874–1896, 1–4; Letter, Frederic S. Dennis M.D. Carnegie Lboratory [*sic*] Bellevue Hospital Medical College New York to Dr. Hamilton, Surgeon General M.H. Service, 16 March 1886.

Chapter II

1. *Official List of Medical Officers and Acting Assistant Surgeons of the United States Marine-Hospital Service, with Their Stations* (Treasury Department: 1 July 1881).
2. Letter, Joe J. Kinyoun to John B. Hamilton, 15 February 1886.
3. *Ibid.*
4. *Ibid.*
5. Ezra J. Warner, *Generals in Gray* (Baton Rouge: Louisiana State University Press, 1959, 1987), 57–58.
6. Letter, F.M. Cockrell to Dr. Joe J. Kinyoun, 23 February 1886.
7. *Ibid.*
8. Letter, Jos. J. Kinyoun to Hon. T.T. Crittenden, 27 February 1886.
9. *Ibid.*

10. Letter, Thos. T. Crittenden, Ex. Gov. of Mo., to Dr. John B. Hamilton, Sup Surgeon Gen'l, Undated.

11. Floyd Calvin Shoemaker, LL.D., *Missouri and Missourians* (Chicago: Lewis Publishing, 1943), 76, 78–83; WM. Rufus Jackson, *Missouri Democracy Volume I* (Chicago: S.J. Clarke, 1935), 221, 229; *Missouri Democracy Volume III* (Chicago: S.J. Clarke, 1935), 66, 69–72.

12. Wedding Invitation, Francis Marion Cockrell to Dr. & Mrs. Kinyoun, 14 February 1903.

13. Letter, Herman M. Biggs to Dr. Hamilton Surgeon General Marine Hospital Service, 8 March 1886; Letter, Frederic S. Dennis M.D. Carnegie Lboratory [*sic*] Bellevue Hospital Medical College, New York, to Dr. Hamilton Surgeon General M.H. Service, 16 March 1886; Letter, A. Flint Jr., to the Supervising Surgeon General of the U.S. Marine Hosp. Service, 11 March 1886; Letter, Frank L. James Ph.D. M.D., Editor of the M. & L. Journal Pres. St. L. Society of Microscopy, To whom it may Concern, 19 March 1886.

14. Letter, John B. Hamilton Supervising Surgeon-General, M.H.S. to Joseph J. Kinyoun, M.D. 23 March 1886.

15. Letter, F.M. Cockrell to Gen'l John B. Hamilton, Supervising Surgeon General, U.S. M.H. S., 10 April 1886.

16. *Ibid.*

17. *Ibid.*

18. Letter, John B. Hamilton Supervising Surgeon-General, M.H.S. to J.J. Kinyoun, M.D., 12 April 1886.

19. *Ibid.*

20. *Ibid.*

21. Letter, John B. Hamilton to Hon. F.M. Cockrell, 12 April 1886.

22. *Ibid.*

23. Wedding Invitation, Francis Marion Cockrell to Dr. & Mrs. Kinyoun, 14 February 1903; Letter, F.M. Cockrell to Dr. Kinyoun 14 January 1901.

24. Bess Furman, *A Profile of the United States Public Health Service 1798–1948* (Washington, D.C.: National Library of Medicine, 1973), 391–392.

25. *Ibid.*, 393.

26. *Official List of Medical Officers of the U.S. Marine-Hospital Service Including Acting Assistant Surgeons and Hospital Stewards: Also, Lists of U.S. Marine Hospitals and Quarantine Stations* (Washington, D.C.: Government Printing Office, January 1, 1887), 5, 9.

27. Ralph Chester Williams, *The United States Public Health Service 1798–1950* (Washington, D.C.: Commissioned Officers Association of the United States Public Health Service, 1951), 23.

28. *Ibid.*, 23–24.

29. *Ibid.*, 25.

30. Furman, *A Profile of the United States Public Health Service 1798–1948*, 3–4.

31. Williams, *The United States Public Health Service 1798–1950*, 28–29.

32. *Ibid.*, 31.

33. *Ibid.*, 30.

34. *Ibid.*, 29–30.

35. *Ibid.*, 31–32.

36. *Ibid.*, 32.

37. *Ibid.*, 32–37.

38. Furman, *A Profile of the United States Public Health Service 1798–1948*, 3.

39. Williams, *The United States Public Health Service 1798–1950*, 46–47.

40. *Ibid.*, 472–475.

41. Furman, *A Profile of the United States Public Health Service 1798–1948*, 109.

42. Williams, *The United States Public Health Service 1798–1950*, 63–65.

43. Furman, *A Profile of the United States Public Health Service 1798–1948*, 9–10.

44. *Ibid.*, 10–11.

45. *Ibid.*, 12.

46. Williams, *The United States Public Health Service 1798–1950*, 72–74.

47. *Ibid.*, 74–75.

48. Furman, *A Profile of the United States Public Health Service 1798–1948*, xi.

49. Williams, *The United States Public Health Service 1798–1950*, 72–76.

50. Furman, *A Profile of the United States Public Health Service 1798–1948*, xi.

51. National Board of Health Bill, Sec. 2; Memorandum concerning proposed National Board of Health Bill, 1–3, Kinyoun Family Papers; Williams, *the United States Public Health Service 1798–1950*, 76–79.

52. Williams, *the United States Public Health Service 1798–1950*, 76–79.

53. *Ibid.*, 82–85.

54. *Ibid.*, 84–85.

55. *Ibid.*, 476.

56. *Ibid.*, 102–104.

57. *Ibid.*, 100–104.

58. *Ibid.*, 102, 104–105.

59. *Ibid.*, 104–105.

60. *Ibid.*, 166–167.

Chapter III

1. Irving Robbin and Samuel Nisenson, *Giants of Medicine* (New York: Grosset & Dunlap, 1962), 41–42, 61, 68, 71.

2. Ralph Chester Williams, *The Unites States Public Health Service 1798–1950* (Washington, D.C.: Commissioned Officers Association of the United States Public Health Service, 1951), *1798–1950*, 249.

3. Joseph J. Kinyoun, *Biographical Sketch*, 1–2; Joseph James Kinyoun, *Memorandum, 1874–1896*, 1–4; Letter, Frederic S. Dennis M.D. Carnegie Lboratory [*sic*] Bellevue Hospital Medical College New York to Dr. Hamilton Surgeon General M.H. Service, 16 March 1886.

4. Bess Furman, *A Profile of the United States Public Health Service* (Washington, D.C.: National Library of Medicine, 1973), 114; Williams, *The United States Public Health Service 1798–1950*, 249.

5. Kinyoun Family Papers.

6. Williams, *The United States Public Health Service 1798–1950*, 178, 249.

7. Centre View Academy Brochure, Centreview, Mo., 1 September 1884.

8. Williams, *The United States Public Health Service 1798–1950*, 178, 249.

9. Joseph J. Kinyoun, *Biographical Sketch*, 1–2; Joseph James Kinyoun, *Memorandum, 1874–1896*, 1–4; Letter, Frederic S. Dennis M.D. Carnegie Lboratory [*sic*] Bellevue Hospital Medical College New York to Dr. Hamilton Surgeon General M.H. Service, 16 March 1886.

10. Williams, *The United States Public Health Service 1798–1950*, 176–178.

11. Williams, *The United States Public Health Service 1798–1950*, 178.

12. *Ibid.*, 177.

13. *Ibid.*, 177–178.

14. Dr. David M. Morens, NIAID, NIH, Abutment Joseph James Kinyoun, MD, PhD, America's First Microbiologists: Founder of the National Institutes of Health (and Almost-Founder of CDC & FDA?) Presented to the colleagues in the National Institute of Allergy & Infectious Diseases, NIH (Bethesda, MD: 28 May 2009), 17.

15. Furman, *A Profile of the United States Public Health Service 1798–1948*, 194.

16. *Ibid.*

17. Furman, *A Profile of the United States Public Health Service 1798–1948*, 194; Williams, *The United States Public Health Service 1798–1950*, 76–79.

18. Furman, *A Profile of the United States Public Health Service 1798–1948*, 194.

19. *Ibid.*, 194.

20. *Ibid.*, 195.

21. *Ibid.*

22. *Ibid.*

23. Williams, *The United States Public Health Service 1798–1950*, 177.

24. *Ibid.*, 177–180.

25. *Ibid.*

26. Notation: Alice Kinyoun Houts to Joseph Kinyoun Houts, Jr., 5 January 1963.

27. Furman, *A Profile of the United States Public Health Service 1798–1948*, 217.

28. Letter, Prof. Dr. Kitasato to Dr. Kinyoun, 17 August 1901.

29. Robbin and Nisenson, *Giants of Medicine*, 65.

30. Robbin and Nisenson, *Giants of Medicine*, 41–45, 66–67.

31. *Ibid.*, 41–44, 66–68.

32. *Ibid.*, 73.

33. *Ibid.*, 73–74.

34. *Ibid.*, 74.

35. *Ibid.*, 76.

36. *Ibid.*, 74–77.

37. *Ibid.*, 79–81.

38. Philip Cane and Samuel Nisenson, *Giants of Science* (New York: Grosset & Dunlap, 1959), 149; Robbin and Nisenson, *Giants of Medicine*, 79–81.

39. Notation: Alice Kinyoun Houts to Joseph Kinyoun Houts, Jr., 5 January 1963.

39. Robbin and Nisenson, *Giants of Medicine*, 61.

40. *Ibid.*

41. *Ibid.*

42. *Ibid.*

43. *Ibid.*

44. *Ibid.*, 73–74.

45. *Ibid.*, 61–63.

46. Notation: Alice Kinyoun Houts to Joseph Kinyoun Houts, Jr., 5 January 1963.

47. Robbin and Nisenson, *Giants of Medicine*, 87–88.

48. *Ibid.* 88–89.

49. *Ibid.*, 90–91.

50. *Ibid.*

51. *Ibid.*

52. *Ibid.*, 91.

53. *Ibid.*

54. *Ibid.*

55. *Ibid.*, 90.

56. Notation: Alice Kinyoun Houts to Joseph Kinyoun Houts, Jr., 5 January 1963; Letter, John B. Hamilton, Supervising Surgeon-General, M.H.S. to Passed assistant Surgeon J.J. Kinyoun, U.S. Marine-Hospital Service, Berlin, Germany 20 January 1891.

57. Biographical Sketch, Joseph J. Kinyoun, 1–2; Joseph James Kinyoun, *Memorandum 1874–1896*, 1–4; Letter, Frederic S. Dennis M.D., Carnegie Lboratory [*sic*] Bellevue Hospital Medical College, New York, to Dr. Hamilton Surgeon General M.H. Service, 16 March 1886.

58. Williams, *The United States Public Health Service 1798–1950*, 178–179; Furman, *A Profile of the United States Public Health Service 1798–1948*, 114, 194–195, 202–203, 213.

59. Williams, *The United States Public Health Service 1798–1950*, 178–179; Furman, *A Profile of the United States Public Health Service 1798–1948*, 114, 194–195, 202–203, 213.

Chapter IV

1. Ralph Chester Williams, *The United States Public Health Service 1798–1950* (Washington, D.C.: Commissioned Officers Association of the United States Public Health Service, 1951), 177, 249–250.

2. *Ibid.*

3. "Genesis of a National Treasure: The NIH." *Mayo Clinic Proceedings*, Vol. 62, No. 2, 1987, 30–35.

4. Bess Furman, *A Profile of the United States Public Health Service 1798–1948* (Washington, D.C.: U.S. Department of Health, Education and Welfare, National Institutes of Health, National Library of Medicine, 1973), 114 and Williams, *The United States Public Health Service 1798–1950*, 177, 408.

5. *Ibid.*

6. Williams, *The United States Public Health Service 1798–1950*, 177.

7. Dr. S.T. Armstrong, M.D. and Dr. J.J. Kinyoun, *Observations on the Cholera Bacillus as a Means of Positive Diagnosis* (New York Medical Journal, 6 November 1887), 546–547.

8. *Ibid.*

9. Williams, *The United States Public Health Service 1798–1950*, 177.
10. Armstrong and Kinyoun, *Observations on the Cholera Bacillus as a Means of Positive Diagnosis*, 546–547.
11. *Ibid.*
12. *Ibid.*
13. *Ibid.*
14. Assistant Surgeon J.J. Kinyoun, *Weekly Assistant of Sanitary Reports* (Medical News, 3 February 1888), 164–165.
15. *Ibid.*
16. "Sea Water a Pest Carrier," *The Daily Light* (San Antonio, 25 June 1888).
17. Furman, *A Profile of the United States Public Health Service 1798–1948*, 194–195.
18. *Ibid.*
19. "Phosphorus Not a Disinfectant," *The Daily Light* (San Antonio, 19 March 1888).
20. *Ibid.*
21. *Ibid.*
22. *Annual Report of the Supervising Surgeon-General of the Marine-Hospital Service of the United States for the Fiscal Year 1889* (Washington, D.C.: Government Printing Office, 1889), 104–105.
23. *Ibid.*, 104.
24. *Ibid.*
25. *Ibid.*
26. *Ibid.*, 104–105.
27. *Ibid.*, 105.
28. *Annual Report of the Supervising Surgeon-General of the Marine-Hospital Service of the United States for the Fiscal Year 1890* (Washington, D.C.: Government Printing Office, 1890), 7.
29. *Ibid.*, 11–27.
30. *Ibid.*, 11.
31. *Ibid.*, 13.
32. *Ibid.*, 13–15.
33. *Ibid.*, 18.
34. *Ibid.*, 15.
35. *Ibid.*
36. *Ibid.*, 19–20.
37. *Ibid.*, 17–19.
38. *Ibid.*, 19.
39. *Ibid.*, 18.
40. *Ibid.*, 19–20.
41. *Ibid.*, 20.
42. Hemotoxin, http://en.wikipedia.org/wiki/Hemotoxin, accessed 23 August 2010, 1; Neurotoxin, http://en.wikipedia.org/wiki/Neurotoxin, 23 August 2010, 1–3.
43. *Annual Report of the Supervising Surgeon-General of the Marine-Hospital Service of the Unites States for Fiscal Year 1890*, 17.
44. *Ibid.*, 20.
45. *Ibid.*, 21–26.
46. *Ibid.*, 26–27.
47. The Western Union Telegraph Company, J.J. Kinyoun to NW Perry, 920 AM 2/26 1888.
48. The Western Union Telegraph Company, J.J. Kinyoun to NW Perry, 1220 PM 2/26 1888.
49. The Western Union Telegraph Company, J.J. Kinyoun to Col NW Perry, 1015 AM 2/27 1888.
50. The Western Union Telegraph Company, J.J. Kinyoun to NW Perry, 707 PM 2/27 1888.
51. The Western Union Telegraph Company, J.J. Kinyoun to NW Perry, February 28 1888.
52. The Western Union Telegraph Company, Jos J Kinyoun to Dr Jno H Kinyoun, 920 AM 2/26 1888.
53. Interview with Dr. Daivd Morens.
54. "A Startling Meeting," *The Baltimore Sun* (Baltimore, MD: 29 December 1888).
55. *The Mears Genealogical Questionnaire*, 2.
56. "A Startling Meeting," *The Baltimore Sun* (Baltimore, MD: 29 December 29, 1888).
57. *Ibid.*
58. "News of the Ships," *The Baltimore Sun* (Baltimore, MD: 10 January 1889).
59. Letter, J.J. Kinyoun to Papa (Dr. John Hendricks Kinyoun), 14 January 1889.
60. *Ibid.*
61. *Ibid.*
62. *Ibid.*
63. *Ibid.*
64. *Ibid.*
65. *Ibid.*
66. *Ibid.*
67. *Ibid.*
68. Williams, *The United States Public Health Services 1798–1950*, 177–178.
69. "News of the Ships," *The Baltimore Sun* (Baltimore, MD: 10 January 1889).
70. Letter, John B. Hamilton Supervising Surgeon-General, M.H.S. to Assistant Surgeon J.J. Kinyoun, 19 March 1889.
71. "Surgeons and Assistants," *The Baltimore Sun* (Baltimore, MD: 16 January 1889).
72. Letter, Bettie (Perry) to Husband (Nathan W. Perry), 19 May 1889.
73. *Ibid.*
74. Letter, Bettie (Perry) to Husband (Nathan W. Perry), 20 May 1889.
75. *Ibid.*

Chapter V

1. Letter, Walter Wyman, Surgeon, M.H.S. to Surgeon General U.S. Marine Hospital Service, 7 October 1890.
2. *Official List of the Medical Officers of the U.S. Marine-Hospital Service, Including Acting Assistant Surgeons and Hospital Stewards; Also, Lists of U.S. Marine Hospitals and Quarantine Stations* (Washington, D.C.: Government Printing Office, January 1, 1887), 3–5.
3. Letter, John B. Hamilton SupervisingSurgeon-General, M.H.S. to Joe J. Kinyoun, 18 February 1886.
4. Letter, Walter Wyman, Surgeon, M.H.S. to Surgeon General U.S. Marine Hospital Service, 7 October 1890.
5. *Ibid.*
6. Letter, John Godfrey, Surgeon, M.H.S. to U.S. Marine Hospital Service, 8 October 1890; Letter, Geo. Purviance. Surgeon, M.H.S. to Board of Examiners, 12 October 1890.

7. Letter, A.B. Nettleton, Acting Secretary Treasury Department to Supervising Surgeon-General, 20 November 1890.

8. *Ibid.*

9. John B. Hamilton Supervising Surgeon-General, M.H.S. to Assistant Surgeon J.J. Kinyoun 20 November 1890.

10. BENJAMIN HARRISON, *President of the United States of America*, appoints Joseph J. Kinyoun Passed assistant Surgeon in the Marine-Hospital Service of the United States, Benjamin Harrison, by the President: A.B. Nettleton, Acting Secretary of the Treasury. Entered in Book No. 1, page 203. John B. Hamilton Supervising Surgeon-General, M.H.S. 21 November 1890.

11. *Ibid.*

12. Letter, John B. Hamilton Supervising Surgeon-General, M.H.S. to Passed Assistant Surgeon Joseph J. Kinyoun, 8 December 1890.

13. Letter, A.B. Nettleton Acting Secretary to Passed Assistant Surgeon J.J. Kinyoun, 11 December 1890.

14. Letter, James G. Blaine to Diplomatic and Consular Office of the United States, 17 December 1890.

15. William T. Wharton, Acting Secretary to William Walter Phelps, Esquire, Envoy Extraordinary and Minister Plenipotentiary of the United States, Berlin, 20 December 1890.

16. *Ibid.*

17. Letter, A.B. Nettleton Acting Secretary to Passed Assistant Surgeon J.J. Kinyoun, 11 December 1890.

18. Letter, Secretary of the Treasury to House of Representatives. 51st Congress, 2nd Session, Ex. Doc. No. 294, 23 January 1891.

19. *Ibid.*

20. *Ibid.*

21. *Ibid;* Bess Furman, *A Profile of the United States Public Health Service 1798–1948* (Washington, D.C.: National Library of Medicine, 1973), 202.

22. Letter, Lizzie to Papa (Dr. John Hendricks Kinyoun), 26 January 1891.

23. *Ibid.*

24. *The Mears Genealogical Questionnaire*, Alice Eccles Kinyoun Houts, 1.

25. Letter, to Papa (Dr. John Hendricks Kinyoun), 26 January 1891.

26. *Ibid.*

27. *Ibid.*

28. Interview Alice Kinyoun Houts, 16 June 1974.

29. Letter, Lizzie to Mamma (Betty Rice Moore Perry), 28 January 1891.

30. *Ibid.*

31. *Ibid.*

32. Letter, John B. Hamilton, Supervising Surgeon-General to Passed Assistant Surgeon J.J. Kinyoun, 26 January 1891.

33. Letter, John B. Hamilton to the Honorable F.M. Cockrell, U.S. S., 19 February 1891.

34. *Ibid;* Letter, John B. Hamilton Supervising Surgeon-General, M.H.S. to Passed Assistant Surgeon J.J. Kinyoun, 26 January 1891.

35. Letter, John B. Hamilton to the Honorable F.M. Cockrell, U.S. S., 19 February 1891.

36. *Ibid.*

37. *Ibid.*

38. Letter, Secretary of the Treasury to House of Representatives. 51st Congress, 2nd Session, Ex Doc. No. 294, 23 January 1891.

39. *Ibid.*

40. Letter, (Weekly Report) Jos Kinyoun P.A. Surgeon M.H.S. to Dr. John B. Hamilton Surgeon General Marine Hospital Service, 28 February 1891.

41. *Ibid.*

42. *Ibid.*

43. *Ibid.*

44. *Ibid.*

45. *Ibid.*

46. *Ibid.*

47. *Ibid.*

48. *Ibid.*

49. *Ibid.*

50. *Ibid.*

51. *Ibid.*

52. *Ibid.*

53. Dr. Joseph James Kinyoun Case Chart.

54. *Ibid.*, H.H. Cunningham, *Doctors in Gray* (Baton Rouge: Louisiana State University Press, 1993), 242–243, 260–261.

55. *Annual Report of the Supervising Surgeon-General of the Marine Hospital Service of the United States for the Fiscal Year 1891*, 58; Irving Robbin and Samuel Nisenson, *Giants of Medicine* (New York: Grosset & Dunlap, 1962), 76–77.

56. *Annual Report of the Supervising Surgeon-General of the Marine Hospital Service of the United States for the Fiscal Year 1891*, 58.

57. *Ibid.*

58. *Ibid.*

59. *Ibid.*

60. *Ibid.*

61. *Ibid.*

62. *Ibid.*

63. *Ibid.*

64. *Ibid.*

65. *Ibid.*, 59.

66. Robbin and Nisenson, *Giants of Medicine*, 61.

67. *Annual Report of the Supervising Surgeon-General of the Marine Hospital Service of the United States for the Fiscal Year 1891*, 59.

68. Robbin and Nisenson, *Giants of Medicine*, 61–63.

69. *Annual Report of the Supervising Surgeon-General of the Marine Hospital Service of the United States for the Fiscal Year 1891*, 59.

70. *Ibid.*

71. *Ibid.*

72. *Ibid.*

73. *Ibid.*

74. *Ibid.*

75. *Ibid.*

76. *Ibid.*

77. *Ibid.*, 60.

78. *Ibid.*

79. *Ibid.*

80. *Ibid.*
81. *Ibid.*
82. *Ibid.*
83. *Ibid.*
84. *Ibid.*
85. *Ibid.*, 60–61.
86. *Ibid.*, 61.
87. Letter, Dr. Roux to Mousier (Dr. Joseph James Kinyoun), 24 April Note 1891:
88. Letter, Bailly-Blanchard, Rte Secretary to Passed Assistant Surgeon Joseph J. Kinyoun M.D., 29 April 1891.
89. *Annual Report of the Supervising Surgeon-General of the Marine Hospital Service of the United States for the Fiscal Year 1891*, 61.
90. *Ibid.*
91. Weekly Report, Dr. Joseph James Kinyoun to Dr. John B. Hamilton, Undated (Likely May 1891).
92. *Ibid.*
93. *Ibid.*
94. *Ibid.*
95. *Ibid.*
96. *Ibid.*
97. *Ibid.*
98. *Ibid.*
99. *Ibid.*
100. Furman, *A Profile of the United States Public Health Service 1798*–1948, 203; *Annual Report of the Supervising Surgeon-General of the Marine Hospital Service of the United States for the Fiscal Year 1891*, 61.
101. Furman, *A Profile of the United States Public Health Service 1798–1948*, 203.
102. *Annual Report of the Supervising Surgeon-General of the Marine Hospital Service of the United States for the Fiscal Year 1891*, 61.
103. *Ibid.*
104. Robbin and Nisenson, *Giants of Medicine*, 79–81.
105. *Annual Report of the Supervising Surgeon-General of the Marine Hospital Service of the United States for the Fiscal Year 1891*, 61; Robbin and Nisenson, *Giants of Medicine*, 79–81.
106. Furman, *A Profile of the United States Public Health Service 1798–1948*, 202.
107. David M. Morens, M.D., National Institute of Allergy & Infectious Diseases, NIH, "The Forgotten Indispensable Man: Joe Kinyoun & the Birth of NIH," Presentation: History of Medicine Seminar, 26 September 2011, 5.
108. *Annual Report of the Supervising Surgeon-General of the Marine Hospital Service for the Fiscal Year 1891*, 62.
109. *Ibid.*
110. Furman, *A Profile of the United States Public Health Service 1789–1948*, 202.
111. *Ibid.*, 203.
112. Letter, Walter Wyman, Supervising Surgeon-General, M.H.S. to Passed Assistant Surgeon J.J. Kinyoun, 8 October 1891.

Chapter VI

1. Ralph Chester Williams, *The United States Public Health Service 1798–1950* (Washington, D.C.: Commissioned Officers Association of the United States Public Health Service, 1951), 18.
2. Kinyoun Family Papers.
3. "Koch's Celebrated Lymph," *The Atlantic Constitution* (13 May 1891). National Library of Medicine, National Institutes of Health.
4. *Ibid.*
5. *Ibid.*
6. *Ibid.*
7. Proceeding and Discussions At the Nineteenth *Annual* Meeting (Kansas City, MO: October 20–23, 1891), 243.
8. *Ibid.*, 251–252.
9. *Ibid.*
10. *Ibid.*, 304.
11. *Ibid.*
12. *Ibid.*
13. *The American Heritage Dictionary, Fourth Edition* (New York: Random House, 2007), 617.
14. Proceedings and Discussions At the Nineteenth *Annual* Meeting, 304.
15. Assignment Order (National Library of Medicine, National Institutes of Health, 7 March 1892).
16. *Miscellany* (National Library of Medicine, National Institutes of Health, 30 April 1892), 570.
17. *Ibid.*
18. Birth Announcement, 13 August 1892.
19. *Boston Medical and Surgical Journal* (6 October 1892), 348.
20. *Abstract of Sanitary Reports, Vol. Vii., No. 37* (Washington, D.C.: National Library of Medicine, National Institutes of Health, 9 September 1892), 466–467.
21. *Ibid.*
22. *Ibid.*
23. *Ibid.*
24. *Ibid.*
25. George Worthington Adams, *Doctors in Blue* (Baton Rouge: Louisiana State University Press, 1996), 3, 194–195; H. H, Cunningham, *Doctors in Gray* (Baton Rouge: Louisiana State University Press, 1993), 3–8.
26. *The American Heritage Dictionary, Fourth Edition*, 689.
27. J.J. Kinyoun, M.D., *Rabies—Its Prevention and Treatment* (Bethesda, MD: National Library of Medicine, National Institutes of Health, 1892), 162–163, 165–166.
28. *Ibid.*, 162.
29. *Ibid.*, 163–164.
30. *Ibid.*, 164.
31. *Ibid.*
32. *Ibid.*, 164–165.
33. *Ibid.*, 163, 167–168.
34. *Ibid.*
35. *Ibid.*, 168.
36. *Ibid.*, 166–167.
37. *Ibid.*, 166.
38. *Ibid.*

39. *Operations of the United States Marine-Hospital Service* (National Library of Medicine, 1892), 96; *Abstract of Sanitary Reports, Vol. Vii., No. 40* (Washington, D.C.: National Library of Medicine, National Institutes of Health, 30 September 1892); *Abstract of Sanitary Reports, Vol. Vii., No. 42* (Washington, D.C.: National Library of Medicine, National Institutes of Health, 14 October 1892).

40. *Operations of the United States Marine-Hospital Service*, 96.

41. *Ibid.*, 96–97.

42. *Ibid.*, 98.

43. *Ibid.*, 98–99.

44. *Ibid.*

45. *Ibid.*, 99.

46. *Ibid.*, 99.

47. *Ibid.*, 99–100.

48. Dr. Joseph James Kinyoun, *Animal Immunity Against Diptheria* (Berlin: From the Hygienische Resndeschau, 15 October 1892), 1–2.

49. *Ibid.*

50. Letter, John H. Kinyoun to Joe, 20 December 1892.

51. *Ibid.*

52. Letter, John H. Kinyoun to Joe, 26 January 1893.

53. Letter, John H. Kinyoun to Joe, 20 December 1892.

54. The White House, Grover Cleveland, www.whitehouse.gov/about/presidents/grovercleveland 22, accessed 25 February 2012.

55. Letter, John H. Kinyoun to Joe, 26 January 1893.

56. Letter, John H. Kinyoun to Joe, 26 March 1893.

57. Letter, John H. Kinyoun to Dr. J.J. Kinyoun, 14 August 1893.

58. Letter, John H. Kinyoun to Lizzie, 22 September 1893.

59. *Ibid.*

60. Letter, Walter Wyman, Supervising Surgeon General, M.H.S. to Passed Assistant Surgeon J.J. Kinyoun, U.S. Marine Hospital Services, Washing ton, D.C., 16 February 1893.

61. *Ibid.*

62. *Memorandum*. Senate Bill 4895 (House 13247), February 15, 1893.

63. *Ibid.*

64. *Ibid.*

65. *Ibid.*

66. *Ibid.*

67. *Ibid.*

68. *Ibid.*

69. *Ibid.*

70. *Ibid.*

71. *Ibid.*

72. *Ibid.*

73. Letter, Walter Wyman, Supervising Surgeon-General, M.H.S. to Passed Assistant Surgeon J.J. Kinyoun U.S. Marine Hospital Service, Washington, D.C., 4 April 1893.

74. *State Medicine*, Walter Wyman to 44th *Annual* American Medical Association Meeting, *Address on State Medicine* (Milwaukee: 8 July 1903), 52–54.

75. *Ibid.*

76. *Domestic Correspondence* (National Library of Medicine, National Institutes of Health, 22 July 1893), 139.

77. *Ibid.*

78. *Ibid.*

79. *Ibid.*

80. Letter, Joe to Lizzie, 18 June 1893.

81. Thomas Edison, en.wikipedia.org/wiki/Thomas_Edison, accessed 26 February 2012, 1–21.

82. Letter, Walter Wyman, Supervising Surgeon-General, M.H.S. to Passed Assistant Surgeon J.J. Kinyoun, Marine Hospital Service, Stapleton, Staten Island, N.Y., 26 August 1893.

83. Ellis Island History-a Brief Look, accessed 13 December 2011. www.nps.gov/elis/contacts.htm.

84. *Ibid.*

85. *Ibid.*

86. *Ibid.*

87. *Ibid.*

88. *Ibid.*

89. *Ibid.*

90. *Abstract of Sanitary Reports, Vol. Viii., No. 32* (Washington, D.C.: National Library of Medicine, National Institutes of Health, August 11, 1893), 681.

91. *Ibid.*

92. *Annual Report of the Supervising Surgeon-General of the Marine-Hospital Service of the United States for the Fiscal Year 1893, Volume II.* (Washington, D.C.: Government Printing Office, 1895), 8.

93. *Ibid.*, 9.

94. *Ibid.*

95. *Ibid.*, 9–10.

96. *Ibid.*, 10.

97. *Ibid.*

98. *Ibid.*, 9–10.

99. *Ibid.*, 8–10. 103. Letter, Walter Wyman, Supervising Surgeon-General, M.H.S. to Passed Assistant Surgeon J.J. Kinyoun, Marine-Hospital Service, Stapleton, Staten Island, N.Y., 26 August 1893.

100. *Abstract of Sanitary Reports, Vol. Viii., No. 35* (Washington, D.C.: National Library of Medicine, National Institutes of Medicine, 1 September 1893), 785–786; *Abstract of Sanitary Reports, Vol. Viii., No. 41* (Washington, D.C.: National Library of Medicine, National Institutes of Health, 993.

101. *Abstract of Sanitary Reports, Vol. Viii., No. 42* (Washington, D.C.: National Library of Medicine, National Institutes of Health), 1035–1036.

102. *Miscellany* (Washington, D.C.: National Library of Medicine, National Institutes of Health, 11 November 1893), 50.

103. *Miscellany* (Washington, D.C.: National Library of Medicine, National Institutes of Health, 30 December 1893), 1024.

104. The Western Union Telegraph Company, Kate Houx to Mrs. J.J. Kinyoun, care of Dr. C.J. Atkins, 30 December 1893.

105. *Annual Report of the Supervising Surgeon-General of the Marine-Hospital Service of the United*

States for the Fiscal Year 1894. (Washington, D.C.: Government Printing Office, 1895), 187.

106. *Ibid.*

107. *Ibid.*

108. Letter, Joe to Dad, 4 February 1894.

109. Letter, Rich. H. Lewis to Doctor Kinyoun, 24 January 1894.

110. Letter, G.W. Shell to Dr. Walter Wyman, 13 February 1894; Return, Walter Wyman, Surgeon General M.H.S. to Hon. G.W. Shell H.R. 14 February 1894.

111. Letter, Walter Wyman, Supervising Surgeon-General, M.H.S. to Passed Assistant Surgeon J.J. Kinyoun, Washington, D.C., 21 February 1894; *Annual Report of the Supervising Surgeon-General of the Marine-Hospital Service of the United States for the Fiscal Year 1894,* 189.

112. *Annual Report of the Supervising Surgeon-General of the Marine-Hospital Service of the United States for the Fiscal Year 1894,* 189–190.

113. *Ibid.*, 190–193.

114. Letter, J.J. Kinyoun Passed Assistant Surgeon, M.H.S. to the Supervising Surgeon-General, M.H.S., Washington, D.C., 20 February 1894, 1–3.

115. *Ibid.*, 2.

116. *Ibid.*, 3.

117. *Ibid.*

118. *Ibid.*

119. *Ibid.*, 3–4.

120. *Ibid.*, 5.

121. Letter, J.J. Kinyoun P.A. Surgeon, M.H.S. to Supervising Surgeon-General, U.S. Marine-Hospital Service, Washington, D.C., 18 June 1894.

122. *Ibid.*, 3.

123. *Ibid.*, 4.

124. Letter, Walter Wyman, Supervising Surgeon-General, M.H.S. to Passed Assistant Surgeon J.J. Kinyoun, U.S. Marine-Hospital Service, Washington, D.C., 26 April 1894.

125. *Ibid.*

126. *Ibid.*

127. *Ibid.*

128. *Annual Report of the Supervising Surgeon General of the Marine-Hospital Service of the United States for the Fiscal Year 1894,* 224–228.

129. Letter, Walter Wyman, Supervising Surgeon-General, M.H.S. to Passed Assistant Surgeon J.J. Kinyoun, U.S. Marine-Hospital Service, Washington, D.C., 11 May 1894.

130. *The American Heritage Dictionary, Fourth Edition,* 244.

131. Letter, J.J. Kinyoun, Passed Assistant Surgeon, M.H.S. to the Supervising Surgeon-General, U.S. Marine-Hospital Service, Washington, D.C., 18 June 1894.

132. Letter, Emill Boas, General Passenger Manager Hamburg-American Line, to Mr. J.J. Kinyoun, c/o Dr. Geo. O. Glavis, Washington Post Building, Washington, D.C., 19 June 1894.

133. Letter, J.J. Kinyoun Passed Assistant Surgeon, M.H.S. to the Supervising Surgeon-General, U.S. Marine-Hospital Service, Washington, D.C., 18 June 1894.

134. *Ibid.*

135. Letter, Walter Wyman, Supervising Surgeon-General, M.H.S. to the Honorable Secretary of the Treasury, July 1894.

136. *Ibid.*

137. *Annual Report of the SupervisingSurgeon-General of the Marine-Hospital Service of the Unites States for the Fiscal Year 1894,* 13–18.

138. *Ibid.*, 16.

139. *Ibid.*, 16–17.

140. *Ibid.*, 16.

141. *Ibid.*

142. *Ibid.*

143. *Ibid.*

144. Letter, Walter Wyman, Supervising Surgeon-General, M.H.S. to the Honorable Secretary of the Treasury. 9 July 1894.

145. *Annual Report of the Supervising Surgeon-General of the Marine-Hospital Service of the United States for the Fiscal Year 1894,* 17.

146. *Ibid.*

147. *Annual Report of the Supervising Surgeon-General of the Marine-Hospital Service of the United States for the Fiscal Year 1897* (Washington, D.C.: Government Printing Office, 1899), 711–712.

148. Dr. David M. Morens, Senior Advisor to the Director, National Institute of Allergy and Infectious Diseases, National Institutes of Health, Kinyoun Time Line 1887–1896, undated.

149. *Ibid.*

150. *Annual Report of the Supervising Surgeon-General of the Marine-Hospital Service of the United States for the Fiscal Year 1894,* 17.

151. *Ibid.*

152. *Ibid.*

153. Passed Assistant Surgeon J.J. Kinyoun, *Report on the Treatment of Diphtheria by Antitoxic Serum, and Notes on the Prevention of Diphtheria* (Washington, D.C.: Government Printing Office, 1894), 3, 11; "The Serum Therapy of Diphtheria," *Abstract of Sanitary Reports, Vol IX, No 47* (Washington, D.C.: National Library of Medicine, National Institutes of Health, 23 November 1894), 1113–114.

154. Passed Assistant Surgeon J.J. Kinyoun, *Report on the Treatment of Diphtheria by Antitoxic Serum, and Notes on the Prevention of Diphtheria* (Washington, D.C.: Government Printing Office, 1894), 3, 11; "The Serum Therapy of Diphtheria," *Abstract of Sanitary Reports, Vol IX, No 47* (Washington, D.C.: National Library of Medicine, National Institutes of Health, 23 November 1894), 1113–114.

155. Passed Assistant Surgeon J.J. Kinyoun, *Report on the Treatment of Diphtheria by Antitoxic Serum, and Notes on the Prevention of Diphtheria* (Washington, D.C.: Government Printing Office, 1894), 3, 11; "The Serum Therapy of Diphtheria," *Abstract of Sanitary Reports, Vol IX, No 47* (Washington, D.C.: National Library of Medicine, National Institutes of Health, 23 November 1894), 1113–114.

156. "The Serum Therapy of Diphtheria," *Abstract of Sanitary Reports, Vol IX, No 47*, (Washington, D.C.: National Library of Medicine, National Institutes of Health, 23 November 1894), 1117.

157. *Abstract of Sanitary Reports, Vol. IX, No. 47*, 1118–1119.
158. *St. Louis Post-Dispatch*, 7 December 1899; the *New York Times*, 17 October 1894; the *Argus*, 18 October 1894; *Daily State Press*, 27 October 1894; *Fort Wayne News* 29 November 1894; the *Washington Post*, 27 October 1894; *Logan Sport Reporter*, 27 October 1894; the *Daily Gazette*, 30 October 1894; *Daily State* Press, 27 October 1894; *Daily Republican*, 30 November 1894; *Weekly Wisconsin Cousin*, 15 December 1894; the *Daily Northwestern*, 30 November 1894; *Chicago Daily Tribune*, 30 November 1894 (All articles listed in this endnote: National Library of Medicine, National Institutes of Health).
159. *Abstract of Sanitary Reports, Vol. IX, No. 47*, 1113.
160. Letter, Kinyoun to Geddings, Undated (1894), 1.
161. *Ibid.*
162. *Ibid.*
163. *Ibid.*, 2–4.
164. *Ibid.*, 4–5.
165. *Ibid.*
166. *Ibid.*
167. *Ibid.*, 4.
168. Letter, Kinyoun to Geddings, Entitled Postscript, Undated (1894).
169. *Ibid.*, 1.
170. *Ibid;* Passed Assistant Surgeon J.J. Kinyoun, *Report on the Treatment of Diphtheria by Antitoxic Serum, and Notes on the Prevention of Diphtheria* (Washington, D.C.: Government Printing Office, 1894); Letter, Kinyoun to Geddings, Entitled Postscript Undated, 1.
171. Letter, Kinyoun to Geddings, Undated, 5.
172. *Ibid.*
173. Letter, Kinyoun to Geddings, Entitled Postscript, Undated, 1–2.
174. *Ibid.*, 2
175. *Ibid.*
176. *Public Health* (National Library of Medicine, National Institutes of Health, 22 December 1894), 956–960.
177. Williams, the *United States Public Health Service 1798–1950*, 179.
178. *Ibid.*
179. Letter, Kinyoun to Dr. Geddings, Entitled Postscript, 2–3.
180. *Public Health* (National Library of Medicine, National Institutes of Health, 22 December 1894), 956–960; Letter, Kinyoun to Dr. Geddings, Entitled Postscript, 2–3.
181. Williams, the *United States Public Health Service 1798–1950*, 179.
182. Interview with David M. Morens, M.D., Senior Advisor to the Director, Office of the Director, National Institute of Allergy and Infectious Diseases, National Institutes of Health, St. Joseph, Missouri, 13 May 2010.

Chapter VII

1. *Annual Report of the Supervising Surgeon-General of the Marine-Hospital Service of the United States for the Fiscal Year 1896* (Washington, D.C.: Government Printing Office, 1896), 994, 999.
2. *Ibid.*
3. *Ibid.*, 1000.
4. *Ibid.*, 1001.
5. *Ibid.*, 1002, 1004.
6. *The American Heritage Dictionary, Fourth Edition* (New York: Random House, 2007), 781.
7. *Annual Report of the Supervising Surgeon-General of the Marine-Hospital Service of the United States for the Fiscal Year 1895* (Washington, D.C.: Government Printing Office, 1896), 367–368.
8. *Ibid.*, 368.
9. J.J. Kinyoun, M.D. Passed Assistant Surgeon, M.H.S. "Treatment of Variola by Its Antitoxin," *Abstract of Sanitary Reports, Vol. X, No. 3* (Washington, D.C.: National Library of Medicine, National Institutes of Medicine, 18 January 1895), 87.
10. *Ibid.*, 87–89.
11. *Ibid.*
12. *Ibid.*, 87.
13. *Ibid.*
14. *Ibid.*
15. Maurice Raynaud, http://en.wikipedia.org/wiki/Maurice Raynaud, accessed 10 March 2012, 1.
16. George Miller Sternberg, http://wikipedia.org/wiki/George_Sternberg, accessed 10 March 2012, 1.
17. *Ibid.*
18. *Ibid.*
19. *Ibid.*, 1–6.
20. Surgeon General of the United States Army, http://en.wikipedia.org/wiki/Surgeon_General_of_the_United_States_Army, accessed 4 July 2012, 1–6 and; Ralph Chester Williams, *The United States Public Health Service 1798–1950* (Washington, D.C.: Commissioned Officers Association of the Unites States Public Health Service, 1951), 471–472.
21. *The American Heritage Dictionary, Fourth Edition*, 504.
22. Kinyoun, "Treatment of Variola by Its Antitoxin," 87.
23. *Ibid.*
24. *Ibid.*, 88–89.
25. *Ibid.*
26. *Ibid.*, 89.
27. *Ibid.*
28. *Ibid.*
29. *Ibid.*
30. "To Cure Dread Smallpox," *Washington News*, 22 January 1895; (National Library of Medicine, National Institutes of Health), "Antitoxin for Smallpox," *Philadelphia Record*, 24 January 1895. (National Library of Medicine, National Institutes of Health).
31. "To Cure Dread Smallpox," *Washington News*, 22 January 1895. (National Library of Medicine, National Institutes of Health).
32. "Antitoxin for Smallpox," *Philadelphia*

Record, 24 January 1895. (National Library of Medicine, National Institutes of Health).

33. "A Serum Remedy for Smallpox?" *New York Times*, 23 January 1895. (National Library of Medicine, National Institutes of Health).

34. *Ibid.*

35. *Annual Report of the Supervising Surgeon-General of the Marine-Hospital Service of the United States for the Fiscal Year 1896*, 1004–Note 1005:

36. "Antitoxin for Smallpox," *Philadelphia Record*, 24 January 1895. (National Library of Medicine, National Institutes of Health).

37. David. M. Morens, M.D., National Institute of Allergy & Infectious Disease, NIH, "The Forgotten Indispensable Man: Joe Kinyoun & the Birth of NIH," Presentation: History of Medicine Seminar, 26 September 2011, 7.

38. Interview with David M. Morens, M.D., Senior Advisor to the Director, National Institute of Allergy and Infectious Diseases, National Institutes of Health, St. Joseph, Missouri, 13 May 2010.

39. *Miscellany* (Washington, D.C.: National Library of Medicine, National Institutes of Health, 19 January 1895), 105.

40. Walter Reed. http://en.wikipedia.org/wiki/Walter_Reed, 10 March 2012, 1.

41. *Annual Report of the Supervising Surgeon-General of the Marine-Hospital Service of the United States for the Fiscal Year 1897* (Washington, D.C.: Government Printing Office, 1899), 468–472.

42. Bess Furman, *A Profile of the United States Public Health Service 1798–1948* (Washington, D.C.: National Library of Medicine, 1973), 234–244.

43. *Ibid.*, 241.

44. Letter, Walter Read to Dr. Kinyoun, 20 June 1902, 1–4.

45. George Miller Sternberg. http://en.wikipedia.org/wiki/George_Sternberg, accessed 11 October 2016.

46. Interview with David M. Morens, M.D., Senior Advisor to the Director, National Institute of Allergy and Infectious Diseases, National Institutes of Health, St. Joseph, Missouri, 13 May 2010.

47. *Ibid.*

48. *Miscellany* (Washington, D.C.: National Library of Medicine, National Institutes of Health, 19 January 1895), 105.

49. "Program … Forty-Fifth *Annual* Meeting of the Illinois State Medical Society at Springfield, Illinois May 21st, 22nd and 23rd, 1895." Gentral Music Hall (Chicago: American Medical Association Press: 1895), 3, 13.

50. *Ibid.*, 2.

51. Letter, Walter Wyman, Supervising Surgeon-General, M.H.S. to Passed Assistant Surgeon J.J. Kinyoun, U.S. Marine Hospital Service, Washington, D.C., 13 June 1895; Letter, Acting Secretary Treasury Department to Passed Assistant Surgeon Joseph J. Kinyoun, U.S. Marine-Hospital Service, 24 September 1895; Letter, Walter Wyman, Supervising Surgeon-General M.H.S., to Passed Assistant Surgeon J.J. Kinyoun U.S. Marine Hospital Service, Washington, D.C., 26 September 1895.

52. *Annual Report of the Supervising Surgeon-General of the Marine-Hospital Service of the United States for the Fiscal Year 1895*, 12.

53. *Ibid.*

54. Letter, Jose Andrade to Doctor J.J. Kinyoun, 20 July 1895.

55. A Bill, S. 3214. In the Senate of the United States, by Mr. Cockrell, 23 May 1896.

56. *Annual Report of the Supervising Surgeon-General of the Marine-Hospital Service of the United States for the Fiscal Year 1895*, 335–339.

57. Interview with Alice Kinyoun Houts, Kansas City, Missouri, 16 June 1974.

58. Letter, Jose Andrade to Dr. J.J. Kinyoun, 20 July 1895.

59. *The American Heritage Dictionary, Fourth Edition*, 268, 288, 878.

60. *Annual Report of the Supervising Surgeon-General of the Marine-Hospital Service of the United States for the Fiscal Year 1895*, 310.

61. *Annual Report of the Supervising Surgeon-General of the Marine-Hospital Service of the United States for the Fiscal Year 1896*, 1005, 1009, 1011.

62. *Ibid.*, 1007.

63. *Ibid.*

64. *Ibid.*, 1011.

65. *Ibid.*

66. *Ibid.*, 1008.

67. *Ibid.*, 1008–1010.

68. *Ibid.*, 1009–1010.

69. "Report on the Water Supply of Washington, D.C.," *Abstract, No. 52.* (National Library of Medicine, National Institutes of Health, 27 December 1895), 1183.

70. *Annual Report of the Supervising Surgeon-General of the Marine-Hospital Service of the United States for the Fiscal Year 1896*, 1010.

71. "Report on the Water Supply of Washington, D.C.," 1083.

72. *Ibid.*

73. *Annual Report of the Supervising Surgeon-General of the Marine-Hospital Service of the United States for the Fiscal Year 1896*, 1011.

74. *Ibid.*

75. Letter, Walter Wyman, Supervising Surgeon-General M.H.S., to the Secretary of the Treasury, 9 July 1894; *Annual Report of the Supervising Surgeon-General of the Marine-Hospital Service of the United States for the Fiscal Year 1894.* (Washington, D.C.: Government Printing Office, 1895), 17.

76. 1020–1022.

77. "Washington Notes," *Miscellany* (Washington, D.C.: National Library of Medicine, National Institutes of Health, 8 February 1896), 297.

78. *Ibid.*

79. *Annual Report of the Supervising Surgeon-General of the Marine-Hospital Service of the United States for the Fiscal Year 1896*, 1014.

80. *Ibid.*

81. *Ibid.*

82. *Ibid.*

83. *Ibid.*

84. *Ibid.*

85. *Ibid.*, 1014–1015.
86. *Ibid.*, 1016.
87. *Ibid.*
88. *Ibid.*
89. *Ibid.*
90. *Ibid.*
91. *Ibid.*
92. *Ibid.*
93. *Ibid.*
94. *Ibid.*
95. *Ibid.*
96. *Ibid.*, 1016–1017.
97. *Ibid.*, 34.
98. *Ibid.*
99. *Ibid.*
100. *Ibid.*
101. *Ibid.*, 34–35.
102. *Ibid.*
103. A Bill, S. 3214. In the Senate of the United States, by Mr. Cockrell, 23 May 1896.
104. *Ibid.*
105. Memorandum (Copy), 54th Congress Second Session Calendar No. 1259 S. 3214, 21 December 1896.
106. A Bill, S. 3214. In the Senate of the United States, by Mr. Cockrell, 23 May 1896.
107. Order of the Liberator. http://en.wikipedia.org/wiki/Order_of_the_Librator, 6 May 2012, 1, 4–5.
108. "Mr. Cleveland to Attend," *The Washington Post*, 20 June 1896. (National Library of Medicine, National Institutes of Health).
109. Letter, J. Havens Richard, President, Georgetown College to Dr. J.J. Kinyoun, M.D., Ph.D., 14 July 1896.
110. *Ibid.*
111. *Annual Report of the Supervising Surgeon-General of the Marine-Hospital Service of the United States for the Fiscal Year 1896*, 1011–1012.
112. *Ibid.*, 1011.
113. *Ibid.*, 1012.
114. *Ibid.*
115. *Ibid.*, 1012–1013.
116. *Ibid.*, 1013.
117. *Ibid.*, 1012.
118. *Ibid.*, 1012–1013.
119. Letter, Walter Wyman, Supervising Surgeon-General, M.H.S. to Passed Assistant Surgeon J.J. Kinyoun, 24 August 1896.
120. Letter, John H. Kinyoun to Dr. Joseph J. Kinyoun, 3 September 1896.
121. "Society Proceedings," *Miscellany* (Washington, D.C.: National Library of Medicine, National Institutes of Health, 3 October 1896), 754.
122. *Ibid.*
123. *Ibid.*
124. *The Washington Post*, 30 November 1896. (National Library of Medicine, National Institutes of Health).
125. *Ibid.*
126. *Ibid.*

Chapter VIII

1. *Annual Report of the Supervising Surgeon-General of the Marine-Hospital Service of the United States for the Fiscal Year 1897* (Washington, D.C.: Government Printing Office, 1899), 714.
2. *Ibid.*
3. *Ibid.*
4. *Ibid.*
5. *Ibid.*
6. *Ibid.*
7. *Ibid.*
8. *Ibid.*
9. *Ibid.*, 715.
10. *Ibid.*
11. *Ibid.*
12. *Ibid.*
13. *Ibid.*
14. *Ibid.*
15. *Ibid.*, 715–716.
16. *Ibid.*, 716.
17. *Ibid.*, 714.
18. Ralph Chester Williams, *The United States Public Health Service 1798–1950* (Washington, D.C.: Commissioned Officers Association of the United States Public Health Service, 1951), 180.
19. Letter, JH Kinyoun to Dr. J.J. Kinyoun, 24 January 1897, 1.
20. *Ibid.*
21. *Ibid.*
22. Letter, Father to Dr. Joseph J. Kinyoun, 16 November 1896, 1.
23. Syringe. http://en.wikipedia.org/wiki/Syringes, accessed 18 November 2012, 1–7.
24. Letter, Walter Wyman, Surgeon-General, M.H.S. to Surgeon Fairfax Irwin, Chairman, Passed Assistant Surgeon J.J. Kinyoun, Passed Assistant Surgeon H.D. Geddings, Passed Assistant Surgeon W.J. Stewart, Recorder, 25 January 1897, 1–2.
25. *Ibid.*, 1–2.
26. *The American Heritage Dictionary, Fourth Edition* (New York, NY: Random House, 2007), 115.
27. *Miscellany* (Washington, D. C.: National Library of Medicine, National Institutes of Health, 27 March 1897), 623.
28. *Ibid.*
29. *Ibid.*
30. "The Plague to Be Investigated." *Correspondence, Vol. 28, No. 6*, (Washington, D.C.: National Library of Medicine, National Institutes of Health, 6 February 1897).
31. *Ibid.*
32. *Ibid.*
33. *Ibid.*
34. *Ibid.*
35. *Ibid.*
36. *Ibid.*
37. *Ibid.*
38. *Ibid.*
39. *Ibid.*
40. *Ibid.*
41. *Ibid.*
42. *Annual Report of the Supervising Surgeon-

General of the Marine-Hospital Service of the United States for the Fiscal Year 1897, 744.

43. *Ibid.*

44. *Ibid.*, Letter, John B. Hamilton, Supervising Surgeon-General, M.H.S. to Passed Assistant Surgeon Joseph J. Kinyoun, 8 December 1890.

45. *Annual Report of the Supervising Surgeon-General of the Marine-Hospital Service of the United States for the Fiscal Year 1897*, 744.

46. *Ibid.*, 747.

47. *Ibid.*, 745.

48. *Ibid.*, 747.

49. *Ibid.*, 746–748.

50. *Ibid.*, 744–746.

51. *Ibid.*, 749.

52. *Ibid.*

53. *Ibid.*

54. Bess Furman, *A Profile of the United States Public Health Service 1798–1948* (Washington, D.C.: National Library of Medicine, 1973), 216–218, 229–232; Ralph Chester Williams, *The United States Public Health Service 1798–1950*, 123–125.

55. J.J. Kinyoun, M.D., *Bubonic Plague*, 4–5; Bubonic Plague, accessed July 11, 2006, *Infection/Transportation*; National Park Service, U.S. Department of the Interior, Public Health Program, accessed 16 July 2006.

56. *Annual Report of the Supervising Surgeon-General of the Marine-Hospital Service of the United States for the Fiscal Year 1897*, 750.

57. *Ibid.*

58. *Ibid.*

59. *Ibid.*

60. *Ibid.*

61. *Ibid.*

62. *Ibid.*, 749–751.

63. *Ibid.*, 751.

64. *Ibid.*

65. *Ibid.*

66. *Ibid.*

67. *Ibid.*

68. *Ibid.*

69. *Ibid.*, 752.

70. *Ibid.*

71. Bess Furman, *A Profile of the United States Public Health Service 1798–1948*, 234–244. Interview with David M. Morens, M.D., Senior Advisor to the Director, National Institute of Allergy and Infectious Diseases, National Institutes of Health, St. Joseph, Missouri, 13 May 2010.

72. Furman, *A Profile of the United States Public Health Service 1798–1948*, 229–231.

73. Williams, *The United States Public Health Service 1798–1950*, 97, 121.

74. Letter, Walter Wyman, Supervising Surgeon-General, M.H.S. to the Honorable Secretary of the Treasury, 9 July 1894, *Annual Report of the Supervising Surgeon-General of the Marine-Hospital Service of the United States for the Fiscal Year 1896* (Washington, D.C.: Government Printing Office, 1896), 1011–1012, *Annual Report of the Supervising Surgeon-General of the Marine-Hospital Service of the United States for the Fiscal Year 1897*, 722.

75. *Annual Report of the SupervisingSurgeon-General of the Marine-Hospital Service of the United States for the Fiscal Year 1897*, 722–723.

76. *Ibid.*

77. *Ibid.*, 733–738.

78. *Ibid.*, 709–710.

79. *Ibid.*, 722.

80. *Ibid.*, 739.

81. *Ibid.*, 733–735.

82. *Ibid.*, 738.

83. *Ibid.*

84. Formaldehyde and Cancer Rick. www.cancer.gov/cancertopics/factsheet/Risk/formaldehyde, accessed 18 November 2012.

85. Letter, Walter Wyman, Supervising Surgeon-General, M.H.S. to Passed Assistant Surgeon J.J. Kinyoun, 15 February 1897.

86. *Annual Report of the Supervising Surgeon-General of the Marine-Hospital Service of the United States for the Fiscal Year 1897*, 468–469.

87. *Ibid.*, 469.

88. *Ibid.*

89. *Ibid.*

90. *Ibid.*

91. *Ibid.*, 469–470.

92. *Ibid.*, 470.

93. *Ibid.*, 470–471.

94. *Ibid.*, 471.

95. *Ibid.*, 471–472.

Chapter IX

1. *The American Heritage Dictionary, Fourth Edition* (New York: Random House, 2007), 185–186, 466.

2. *Ibid.*, 173.

3. *Ibid.*, 185–186, 466.

4. *Annual Report of the Supervising Surgeon-General of the Marine-Hospital Service of the United States for the Fiscal Year 1897* (Washington, D.C.: Government Printing Office, 1899), 20–24.

5. *Ibid.*, 20–21.

6. *Ibid.*, 21.

7. *Ibid.*, 20–21.

8. *Ibid.*

9. *Ibid.*, 21.

10. *Ibid.*

11. *Ibid.*

12. *Ibid.*

13. *Ibid.*, 23–24.

14. *Ibid.*, 24.

15. *Ibid.*

16. *Ibid.*

17. *Annual Report of the Supervising Surgeon-General of the Marine-Hospital Service of the United States for the Fiscal Year 1897*, 24.

18. *Ibid.*

19. *Ibid.*

20. *Ibid.*

21. *Ibid.*

22. *Ibid.*

23. Letter, Unsigned to My dear ones, 5 Sep-

tember 1897 & 9 September (Grand Hotel Mengelle), 24.

24. *Ibid.*

25. *Ibid.*

26. *Ibid.*, 25–26.

27. Track gauge. http://en.wikipedia.org/wiki/Track_gauge, accessed 8 December 2012, 1–2, 4–9.

28. *Ibid.*, 9.

29. *Ibid.*, 2, 4, 5.

30. Letter, Unsigned to My dear ones, 5 September 1897 & 9 September (Grand Hotel Mengelle), 25–26.

31. *The American Heritage Dictionary, Fourth Edition* (New York: Random House, 2007), 486.

32. *Annual Report of the Supervising Surgeon-General of the Marine-Hospital Service of the United States for the Fiscal Year 1897*, 25.

33. *Ibid.*, 25.

34. *Ibid.*

35. *Ibid.*

36. *Ibid.*, 26.

37. *Ibid.*, 30.

38. *Ibid.*, 31.

39. *Ibid.*

40. *Ibid.*

41. *Ibid.*

42. *Ibid.*

43. *Ibid.*, 31–32.

44. *Ibid.*, 31.

45. *Ibid.*

46. *Ibid.*, 31–33.

47. *Ibid.*, 32.

48. *Ibid.*

49. *Annual Report of the Supervising Surgeon-General of the Marine-Hospital Service of the United States for the Fiscal Year 1897*, 710–711.

50. *Ibid.*, 718–720.

51. *Ibid.*, 712–713, 752–756.

52. *Ibid.*, 716.

53. *Ibid.*, 717–718.

54. *Ibid.*, 717.

55. *Ibid.*

56. *Ibid.*

57. *Ibid.*

58. *Ibid.*

59. *Ibid.*

60. *Ibid.*

61. *Ibid.*

62. *Ibid.*

63. *Ibid.*

64. *Ibid.*

65. *Ibid.*

66. *Ibid.*

67. *Ibid.*

68. *Ibid.*, 717–718.

69. *Ibid.*, 718.

70. *Ibid.*

71. *Ibid.*, 1019.

72. Williams, *The United States Public Health Service 1798–1950*, 181.

73. *Annual Report of the Supervising Surgeon-General of the Marine-Hospital Service of the United States for the Fiscal Year 1897*, 714–718, 1019.

74. Bess Furman, *A Profile of the United States Public Health Service 1798–1948* (Washington, D.C.: National Library of Medicine, 1973), 234–235.

Chapter X

1. Spanish-American War, accessed 30 March 2013. http://en.wikipedia.org/wiki/Spanish-american_war, 6.

2. Spanish-American War, accessed 30 March 2013. http://en.wikipedia.org/wiki/Spanish-american_war, 8; Yellow journalism, accessed 5 July 2014, http://en.wikipedia.org/wiki/Yellow_journalism, 1.

3. Spanish-American War, accessed 30 March 2013. http://en.wikipedia.org/wiki/Spanish-american_war; 6–7.

4. *Ibid.*, 7.

5. *Ibid.*

6. *Ibid.*, 7–8.

7. *Ibid.*

8. *The American Heritage Dictionary, Fourth Edition* (New York: Random House, 2007), 943.

9. Letter, J.J. Kinyoun, Passed Assistant Surgeon, M.H.S. to the President, 23 April 1898.

10. Letter, J.J. Kinyoun, Passed Assistant Surgeon, M.H.S. to the Supervising Surgeon-General.

11. Letter, George M. Sternberg Surgeon General, U.S. Army to Dr. J.J. Kinyoun Passed Asst. Surgeon, M.H.S., 12 May 1898.

12. Letter, W. Wyman, Supervising Surgeon-General, M.H.S. to Passed Assistant Surgeon J.J. Kinyoun, 6 August 1898.

13. Spanish-American War, accessed 30 March 2013. http://en.wikipedia.org/wiki/Spanish-american_war, 14.

14. *Ibid.*

15. *Ibid.*, 15.

16. *Ibid.*

17. *Ibid.*

18. Bess Furman, *A Profile of the United States Public Health Service 1798–1948* (Washington, D.C.: National Library of Medicine, 1973), 9–10.

19. Yellow fever, accessed 30 March 2013. http://en.wikipedia.org/wiki/Yellow_fever, 9–10.

20. Bess Furman, *A Profile of the United States Public Health Service 1798–1948*, 234–244.

21. *Ibid.*, 243.

22. H.C. Francis,to Dr. Walter Wyman, Supervising Surgeon General, 30 July 1898; Letter, H.C. Francis, Chairman to Dr. Walter Wyman, Supervising Surgeon General, 1 August 1898; Letter, H.C. Francis, Chairman to Walter Wyman, Supervising Surgeon General, M.H.S., 2 August, 1898; Letter, W.H. Francis, Secretary & Treasurer, to Walter Wyman, Supervising Surgeon General, 3 August 1898; Second Letter, W.H. Francis, Secretary & Treasurer to Walter Wyman, Supervising Surgeon General, 3 August 1898; Letter, from Kensington Engine Works, Ltd., Francis Bros., to Depot Quartermaster, 3 August 1898; Letter, W.H. Francis, Secretary & Treasurer, to Dr. Walter Wyman, Supervising

Surgeon General, 4 August 1898; Letter, W.H. Francis, Secretary & Treasurer, to Dr. Walter Wyman, Supervising Surgeon General, 18 August 1898; Letter, W.H. Francis, Secretary & Treasurer, to Dr. Walter Wyman, Supervising Surgeon General, 1 September 1898; Letter, W.H. Francis, Secretary & Treasurer, to Dr. Walter Wyman, Supervising Surgeon General, 7 September 1898; Letter, H.C. Francis, Chairman to Dr. Walter Wyman, Supervising Surgeon General, 12 September 1898; Letter, Chas. P. Francis, to Dr. Walter Wyman, Surgeon General [*sic*], 30 September 1898; Letter, W.H. Francis, Secretary & Treasurer, to Dr. J.J. Kinyoun, P.A. Surgeon, 30 September 1898; Letter, W.H. Francis, Secretary & Treasurer, to Dr. Walter Wyman, Supervising Surgeon General, 29 October 1898 (Courtesy Eva Ahren, Washington, D.C.: National Library of Medicine, National Institutes of Health).

23. The Western Union Telegraph Company, Telegraph Kensington Engine Works Ltd to Walter Wyman, Supervising Surgeon-General, 4 August; Letter, W.H. Francis, Secretary & Treasurer, to Dr. Walter Wyman, Supervising Surgeon General, 4 August 1898 (Courtesy Eva Ahren, Washington, D.C.: National Library of Medicine, National Institutes of Health).

24. Letter, W.H. Francis, Secretary & Treasurer, to Dr. Walter Wyman, Supervising Surgeon General, 4 August 1898 (Courtesy Eva Ahren, Washington, D.C.: National Library of Medicine, National Institutes of Health).

25. Letter, W.H. Francis, Secretary & Treasurer, to Dr. J.J. Kinyoun, P.A. Surgeon, 30 September 1898, 1–2 (Courtesy Eva Ahren, Washington, D.C.: National Library of Medicine, National Institutes of Health).

26. Montauk, New York, accessed 27 April 2013. http://en.wikipedia.org/wiki/Montauk,_New_York, 1.

27. *Ibid.*, 3.

28. Montauk, New York, accessed 27 April 2017. http://en.wikipedia.org/wiki/Montauk,_New_York, 3. David. M. Morens, M.D., National Institute of Allergy & Infectious Disease, NIH, "The Forgotten Indispensable Man: Joe Kinyoun & the Birth of NIH," Presentation: History of Medicine Seminar, 26 September 2011, 8.

29. Kinyoun Family Papers, Photographs and Artifacts.

30. *Ibid.*

31. *Centennial Year Annual Report of the Supervising Surgeon-General of the Marine-Hospital Service of the United States for the Fiscal Year 1898*, 632.

32. William H. McNeill, *Plagues and People* (New York: Random House, 1976), 164–165, 199; Bubonic plague, accessed July 11, 2006. http://en.wikipedia.org/wiki/Bubonic_plague; J.J. Kinyoun M.D., *Bubonic Plague* (San Francisco: Occidental Medical Times, Reprint, August 1901),4–6, 8.

33. McNeill, *Plagues and Peoples*, 164–165, 169; Kinyoun, *Bubonic Plague*, 4–6, 8.

34. *Ibid.*

35. *Centennial Year Annual Report of the Supervising Surgeon-General of the Marine-Hospital Service of the United States for the Fiscal Year 1898*, 632.

36. *Ibid.*

37. *Ibid.*

38. *Ibid.*

39. *Ibid.*, 632–633.

40. *Ibid.*, 635.

41. *Ibid.*, 633.

42. *Ibid.*

43. *Ibid.*

44. *Ibid.*

45. *Ibid.*, 633–634.

46. *Ibid.*, 634.

47. *Ibid.*

48. *Ibid.*

49. *Ibid.*

50. *Ibid.*, 634–635.

51. *Ibid.*, 635.

52. *Ibid.*, 634.

53. *Ibid.*, 635.

54. *Ibid.*

55. *Ibid.*

56. *Ibid.*

57. *Ibid.*, 635–636.

58. *Ibid.*

59. *Ibid.*, 637.

60. *Ibid.*

61. *Ibid.*, 633, 638.

62. *Ibid.*, 637.

63. *Ibid.*, 638–639.

64. *Ibid.*

65. *Ibid.*

66. *Ibid.*

67. *Ibid.*

68. *Ibid.*, 640–641.

69. *Ibid.*, 641.

70. *Ibid.*

71. Waldemar Haffkine, accessed 30 March 2013. http://en.Wikipedia.org/wiki/Waldemar_Haffkine. 1–2.

72. *Centennial Year Annual Report of the Supervising Surgeon-General of the Marine-Hospital Service of the United States for the Fiscal Year 1898*, 642.

73. *Ibid.*

74. Waldemar Haffkine, accessed 30 March 2013. http://en.Wikipedia.org/wiki/Waldemar_Haffkine, 2.

75. *Ibid.*

76. *Ibid.*

77. Bubonic plague, accessed July 11, 2016. http://en.wikipedia.org/wiki/Bubonic_plague, 5–6.

78. *Centennial Year Annual Report of the Supervising Surgeon-General of the Marine-Hospital Service of the United States for the Fiscal Year 1898*, 632–642.

Chapter XI

1. *Annual Report of the Supervising Surgeon-General of the Marine-Hospital Service of the United States for the Fiscal Year 1896* (Washington, D.C.:

Government Printing Office, 1896), 419–421. *Centennial Year Annual Report of the Supervising Surgeon-General of the Marine-Hospital Service of the United States for the Fiscal Year 1898* (Washington, D.C.: Government Printing Office, 1899), 632–641.

2. *Annual Report of the Supervising Surgeon-General of the Marine-Hospital Service of the United States for the Fiscal Year 1899* (Washington, D.C.: Government Printing Office, 1901), 395–397.
3. *Ibid.*, 561–562.
4. *Ibid.*, 561.
5. *Ibid.*
6. *Ibid.*
7. *Ibid.*
8. *Ibid.*
9. *Ibid.*, 562.
10. *Ibid.*
11. *Ibid.*
12. *Ibid.*
13. *Ibid.*
14. *Ibid.*, 563.
15. *Ibid.*
16. *Ibid.*
17. *Ibid.*, 563–564.
18. *Ibid.*
19. *Ibid.*, 564.
20. *Ibid.*
21. *Ibid.*
22. R.A. Forrest, M.D., *Echoes of the Plague Scare in San Francisco* (San Francisco: N.p., 17 November 1900), 1.
23. *Annual Report of the Supervising Surgeon-General of the Marine-Hospital Service of the United States for the Fiscal Year 1899*, 564.
24. R.A. Forrest, M.D., *Echoes of the Plague Scare in San Francisco*, 1.
25. *Annual Report of the Supervising Surgeon-General of the Marine-Hospital Service of the United States for the Fiscal Year 1899*, 564.
26. *Ibid.*, 565.
27. *Ibid.*
28. *Ibid.*
29. *Ibid.*
30. *Ibid.*
31. *Ibid.*
32. Letter, Walter Wyman, Supervising Surgeon-General M.H.S. to Passed Assistant Surgeon J.J. Kinyoun, 10 January 1899.
33. Letter, Walter Wyman, SupervisingSurgeon-General M.H.S. to Passed Assistant Surgeon J.J. Kinyoun, Director, Hygienic Laboratory, 4 February 1899.
34. *Ibid.*
35. *Ibid.*
36. *Ibid.*
37. Letter, John H. Kinyoun to Lizzie and all the family, 6 March 1898. 1–2; Letter, Joseph to Diddie, 11 March 99, 1–3; Letter, Alice Kinyoun to mother, 12 March, 1–2; Letter, Mother to My dear child, 13 March 1899; Letter, E.M. Perry to Diddie, 15 March 1898. 1–4; Letter, Jennie Ridly to Lizzie, 15 March 99 [*sic*]; Letter, Joe to Diddie, 15 March, 1; 1–3; Letter, Joseph to Sweetheart 19 March 1–3; Letter, Joe to Sweetheart; Letter, Sly Kinyoun to Mrs. Kinyoun, 20 March, 1–2; Letter, Joe to Gran, undated, 1; Letter, Momma Perry to My dear child, 21 March 1899, 1–3.
38. Letter, Joseph to Diddie, 15 March 1899 (Postmark).
39. Letter, Joseph to Sweetheart, 19 March 1899.
40. *Ibid.*
41. *Ibid.*
42. *Ibid.*
43. *Ibid.*
44. *Ibid.*, 3.
45. *Ibid.*
46. *Ibid.*
47. *Ibid.*
48. Letter, Momma Perry to My dear child, 21 March 1899, 3.
49. *Ibid.*, 1.
50. Letter, Alice Kinyoun to Mother, 19 March, 1–2.
51. *Ibid.*, 2.
52. Letter, E.M. Perry to Diddie, 19 March 1899, 1–4.
53. Letter, Walter Wyman, Surgeon-General, M.H.S. to Passed Assistant Surgeon J.J. Kinyoun, 27 April 1899; Letter, Walter Wyman, Surgeon-General, M.H.S. to Passed Assistant Surgeon J.J. Kinyoun, 27 April 1899.
54. Letter, Walter Wyman, Surgeon-General, M.H.S. to Passed Assistant Surgeon J.J. Kinyoun, 27 April 1899.
55. *Ibid.*
56. Ralph Chester Williams, *The United States Public Health Service 1798–1950* (Washington, D.C.: Commissioned Officers Association of the United States Public Health Service, 1951), 478.
57. *Ibid.*
58. *Ibid.*
59. *Ibid.*, 477.
60. *Ibid.*
61. *Ibid.*, 476–477.
62. *Ibid.*, 478.
63. *Ibid.*
64. *Ibid.*, 477.
65. Furman, *A Profile of the United States Public Health Service 1798–1948* (Washington, D.C.: National Library of Medicine, 1973), 214.
66. *Ibid.*
67. *Ibid.*
68. *Ibid.*, 214–215.
69. *Ibid.*, 215–216.
70. *Ibid.*, 216.
71. *Ibid.*, 220.
72. *Ibid.*
73. David M. Morens, M.D., Victoria A. Harden, Ph.D., Joseph Kinyoun Houts, Jr., Anthony S. Fauci, M.D., *The Indispensable Forgotten* Man, 26–27.
74. Furman, *A Profile of the United States Public Health Service 1798–1948*, 220–221.
75. COMPLIMENTARY DINNER TO J.J. KINYOUN, Ph.D. March 20, 1899, 1–2.
76. *Ibid.*, 2.

77. *Ibid.*
78. *Ibid.*
79. *Ibid.*
80. *Ibid.*
81. *Ibid.*
82. *Ibid.*
83. *Ibid.*
84. *Ibid.*
85. *Ibid.*
86. *Ibid.*
87. Furman, *A Profile of the United States Public Health Service 1798–1948*, 221.
88. *Ibid.*
89. Letter, G. Burkwell to Doctor, 17 May 1899.
90. Letter, William H. Welch to Jno. F. Moran, 18 May 1899, 1–2.
91. *Ibid.*
92. Letter, Walter Wyman to Doctor Moran, 17 May 1899, 1–2.
93. *Ibid.*, 1.
94. *Ibid.*
95. Letter, Walter Wyman, Surgeon-General, M.H.S. to Passed Assistant Surgeon J.J. Kinyoun, 22 May 1899.
96. Letter, Walter Wyman, Surgeon-General, M.H.S. to Passed Assistant Surgeon J.J. Kinyoun, 29 May 1899.

Chapter XII

1. COMPLIMENTARY DINNER TO J.J. KINYOUN, Ph.D. March 20, 1899, 2.
2. Ralph Chester Williams, *The United States Public Health Service 1798–1950* (Washington, D.C.: The Commissioned Officers Association of the United States Public Health Service, 1951), 97; Bess Furman, *A Profile of the United States Public Health Service 1798–1948* (Washington, D.C.: National Library of Medicine, 1973), 97.
3. *Annual Report of the Supervising Surgeon-General of the Marine-Hospital Service of the United States for the Fiscal Year 1899* (Washington, D.C.: Government Printing Office, 1901), 564.
4. Marilyn Chase, *The Barbary Plague* (New York: Random House Trade Paperbacks, 2003), 12–13, 23.
5. *Annual Report of the Supervising Surgeon-General of the Marine-Hospital Service of the United States for the Fiscal Year 1899*, 564.
6. Robert Barde, *Prelude to the Plague: Health and Politics at America's Pacific Gateway, 1899* (Oxford: Oxford University Press, Volume 58, 2003), 162–163.
7. *Ibid.*
8. *Ibid.*, 163–164.
9. *Annual Report of the Supervising Surgeon-General of the Marine-Hospital Service of the United States for the Fiscal Year 1899*, 564.
10. Letter, Secretary Gage, Treasury Department to Passed Assistant Surgeon J.J. Kinyoun, 12 June 1899.
11. *Ibid.*
12. Letter, Secretary Gage, Treasury Department to Passed Assistant Surgeon J.J. Kinyoun, 14 June 1899.
13. Angel Island (California), accessed 27 December 2013. http://en.wikipedia.org/wiki/Angel_Island_(California), 1–2.
14. *Ibid.*, 3.
15. Chase, *The Barbary Plague*, 3–6.
16. Williams, *The United States Public Health Service 1798–1950*, 102–103.
17. "The Lessons of Kinyounism," *San Francisco Bulletin*, 1900; Barde, *Prelude to the Plague: Health and Politics at America's Pacific Gateway, 1899*, 160; Chase, *The Barbary Plague*, 7–11.
18. Barde, *Prelude to the Plague: Health and Politics at America's Pacific Gateway, 1899*, 165–167; Henry Gage, accessed 19 January 2014. http://en.wikipedia.org/wiki/Henry_T._Gage, 1–2; San Francisco plague of 1900, accessed 27 December 2013. http://en.wikipedia.org/wiki/San_Francisco_plague_of_1900, 1.
19. *The World Almanac and Encyclopedia* New York World (New York: The Press Publishing Company, 1901).
20. Spanish-American War, accessed 30 March 2013. http://en.wikipedia.org/wiki/Spanish-american_war, 8.
21. *Ibid.*, 6.
22. Furman, *A Profile of the United States Public Health Service 1798–1948*, 214–216.
23. Henry Gage, accessed 19 January 2014. http://en.wikipedia.org/wiki/Henry_T._Gage, 2.
24. List of people associated with rail transport, accessed 20 January 2014. http://en.wikipeda.org/wiki/List_of_people_associated_with_rail_transport. 1.
25. Henry Gage, accessed 19 January 2014. http://en.wikipedia.org/wiki/Henry_T._Gage. 2.
26. Barde, *Prelude to the Plague: Health and Politics at America's Pacific Gateway, 1899*, 165–169.
27. Barde, *Prelude to the Plague: Health and Politics at America's Pacific Gateway, 1899*, 166; *The Wasp*, Volume No. 27. San Francisco: 8 July 1899.
28. Barde, *Prelude to the Plague: Health and Politics at America's Pacific Gateway, 1899*, 158.
29. *Ibid.*, 160, 164.
30. Furman, *A Profile of the United States Public Health Service 1798–1948*, 97.
31. Furman, *A Profile of the United States Public Health Service 1798–1948*, 97;Barde, *Prelude to the Plague: Health and Politics at America's Pacific Gateway, 1899*, 173.
32. Toyo Kisen Kaisha, Tokyo, Steamship, *Bill of Fare*, June 30, 1899.
33. *Ibid.*
34. *Ibid.*
35. *Ibid.*
36. *Ibid.*
37. Barde, *Prelude to the Plague: Health and Politics at America's Pacific Gateway, 1899*, 173.
38. *Ibid.*, 175.
39. *Ibid.*
40. *Ibid.*, 178.
41. *Ibid.*, 178–179.

42. *The Wasp*, Volume No. 27. San Francisco, 8 July 1899.
43. *Ibid.*
44. *Ibid.*
45. *Ibid.*
46. *Ibid.*
47. *Ibid.*
48. *The Wasp*, Volume No. 27. San Francisco, 15 July 1899.
49. *Ibid.*
50. *Ibid.*
51. *Ibid.*
52. Barde, *Prelude to the Plague: Health and Politics at America's Pacific Gateway, 1899*, 178–179.
53. J.J. Kinyoun M.D., *Bubonic Plague* (San Francisco: Occidental Medical Times, Reprint, August 1901), 8; Furman, *A Profile of the United States Public Health Service 1798–1948*, 231.
54. R.A. Forrest, M.D., *Echoes of the Plague Scare in San Francisco*, 1.
55. *Ibid.*, 1.
56. *Annual Report of the Supervising Surgeon-General of the Marine-Hospital Service of the United States for the Fiscal Year 1899*, 564–565; Barde, *Prelude to the Plague: Health and Politics at America's Pacific Gateway, 1899*, 182.
57. *Annual Report of the Supervising Surgeon-General of the Marine-Hospital Service of the United States for the Fiscal Year 1899*, 564–565.
58. Chase, *The Barbary Plague*, 28.
59. R.A. Forrest, M.D., *Echoes of the Plague Scare in San Francisco*, 1.
60. J.J. Kinyoun M.D., *Bubonic Plague*, 8.
61. *Ibid.*
62. *Annual Report of the Supervising Surgeon-General of the Marine-Hospital Service of the United States for the Fiscal Year 1899 Ibid.*, 566–567.
63. *Ibid.*
64. *Ibid.*, 567.
65. *Ibid.*, 567–570.
66. *Ibid.*, 568.
67. *Ibid.*
68. *Ibid.*, 569.
69. *Ibid.*
70. Barde, *Prelude to the Plague: Health and Politics at America's Pacific Gateway, 1899*, 160.
71. William H. McNeill, *Plagues and People* (New York: Random House, 1976), 137, 156, 171–177, 199.
72. *Annual Report of the Supervising Surgeon-General of the Marine-Hospital Service of the United States for the Fiscal Year 1899*, 569–570.
73. *Ibid.*
74. *Ibid.*
75. *Ibid.*, 567–570.
76. *Annual Report of the Supervising Surgeon-General of the Marine-Hospital Service of the United States for the Fiscal Year 1899*, 819.
77. *Ibid.*, 823.
78. *Ibid.*
79. *Ibid.*
80. *Ibid*; Furman, *A Profile of the United States Public Health Service 1798–1948*, 214–216.
81. *Annual Report of the Supervising Surgeon-General of the Marine-Hospital Service of the United States for the Fiscal Year 1899*, 823.
82. *Ibid.*, 823–824.
83. *Ibid.*, 824.
84. *Ibid.*
85. *Ibid.*
86. *Ibid.*
87. *Ibid.*
88. *Ibid.*
89. *Ibid.*
90. *Ibid.*, 824–825.
91. *Ibid.*, 824.
92. *Ibid.*

Chapter XIII

Author's Note: Since multiple telegrams transpired on the same day, a sequential number has been placed in front of each entry designating its order for the date. These are set forth *Annual Report of the Supervising Surgeon-General of the Marine-Hospital Service of the United States for the Fiscal Year 1900* (Washington, D.C.: Government Printing Office, 1900).

1. Victor H. Hass, *When Bubonic Plague Came to Chinatown.* (Bethesda, MD: National Institutes of Health, 1959), 141.
2. Letter, Walter Wyman, Surgeon-General M.H.S. to Passed Assistant Surgeon J.J. Kinyoun, 27 April 1899.
3. Loreen George Lipson, M.D., *Plague in San Francisco 1900* (Annals of Internal Medicine, Volume 77, August 1972), 304–305.
4. 2nd Telegram, Wyman to Surgeon General Kinyoun, 30 June 1900, *Annual Report of the Supervising Surgeon-General of the Marine-Hospital Service of the United States for the Fiscal Year 1900* (Washington, D.C.: Government Printing Office, 1900), 570, 676.
5. *Annual Report of the Supervising Surgeon-General of the Marine-Hospital Service of the United States for the Fiscal Year 1900*, 530–531; Hass, *When Bubonic Plague Came to Chinatown*, 141; Lipson, *Plague in San Francisco 1900*, 304.
6. Lipson, *Plague in San Francisco 1900*, 304; Hass, *When Bubonic Plague Came to Chinatown*, 141.
7. Hass, *When Bubonic Plague Came to Chinatown*, 141.
8. Telegram, Wyman to Cassaway, 8 March 1900, *Annual Report of the Supervising Surgeon-General of the Marine-Hospital Service of the United States for the Fiscal Year 1900*, 531; Lipson, *Plague in San Francisco 1900*, 304.
9. Telegram, Wyman to Cassaway, 8 March 1900, *Annual Report of the Supervising Surgeon-General of the Marine-Hospital Service of the United States for the Fiscal Year 1900*, 351.
10. Telegram, Cassaway to Wyman, March 8, 1900, *Annual Report of the Supervising Surgeon-General of the Marine-Hospital Service of the United States for the Fiscal Year 1900*, 351.

11. Telegram, Kinyoun to Wyman, 8 March 1900, *Annual Report of the Supervising Surgeon-General of the Marine-Hospital Service of the United States for the Fiscal Year 1900*, 351.

12. Telegram, Cassaway to Surgeon-General Wyman, 11 March 1900, *Annual Report of the Supervising Surgeon-General of the Marine-Hospital Service of the United States for the Fiscal Year 1900*, 532.

13. Telegram, Cassaway to Surgeon-General Wyman, 11 March 1900, *Annual Report of the Supervising Surgeon-General of the Marine-Hospital Service of the United States for the Fiscal Year 1900*, 532–533.

14. *Ibid.*

15. Lipson, *Plague in San Francisco 1900*, 305; Telegram, Cassaway to Surgeon-General Wyman, 21 March 1900, *Annual Report of the Supervising Surgeon-General of the Marine-Hospital Service of the United States for the Fiscal Year 1900*, 534.

16. *Ibid.*

17. *Associated Press* dispatch to Marine Hospital Service, 21 March 1900, *Annual Report of the Supervising Surgeon-General of the Marine-Hospital Service of the United States for the Fiscal Year 1900*, 534.

18. *Ibid.*

19. Lipson, *Plague in San Francisco 1900*, 304; *Scripps-McRae* dispatch to Marine Hospital Bureau, 22 March 1900, *Annual Report of the Supervising Surgeon-General of the Marine-Hospital Service of the United States for the Fiscal Year 1900*, 534.

20. Telegram, Cassaway to Surgeon-General Wyman, 22 March 1900, *Annual Report of the Supervising Surgeon-General of the Marine-Hospital Service of the United States for the Fiscal Year 1900*, 534–535.

21. "Health Gang Wants Cash," *Chronicle*, 25 March 1900.

22. *Ibid.*

23. *Ibid.*

24. Telegram, Kinyoun to Surgeon-General Wyman, 23 March 1900, *Annual Report of the Supervising Surgeon-General of the Marine-Hospital Service of the United States for the Fiscal Year 1900*, 535.

25. *Ibid.*

26. Lipson, *Plague in San Francisco in 1900*, 304; Hass, *When Bubonic Plague Came to Chinatown*, 142.

27. Telegram, Kinyoun to Surgeon-General Wyman, 23 March 1900, *Annual Report of the Supervising Surgeon-General of the Marine-Hospital Service of the United States for the Fiscal Year 1900*, 535.

28. "Phelan Fears His Specter," *Chronicle*, 27 March 1900.

29. *Ibid.*

30. *Ibid.*

31. Hass, *When Bubonic Plague Came to Chinatown*, 142; Lipson, *Plague in San Francisco 1900*, 304; *Annual Report of the Supervising Surgeon-General of the Marine-Hospital Service of the United States for the Fiscal Year 1900*, 536.

32. Interview with Alice Kinyoun Houts, Kansas City, Missouri, 16 June 1974.

33. Hass, *When Bubonic Plague Came to Chinatown*, 142.

34. Marilyn Chase, *The Barbary Plague* (New York: Random House, 2003), 6–11.

35. Ralph Chester Williams, *The United States Public Health Service 1798–1950* (Washington, D.C.: Commissioned Officers Association of the United States Public Health Service, 1951), 102–104.

36. Chase, *The Barbary Plague*, 19, 57–60.

37. Bess Furman, *A Profile of the United States Public Health Service 1798–1948* (Washington, D.C.: National Library of Medicine, 1973), 229–231.

38. Telegram, Glennan to Surgeon-General Wyman, 26 April 1900, *Annual Report of the Supervising Surgeon-General of the Marine-Hospital Service of the United States for the Fiscal Year 1900*, 537.

39. Telegram, Kinyoun to Surgeon-General Wyman, 26 April 1900, *Annual Report of the Supervising Surgeon-General of the Marine-Hospital Service of the United States for the Fiscal Year 1900*, 537.

40. Telegram, Kinyoun to Surgeon-General Wyman, 13 May 1900, *Annual Report of the Supervising Surgeon-General of the Marine-Hospital Service of the United States for the Fiscal Year 1900*, 537.

41. 1st Telegram, Kinyoun to Surgeon-General Wyman, 15 May 1900, *Annual Report of the Supervising Surgeon-General of the Marine-Hospital Service of the United States for the Fiscal Year 1900*, 537.

42. *Ibid.*

43. *Ibid.*

44. *Ibid.*

45. *Ibid.*

46. *Ibid.*

47. 1st Telegram, Wyman to Kinyoun, 15 May 1900, *Annual Report of the Supervising Surgeon-General of the Marine-Hospital Service of the United States for the Fiscal Year 1900*, 538.

48. 2nd Telegram, Wyman to Kinyoun, 15 May 1900, *Annual Report of the Supervising Surgeon-General of the Marine-Hospital Service of the United States for the Fiscal Year 1900*, 538.

49. 3rd Telegram, Wyman to Surgeon Kinyoun, 15 May 1900, *Annual Report of the Supervising Surgeon-General of the Marine-Hospital Service of the United States for the Fiscal Year 1900*, 538.

50. *Ibid.*

51. Telegram, Cassaway to Surgeon-General Wyman, 17 May 1900, *Annual Report of the Supervising Surgeon-General of the Marine-Hospital Service of the United States for the Fiscal Year 1900*, 538.

52. Telegram, Kinyoun to Surgeon-General Wyman, 17 May 1900, *Annual Report of the Supervising Surgeon-General of the Marine-Hospital Service of the United States for the Fiscal Year 1900*, 538.

53. Chase, *The Barbary Plague*, 7.

54. Telegram, Kinyoun to Surgeon-General Wyman, 17 May 1900, *Annual Report of the Supervising Surgeon-General of the Marine-Hospital Service of the United States for the Fiscal Year 1900*, 538.

55. 1st Telegram, Wyman to Surgeon Kinyoun, 17 May 1900, *Annual Report of the Supervising Surgeon-General of the Marine-Hospital Service of the United States for the Fiscal Year 1900*, 538.

56. *Annual Report of the Supervising*

Surgeon-General of the Marine-Hospital Service of the United States for the Fiscal Year 1900, 539–541.

57. 3rd Telegram, Wyman to Surgeon Kinyoun, 17 May 1900, *Annual Report of the Supervising Surgeon-General of the Marine-Hospital Service of the United States for the Fiscal Year 1900*, 539.

58. 4th Telegram, Wyman to Assistant Surgeon Cofer, 17 May 1900, *Annual Report of the Supervising Surgeon-General of the Marine-Hospital Service of the United States for the Fiscal Year 1900*, 539.

59. 5th Telegram, Wyman to Harris, 17 May 1900, *Annual Report of the Supervising Surgeon-General of the Marine-Hospital Service of the United States for the Fiscal Year 1900*, 539.

60. 6th Telegram, Wyman to Frary, 17 May 1900, *Annual Report of the Supervising Surgeon-General of the Marine-Hospital Service of the United States for the Fiscal Year 1900*, 539.

61. 7th Telegram, Wyman to Foster, 17 May 1900, *Annual Report of the Supervising Surgeon-General of the Marine-Hospital Service of the United States for the Fiscal Year 1900*, 539.

62. 1st Telegram, Wyman to Earle, 18 May 1900, 2nd Telegram, Wyman to Surgeon Cassaway, 18 May 1900, 3rd Telegram, Wyman to Lloyd, 18 May, 1900, *Annual Report of the Supervising Surgeon-General of the Marine-Hospital Service of the United States for the Fiscal Year 1900*, 539.

63. 4th Telegram to Roux, 18 May 1900, *Annual Report of the Supervising Surgeon-General of the Marine-Hospital Service of the United States for the Fiscal Year 1900*, 539.

64. 1st Telegram, Kinyoun to Surgeon-General Wyman, 19 May 1900, *Annual Report of the Supervising Surgeon-General of the Marine-Hospital Service of the United States for the Fiscal Year 1900*, 540.

65. 3rd Telegram, Wyman to Surgeon Kinyoun, 19 May 1900, *Annual Report of the Supervising Surgeon-General of the Marine-Hospital Service of the United States for the Fiscal Year 1900*, 540.

66. 1st Telegram, Kinyoun to Surgeon-General Wyman, 19 May 1900, *Annual Report of the Supervising Surgeon-General of the Marine-Hospital Service of the United States for the Fiscal Year 1900*, 540.

67. 2nd Telegram, Wyman to Surgeon Kinyoun 19 May 1900, *Annual Report of the Supervising Surgeon-General of the Marine-Hospital Service of the United States for the Fiscal Year 1900*, 540.

68. 5th Telegram, Wyman to Surgeon Kinyoun, 19 May 1900, *Annual Report of the Supervising Surgeon-General of the Marine-Hospital Service of the United States for the Fiscal Year 1900*, 541.

69. 6th Telegram, Wyman to Surgeon Cofer, 19 May 1900, *Annual Report of the Supervising Surgeon-General of the Marine-Hospital Service of the United States for the Fiscal Year 1900*, 541.

70. 7th Telegram, Wyman to State Health Officer, Dr. W.F. Blunt, 19 May 1900, *Annual Report of the Supervising Surgeon-General of the Marine-Hospital Service of the United States for the Fiscal Year 1900*, 541.

71. 8th Telegram, Wyman to President State Board of Health, Dr. Edmond Souchon, 19 May 1900, *Annual Report of the Supervising Surgeon-General of the Marine-Hospital Service of the United States for the Fiscal Year 1900*, 541.

72. Telegram, Kinyoun to Surgeon-General Wyman, 20 May 1900, *Annual Report of the Supervising Surgeon-General of the Marine-Hospital Service of the United States for the Fiscal Year 1900*, 541.

73. *Ibid.*

74. *Ibid.*

75. 1st Telegram, Walter Wyman, Supervising Surgeon-General to the Secretary of the Treasury, 21 May 1900, *Annual Report of the Supervising Surgeon-General of the Marine-Hospital Service of the United States for the Fiscal Year 1900*, 542.

76. Telegram, L.J. Gage, Secretary to President William McKinley, 21 May 1900, *Annual Report of the Supervising Surgeon-General of the Marine-Hospital Service of the United States for the Fiscal Year 1900*, 542.

77. 2nd Telegram, Wyman to Surgeon Kinyoun, 21 May 1900, *Annual Report of the Supervising Surgeon-General of the Marine-Hospital Service of the United States for the Fiscal Year 1900*, 542.

78. 3rd Telegram, Wyman, Surgeon-General, M.H.S. to Surgeon Kinyoun, 21 May 1900, *Annual Report of the Supervising Surgeon-General of the Marine-Hospital Service of the United States for the Fiscal Year 1900*, 543.

79. 4th Telegram, Wyman, Surgeon-General, M.H.S. to Surgeon Kinyoun, 21 May 1900, *Annual Report of the Supervising Surgeon-General of the Marine-Hospital Service of the United States for the Fiscal Year 1900*, 543.

80. L.J. Gage, Secretary, Interstate Quarantine Regulation to Prevent the Spread of Plague in the United States (Washington D.C.: Department Circular No. 73 1900. Marine Hospital Service: May 22, 1900), 543.

81. *Ibid.*

82. *Ibid.*

83. *Ibid.*

84. *Ibid.*

85. *Ibid.*

86. 2nd Telegram, Kinyoun to Surgeon-General Wyman, 22 May 1900, *Annual Report of the Supervising Surgeon-General of the Marine-Hospital Service of the United States for the Fiscal Year 1900*, 544.

87. 3rd Telegram, Kinyoun to Surgeon-General Wyman, 22 May 1900, *Annual Report of the Supervising Surgeon-General of the Marine-Hospital Service of the United States for the Fiscal Year 1900*, 544.

88. 4th Telegram, Kinyoun to Surgeon-General Wyman, 22 May 1900, *Annual Report of the Supervising Surgeon-General of the Marine-Hospital Service of the United States for the Fiscal Year 1900*, 544.

89. 1st Telegram, Wyman to Kinyoun, 23 May 1900, *Annual Report of the Supervising Surgeon-General of the Marine-Hospital Service of the United States for the Fiscal Year 1900*, 544.

90. 1st Telegram, Kinyoun to Surgeon-General Wyman, 23 May 1900, *Annual Report of the Supervising Surgeon-General of the Marine-Hospital Service of the United States for the Fiscal Year 1900*, 545.

91. Letter, H.L. Nicholas, Secretary & Health Officer to C.[*sic*]J. Kinyoun, M.D., 23 May 1900.
92. 1st Telegram, Kinyoun to Surgeon-General Wyman, 23 May 1900, *Annual Report of the Supervising Surgeon-General of the Marine-Hospital Service of the United States for the Fiscal Year 1900*, 545.
93. Telegram, Wyman to Kinyoun, 23 May 1900, *Annual Report of the Supervising Surgeon-General of the Marine-Hospital Service of the United States for the Fiscal Year 1900*, 545.
94. 1st Telegram, Kinyoun to Surgeon-General Wyman, 23 May 1900.
95. 2nd Telegram, Kinyoun to Surgeon-General Wyman, 23 May 1900, *Annual Report of the Supervising Surgeon-General of the Marine-Hospital Service of the United States for the Fiscal Year 1900*, 545.
96. 1st Telegram, Kinyoun to Surgeon-General Wyman, 24 May 1900, *Annual Report of the Supervising Surgeon-General of the Marine-Hospital Service of the United States for the Fiscal Year 1900*, 545.
97. 3rd Telegram, Wyman to Surgeon Kinyoun, 24 May 1900, *Annual Report of the Supervising Surgeon-General of the Marine-Hospital Service of the United States for the Fiscal Year 1900*, 545.
98. 2nd Telegram, Kinyoun to Surgeon-General Wyman, 24 May 1900, *Annual Report of the Supervising Surgeon-General of the Marine-Hospital Service of the United States for the Fiscal Year 1900*, 546.
99. *Wong Wai vs. Williamson et al.* (103 F. 384, 1900).
100. 2nd Telegram, Kinyoun to Surgeon-General Wyman, 24 May 1900, *Annual Report of the Supervising Surgeon-General of the Marine-Hospital Service of the United States for the Fiscal Year 1900*, 546.
101. *Ibid.*
102. Telegram, Kinyoun to Surgeon-General Wyman, 25 May 1900, *Annual Report of the Supervising Surgeon-General of the Marine-Hospital Service of the United States for the Fiscal Year 1900*, 546.
103. 2nd Telegram, Kinyoun to Surgeon-General Wyman, 26 May 1900, *Annual Report of the Supervising Surgeon-General of the Marine-Hospital Service of the United States for the Fiscal Year 1900*, 546.
104. 3rd Telegram, Wyman to Kinyoun, 26 May 1900, *Annual Report of the Supervising Surgeon-General of the Marine-Hospital Service of the United States for the Fiscal Year 1900*, 547.
105. 3rd Telegram, Kinyoun to Surgeon-General Wyman, 26 May 1900, *Annual Report of the Supervising Surgeon-General of the Marine-Hospital Service of the United States for the Fiscal Year 1900*, 547.
106. 4th Telegram, Kinyoun to Surgeon-General Wyman, 26 May 1900, *Annual Report of the Supervising Surgeon-General of the Marine-Hospital Service of the United States for the Fiscal Year 1900*, 547.
107. Telegram, Crowninshield to Captain Glass, 26 May 1900, *Annual Report of the Supervising Surgeon-General of the Marine-Hospital Service of the United States for the Fiscal Year 1900*, 547.
108. Telegram, O.L. Spaulding, Acting Secretary to Collector of Customs, 26 May 1900, *Annual Report of the Supervising Surgeon-General of the Marine-Hospital Service of the United States for the Fiscal Year 1900*, 548.
109. Telegram, Kinyoun to Surgeon-General Wyman, 27 May 1900, *Annual Report of the Supervising Surgeon-General of the Marine-Hospital Service of the United States for the Fiscal Year 1900*, 548.
110. 2nd Telegram, Wyman to Kinyoun, 28 May 1900, *Annual Report of the Supervising Surgeon-General of the Marine-Hospital Service of the United States for the Fiscal Year 1900*, 548.
111. *Wong Wai vs. Williamson et al* (103 F. 384, 1900) (Contempt Ruling).
112. *Wong Wai vs. Williamson et al* (103 F. 384, 1900) (Injunction Ruling 28 May 1900).
113. *Ibid.*
114. *Ibid.*
115. *Ibid.*
116. *Ibid.*
117. *Ibid.*
118. *Ibid.*
119. *Ibid.*
120. *Ibid.*
121. *Ibid.*
122. 2nd Telegram, Kinyoun to Surgeon-General Wyman, 28 May 1900, *Annual Report of the Supervising Surgeon-General of the Marine-Hospital Service of the United States for the Fiscal Year 1900*, 549.
123. *Ibid.*
124. *Ibid.*
125. *Ibid.*
126. 3rd Telegram, Wyman to Kinyoun, 28 May 1900, *Annual Report of the Supervising Surgeon-General of the Marine-Hospital Service of the United States for the Fiscal Year 1900*, 550.
127. 1st Telegram, Kinyoun to Surgeon-General Wyman, 29 May 1900, *Annual Report of the Supervising Surgeon-General of the Marine-Hospital Service of the United States for the Fiscal Year 1900*, 550.
128. *Ibid.*
129. 2nd Telegram, Kinyoun to Surgeon-General Wyman, 29 May 1900, *Annual Report of the Supervising Surgeon-General of the Marine-Hospital Service of the United States for the Fiscal Year 1900*, 550.
130. *Ibid.*
131. *Ibid.*
132. Telegram, Kinyoun to Surgeon-General Wyman, 30 May 1900, *Annual Report of the Supervising Surgeon-General of the Marine-Hospital Service of the United States for the Fiscal Year 1900*, 550.
133. 2nd Telegram, Wyman to Kinyoun, 30 May 1900, *Annual Report of the Supervising Surgeon-General of the Marine-Hospital Service of the United States for the Fiscal Year 1900*, 551.
134. Telegram, Wyman to Kinyoun, 3 June 1900, *Annual Report of the Supervising Surgeon-General of the Marine-Hospital Service of the United States for the Fiscal Year 1900*, 558.
135. *Ibid.*
136. *Ibid.*
137. *Ibid.*
138. Telegram, J.J. Kinyoun to Surgeon-General Marine-Hospital Service, 11 June 1900, *Annual Report of the Supervising Surgeon-General of the*

Marine-Hospital Service of the United States for the Fiscal Year 1900, 558–61.

139. *Ibid.*, 559.

140. *Ibid.*

141. *Ibid.*, 560.

142. *Ibid.*

143. *Ibid.*

144. *Ibid.*

145. *Ibid.*

146. *Ibid.*

147. *Wong Wai vs. Williamson et al* (103 Fed 384, 1900) (Injunction Ruling 28 May 1900).

148. Telegram, J.J. Kinyoun to Surgeon-General Marine-Hospital Service, 11 June 1900, *Annual Report of the Supervising Surgeon-General of the Marine-Hospital Service of the United States for the Fiscal Year 1900*, 560.

149. *Ibid.*

150. 1st Telegram, Kinyoun to Surgeon-General Wyman, 31 May 1900, *Annual Report of the Supervising Surgeon-General of the Marine-Hospital Service of the United States for the Fiscal Year 1900*, 561.

151. Link, *A History of Plagues in the United States of America*, 4–5.

152. *Wong Wai vs. Williamson et al* (103 Fed 384, 1900) (Injunction Ruling, 28 May 1900).

153. *Wong Wai vs. Williamson et al* (103 Fed 384, 1900) (Contempt Ruling).

154. 1st Telegram, Kinyoun to Surgeon-General Wyman, 31 May 1900, *Annual Report of the Supervising Surgeon-General of the Marine-Hospital Service of the United States for the Fiscal Year 1900*, 561.

155. 2nd Telegram, Kinyoun to Surgeon-General Wyman, 31 May 1900, *Annual Report of the Supervising Surgeon-General of the Marine-Hospital Service of the United States for the Fiscal Year 1900*, 561.

156. 2nd Telegram, Wyman to Kinyoun, 1 June 1900, *Annual Report of the Supervising Surgeon-General of the Marine-Hospital Service of the United States for the Fiscal Year 1900*, 561.

157. 1st Telegram, Kinyoun to Surgeon-General Wyman, 4 June 1900, *Annual Report of the Supervising Surgeon-General of the Marine-Hospital Service of the United States for the Fiscal Year 1900*, 562.

158. Telegram, Wyman to Kinyoun, 4 June 1900, *Annual Report of the Supervising Surgeon-General of the Marine-Hospital Service of the United States for the Fiscal Year 1900*, 562.

159. 2nd Telegram, Kinyoun to Surgeon-General Wyman, 3 June 1900, *Annual Report of the Supervising Surgeon-General of the Marine-Hospital Service of the United States for the Fiscal Year 1900*, 562.

160. Telegram, Wyman to Kinyoun, 1 June 1900, *Annual Report of the Supervising Surgeon-General of the Marine-Hospital Service of the United States for the Fiscal Year 1900*, 561.

161. 1st Telegram, Kinyoun to Surgeon-General Wyman, 4 June 1900, *Annual Report of the Supervising Surgeon-General of the Marine-Hospital Service of the United States for the Fiscal Year 1900*, 562.

162. 2nd Telegram, Kinyoun to Surgeon-General Wyman, 4 June 1900, *Annual Report of the Supervising Surgeon-General of the Marine-Hospital Service of the United States for the Fiscal Year 1900*, 562.

163. Telegram, Kinyoun to Surgeon-General Wyman, 6 June 1900, *Annual Report of the Supervising Surgeon-General of the Marine-Hospital Service of the United States for the Fiscal Year 1900*, 563; *Jew Ho vs. Williamson et al.*

164. Telegram, Kinyoun to Surgeon-General Wyman, 7 June 1900, *Annual Report of the Supervising Surgeon-General of the Marine-Hospital Service of the United States for the Fiscal Year 1900*, 563.

165. Telegram, Kinyoun to Surgeon-General Wyman, 6 June 1900, *Annual Report of the Supervising Surgeon-General of the Marine-Hospital Service of the United States for the Fiscal Year 1900*, 563.

166. *Ibid.*

167. *Ibid.*

168. Telegram, Kinyoun to Surgeon-General Wyman, 7 June 1900, *Annual Report of the Supervising Surgeon-General of the Marine-Hospital Service of the United States for the Fiscal Year 1900*, 563.

169. Telegram, Kinyoun to Surgeon-General Wyman, 9 June 1900, *Annual Report of the Supervising Surgeon-General of the Marine-Hospital Service of the United States for the Fiscal Year 1900*, 563–564.

170. Telegram, Kinyoun to Surgeon-General Wyman, 12 June 1900, *Annual Report of the Supervising Surgeon-General of the Marine-Hospital Service of the United States for the Fiscal Year 1900*, 564.

171. Telegram, Kinyoun to Surgeon-General Wyman, 13 June 1900, *Annual Report of the Supervising Surgeon-General of the Marine-Hospital Service of the United States for the Fiscal Year 1900*, 564.

172. 1st Telegram, Kinyoun to Surgeon-General Wyman, 14 June 1900, *Annual Report of the Supervising Surgeon-General of the Marine-Hospital Service of the United States for the Fiscal Year 1900*, 564.

173. 2nd Telegram, Kinyoun to Surgeon-General Wyman, 16 June 1900, *Annual Report of the Supervising Surgeon-General of the Marine-Hospital Service of the United States for the Fiscal Year 1900*, 565.

174. *Ibid.*

175. *Ibid.*

176. 3rd Telegram, Kinyoun to Surgeon-General Wyman, 16 June 1900, *Annual Report of the Supervising Surgeon-General of the Marine-Hospital Service of the United States for the Fiscal Year 1900*, 565.

177. 5th Telegram, Kinyoun to Surgeon-General Wyman, 16 June 1900, *Annual Report of the Supervising Surgeon-General of the Marine-Hospital Service of the United States for the Fiscal Year 1900*, 566.

178. 1st Telegram, Wyman to Surgeon Kinyoun, 17 June 1900, *Annual Report of the Supervising Surgeon-General of the Marine-Hospital Service of the United States for the Fiscal Year 1900*, 566.

179. Telegram, Kinyoun to Surgeon-General Wyman, 17 June 1900, *Annual Report of the Supervising Surgeon-General of the Marine-Hospital Service of the United States for the Fiscal Year 1900*, 566.

180. 2nd Telegram, Wyman to Surgeon Kinyoun, 17 June 1900, *Annual Report of the Supervising*

Surgeon-General of the Marine-Hospital Service of the United States for the Fiscal Year 1900, 566.

181. 1st Telegram, Wyman to Surgeon Kinyoun, 18 June 1900, *Annual Report of the Supervising Surgeon-General of the Marine-Hospital Service of the United States for the Fiscal Year 1900*, 566.

182. 2nd Telegram, Wyman to Surgeon Kinyoun, 18 June 1900, *Annual Report of the Supervising Surgeon-General of the Marine-Hospital Service of the United States for the Fiscal Year 1900*, 566.

183. Telegram, O.L. Spaulding, Acting Secretary to the Governor of California, 18 June 1900, *Annual Report of the Supervising Surgeon-General of the Marine-Hospital Service of the United States for the Fiscal Year 1900*, 566.

184. *Ibid.*

185. 3rd Telegram, Wyman to Surgeon Kinyoun, 18 June 1900, *Annual Report of the Supervising Surgeon-General of the Marine-Hospital Service of the United States for the Fiscal Year 1900*, 566.

186. *Ibid.*

187. 2nd Telegram, Kinyoun to Surgeon-General Wyman, 18 June 1900, *Annual Report of the Supervising Surgeon-General of the Marine-Hospital Service of the United States for the Fiscal Year 1900*, 567.

188. *Ibid.*

189. 1st Telegram, Wyman to Surgeon Kinyoun, 19 June 1900, *Annual Report of the Supervising Surgeon-General of the Marine-Hospital Service of the United States for the Fiscal Year 1900*, 567.

190. 2nd Telegram, Wyman to Surgeon Kinyoun, 19 June 1900, *Annual Report of the Supervising Surgeon-General of the Marine-Hospital Service of the United States for the Fiscal Year 1900*, 567.

191. Telegram, Kinyoun to Surgeon-General Wyman, 21 June 1900, *Annual Report of the Supervising Surgeon-General of the Marine-Hospital Service of the United States for the Fiscal Year 1900*, 567.

192. Telegram, Wyman to Surgeon Kinyoun, 22 June 1900, *Annual Report of the Supervising Surgeon-General of the Marine-Hospital Service of the United States for the Fiscal Year 1900*, 567.

193. 1st Telegram, Kinyoun to Surgeon-General Wyman, 22 June 1900, *Annual Report of the Supervising Surgeon-General of the Marine-Hospital Service of the United States for the Fiscal Year 1900*, 567.

194. 2nd Telegram, Kinyoun to Surgeon-General Wyman, 22 June 1900, *Annual Report of the Supervising Surgeon-General of the Marine-Hospital Service of the United States for the Fiscal Year 1900*, 568.

195. Telegram, Kinyoun to Surgeon-General Wyman, 23 June 1900, *Annual Report of the Supervising Surgeon-General of the Marine-Hospital Service of the United States for the Fiscal Year 1900*, 568.

196. Telegram, Wyman to Surgeon Kinyoun, 24 June 1900, *Annual Report of the Supervising Surgeon-General of the Marine-Hospital Service of the United States for the Fiscal Year 1900*, 568.

197. 2nd Telegram, Wyman to Surgeon Kinyoun, 23 June 1900, *Annual Report of the Supervising Surgeon-General of the Marine-Hospital Service of the United States for the Fiscal Year 1900*, 568.

198. 2nd Telegram, Kinyoun to Surgeon-General Wyman, 25 June 1900, *Annual Report of the Supervising Surgeon-General of the Marine-Hospital Service of the United States for the Fiscal Year 1900*, 568.

199. 2nd Telegram, Kinyoun to Surgeon-General Wyman, 26 June 1900, *Annual Report of the Supervising Surgeon-General of the Marine-Hospital Service of the United States for the Fiscal Year 1900*, 569.

200. Letter, Frank L. Coombs, United States Attorney to J.J. Kinyoun M.D. Surgeon M.H.S., 2 July 1900.

201. *Ibid.*

202. *Ibid.*

203. *Ibid.*

204. *Ibid.*

205. Letter, Dr. Jos. J. Kinyoun (Abutment Code Name JJK) to Doctor Bailhache, 9 August 1900.

206. 2nd Telegram, Kinyoun, 26 June 1900, *Annual Report of the Supervising Surgeon-General of the Marine-Hospital Service of the United States for the Fiscal Year 1900*, 569.

207. Telegram, Wyman to Surgeon Kinyoun, 25 June 1900, *Annual Report of the Supervising Surgeon-General of the Marine-Hospital Service of the United States for the Fiscal Year 1900*, 569.

208. Telegram, Wyman to State health officer of Texas, 27 June 1900, *Annual Report of the Supervising Surgeon-General of the Marine-Hospital Service of the United States for the Fiscal Year 1900*, 569.

209. Telegram, Kinyoun to Surgeon-General Wyman, 2 July 1900, *Annual Report of the Supervising Surgeon-General of the Marine-Hospital Service of the United States for the Fiscal Year 1900*, 570.

210. Telegram, H.A. Taylor, Acting Secretary, 3 July 1900, *Annual Report of the Supervising Surgeon-General of the Marine-Hospital Service of the United States for the Fiscal Year 1900*, 570; Telegram, James K. Richards, Acting Attorney General, 3 July 1900, *Annual Report of the Supervising Surgeon-General of the Marine-Hospital Service of the United States for the Fiscal Year 1900*, 570.

211. *Wong Wai vs. Williamson et al.* (103 F. 384), 3 July 1900. Opinion on Order to Show Cause for Contempt, Circuit Judge Morrow and District Judge De Haven.

212. *Ibid.*

213. Affidavit, B.J. Lloyd, July 1900, *Wong Wai vs. Williamson et al*, 103 F. 384, 1900.

214. *Ibid.*

215. *Ibid.*

216. *Ibid.*

217. *Ibid.*

218. *Ibid.*

219. *Ibid.*

220. George Tully Vaughan, Surgeon, United States Marine-Hospital Service in Charge, "Report of the Division of Sanitary Reports and Statistics." *Annual Report of the Supervising Surgeon-General of the Marine-Hospital Service of the United States for the Fiscal Year 1900* (Washington, D.C.: Government Printing Office, 1900), 347.

221. *Ibid.*

222. *Wong Wai vs. Williamson et al*, 103 F. 384, 1900.

223. George Tully Vaughan, Surgeon, United States Marine-Hospital Service, in Charge, "Report of the Division of Sanitary Reports and Statistics." *Annual Report of the Supervising Surgeon-General of the Marine-Hospital Service of the United States for the Fiscal Year 1900*, 347.
224. *Ibid.*

Chapter XIV

1. "The Farcical Side of It." Newspaper Unknown, 30 May 1900.
2. *Ibid.*
3. *Ibid.*
4. "Investigating Experts Inspect Chinatown and Fail to Find a Single Case of Any Illness," *The Call*, 30 May 1900.
5. "No Plague in San Francisco," *The Bulletin*, 14 June 1900.
6. "Governor Officially Brands Bubonic Plague Scare a Fake." *The Bulletin*, 14 June 1900.
7. *Ibid.*
8. *Ibid.*
9. *Ibid.*
10. *Ibid.*
11. *Ibid.*
12. *Ibid.*
13. *Ibid.*
14. "Clip," Kinyoun Newspaper Scrapbook, 25 March 1900–16 December 1902.
15. "Kinyoun's Circular Quarantining State," Newspaper Unknown, 15 June 1900.
16. "Kinyoun Quarantines State." *The Bulletin*, 16 June 1900.
17. "Quarantine of City Just as He Had Hinted." *The Chronicle*, 17 June 1900.
18. "His Recall Is Demanded," *The Chronicle*, 20 June 1900.
19. "Will the Bubonic Board Resign?" *The Bulletin*, Undated.
20. "The Abutment of a Nuisance." *The Chronicle* 23 June 1900.
21. *Ibid.*
22. *Ibid.*
23. *Ibid.*
24. *Ibid.*
25. Chung Sai Yat Po, 22 June 1900.
26. *Ibid.*
27. *Ibid.*
28. "The Lesson of Kinyounism." *The San Francisco Call*, 22 June 1900.
29. *Ibid.*
30. *Ibid.*
31. *Ibid.*
32. *Ibid.*
33. *Ibid.*
34. *Ibid.*
35. "Wedding, Mike De Young's Letter and Kinyoun Lynching." *The Bulletin*, 24 June 1900.
36. *Ibid.*
37. *Ibid.*
38. *Ibid.*
39. "Kinyoun, Enemy of This City, on Trial for Contempt of United Sates Circuit Court." *The Bulletin*, 25 June 1900.
40. *Ibid.*
41. "Kinyoun and His Wirings Evidence of Contumacy Are Read in Court," *The Evening Post*, 26 June 1900.
42. "Kinyoun on the Grill." *The Chronicle*, July 3, 1900.
43. "Quarantine Kinyoun," Newspaper Unknown, Undated.
44. *Ibid.*
45. *Ibid.*
46. "Kinyoun on the Grill." *The Chronicle*, 3 July 1900.
47. *Ibid.*
48. *Ibid.*
49. "Kinyoun Discharged," *The Chronicle*, 4 July 1900.
50. *Ibid.*
51. *Ibid.*
52. *Ibid.*
53. "Dr. Silas Mouser, Whom State Employed, and Surgeon-General Sternberg Say Dread Disease Was Never Here." *The Bulletin*, 31 July 1900.
54. *Ibid.*
55. *Ibid.*
56. George Miller Sternberg, accessed October 11, 2016. https://en.wikipedia.org/wiki/George_Miller_Sternberg.
57. "Surgeon-General Sternberg Here on a Tour of Inspection." *The Chronicle*, 17 July 1900.
58. Letter, G.W. Sternberg, Surgeon General U.S. Army, to Dr. J.J. Kinyoun, 12 May 1898.
59. "Dr. Silas Mouser, Whom the State Employed, and Surgeon-General Sternberg Say Dread Disease Was Never Here." *The Bulletin*, 31 July 1900.
60. *Ibid.*
61. "Dr. Silas Mouser, Whom State Employed, and Surgeon-General Sternberg Say Dread Disease Was Never Here." *The Bulletin*, 31 July 1900; "Expert Says There Was No Plague Here," *The Call*, 31 July 1900.
62. "Expert Says There Was No Plague Here," *The Call*, 31 July 1900.
63. "Suppressing the Truth." *The Chronicle*, 2 August 1900.
64. "Dr. Silas Mouser, Whom State Employed, and Surgeon-General Sternberg Say Dread Disease Was Never Here." *The Bulletin*, 31 July 1900; "Expert Says There Was No Plague Here," *The Call*, 31 July 1900.
65. "Public Records Denied the Public," *The Bee*, 3 August 1900; "The Law Is Above the Governor." *The Bee*, 8 August 1900; "Bubonic Plague Reports Are Public Property." *The Bee*, 13 August 1900.
66. "Dr. Silas Mouser, Whom State Employed, and Surgeon-General Sternberg Say Dread Disease Was Never Here." *The Bulletin*, 31 July 1900.
67. "Has Kinyoun Gone Mad?" Newspaper Unknown, Undated.
68. *Ibid.*
69. *Ibid.*

70. *Ibid.*
71. "Why They Protested," *Town Talk*, Undated, 1.
72. *Ibid.*
73. "Has Kinyoun Gone Mad?" Newspaper Unknown, Undated.
74. *Ibid.*
75. "The Facts Are Not with the Governor." *The Bee*, 19 June 1900.
76. *Ibid.*
77. "Governor Officially Brands Bubonic Plague Scare a Fake." *The Bulletin*, 14 June 1900.
78. *Ibid.*
79. "The Facts Are Not with the Governor." *The Bee*, 19 June 1900.
80. *Ibid.*
81. *Ibid.*
82. "Present Status of the Plague." *The Bee*, 21 June 1900.
83. *Ibid.*
84. *Ibid.*
85. *Ibid.*
86. *Ibid.*
87. *Ibid.*
88. "Why Not Own Up to Truth?" *The Evening Bee*, 23 June 1900.
89. *Ibid.*
90. *Ibid.*
91. *Ibid.*
92. "Vindication of Dr. Kinyoun." Newspaper Unknown, 3 July 1900.
93. *Ibid.*
94. "Fresh Case of the Plague in San Francisco." *The Bee*, 9 July 1900.
95. *Ibid.*
96. *Ibid.*
97. *Ibid.*
98. *Ibid.*
99. "A Swipe at Dr. Henderson." Newspaper Unknown, Undated.
100. *Ibid.*
101. "New Light on Bubonic Plague." *The Evening Bee*, 14 July 1900.
102. *Ibid.*
103. "Governor Gage Should Apologize." *The Evening Bee*, 14 July 1900.
104. *Ibid.*
105. "Wanted to Call It Blood-Poisoning." *The Bee*, 10 July 1900.
106. *Ibid.*
107. *Ibid.*
108. *Ibid.*
109. Victor H. Hass, *When Bubonic Plague Came to Chinatown.* (Bethesda, MD: National Institutes of Health, 1959), 143.
110. *Ibid.*
111. *Ibid.*
112. *Ibid.*
113. *Ibid.*
114. "More Plague in San Francisco." *The Bee*, 17 October 1900.
115. *Ibid.*
116. Letter, J.J. Kinyoun, Surgeon, M.H.S. to Supervising Surgeon-General, U.S. Marine-Hospital Service, Washington, D.C., 19 October 1900, 1–2.
117. "More Plague in San Francisco." *The Bee*, 17 October 1900.
118. *Ibid.*
119. "Finds Hidden Cemetery in Marin Hills," *The Call*, 11 November 1900; "Hunter Finds Three Graves on a Hillside," 11 November 1900.
120. Interview Alice Kinyoun Houts to Joseph Kinyoun Houts, Jr. August 1974.
121. "Reports Sent Out Injurious," *The Bulletin*, 14 November 1900.
122. *Ibid.*
123. *Ibid.*
124. "False Stories of Plague Circulated by the Government," *The Bee*, 10 November 1900.
125. *Ibid.*
126. "The Bubonic Plague at San Francisco." *The Evening Bee*, 14 November 1900.
127. *Ibid.*
128. New York World, *The World Almanac and Encyclopedia* (New York: The Press Publishing Company, 1901), 441.
129. "The Medical Society of Northern California Unanimously Declares That the Bubonic Plague Exists in San Francisco, and Demands That Steps Be Taken for Protection." *The Evening Bee*, 14 November 1900.
130. *Ibid.*
131. *Ibid.*
132. *Ibid.*
133. "State Board on Record Confirming Plague Cases." *The Evening Bee*, 15 November 1900.
134. *Ibid.*
135. *Ibid.*
136. "Kinyoun May Be Replaced," *The Chronicle*, 20 December 1900.
137. *Ibid.*
138. *Ibid.*
139. "Resolution." Department of Public Health, Dr. Buckley Motion, Chief Sullivan, Seconded, Undated.
140. *Ibid.*
141. *Ibid.*
142. *Ibid.*

Chapter XV

1. Letter, Abutment Code Name J.J.K. to Doctor Bailhache, 9 August 1900.
2. *Ibid.*
3. *Ibid.*
4. *Ibid.*
5. *Ibid.*
6. *Ibid.*
7. *Ibid.*
8. *Ibid.*
9. *Ibid.*
10. *Ibid.*, 17.
11. *Ibid.*, 18.
12. *Annual Report of the Supervising Surgeon-General of the Marine-Hospital Service of the United*

States for the Fiscal Year 1901 (Washington, D.C.: Government Printing Office, 1901), 492–501.

13. Telegram, Kinyoun to Surgeon-General Wyman, 29 October 1901, *Annual Report of the Supervising Surgeon-General of the Marine-Hospital Service of the United States for the Fiscal Year 1901*, 493.

14. *Ibid.*

15. Telegram, Kinyoun to Surgeon-General Wyman, 27 October 1901, *Annual Report of the Supervising Surgeon-General of the Marine-Hospital Service of the United States for the Fiscal Year 1901*, 492.

16. Telegram, Kinyoun to Surgeon-General Wyman, 29 October 1901, *Annual Report of the Supervising Surgeon-General of the Marine-Hospital Service of the United States for the Fiscal Year 1901*, 494.

17. *Ibid.*

18. Telegram, Walter Wyman to Hon. Joseph D. Sayers, Governor, Austin, Texas, 27 October 1900, *Annual Report of the Supervising Surgeon-General of the Marine-Hospital Service of the United States for the Fiscal Year 1901*, 494.

19. *Ibid.*

20. *Ibid.*

21. *Ibid.*

22. *Ibid.*

23. Telegram, Kinyoun to Surgeon-General Wyman, 2 November 1900, Telegram, Kinyoun to Surgeon-General Wyman, 6 November 1900, *Annual Report of the Supervising Surgeon-General of the Marine-*Hospital *Service of the United States for the Fiscal Year 1901*, 494–495.

24. Telegram, Kinyoun to Surgeon-General Wyman, 6 November 1900, *Annual Report of the Supervising Surgeon-General of the Marine-Hospital Service of the United States for the Fiscal Year 1901*, 494–495.

25. *Ibid.*, 495.

26. Letter, Abutment Code Name J.J.K. to Doctor Bailhache, 9 August 1900, 11.

27. *Ibid.*, 11–12.

28. *Ibid.*, 12.

29. *Ibid.*

30. *Ibid.*

31. *Ibid.*

32. *Ibid.*

33. *Ibid.*

34. *Ibid.*

35. *Ibid.*

36. *Ibid.*, 12–13.

37. Telegram, Kinyoun to Surgeon-General Wyman, 27 October 1901, *Annual Report of the Supervising Surgeon-General of the Marine-Hospital Service of the United States for the Fiscal Year 1901*, 492.

38. Telegram, J.J. Kinyoun to Wyman, 6 December 1900, *Annual Report of the Supervising Surgeon-General of the Marine-Hospital Service of the United States for the Fiscal Year 1901*, 495–496.

39. *Ibid.*, 497.

40. *Ibid.*, 498.

41. *Ibid.*

42. *Ibid.*, 500.

43. Telegram, Walter Wyman to Surg. J.H. White, 26 December 1900, *Annual Report of the Supervising Surgeon-General of the Marine-Hospital Service of the United States for the Fiscal Year 1901*, 501.

44. Telegram, White to Surgeon-General White, 1 January 1901, *Annual Report of the Supervising Surgeon-General of the Marine-Hospital Service of the United States for the Fiscal Year 1901*, 501.

45. Telegram, White to Surgeon-General White, 8 January 1901, *Annual Report of the Supervising Surgeon-General of the Marine-Hospital Service of the United States for the Fiscal Year 1901*, 501.

46. *Ibid.*

47. Telegram, Walter Wyman to Surgeon White, 9 January 1901, *Annual Report of the Supervising Surgeon-General of the Marine-Hospital Service of the United States for the Fiscal Year 1901*, 502.

48. Telegram, J.H. White to Wyman, 9 January 1901, *Annual Report of the Supervising Surgeon-General of the Marine-Hospital Service of the United States for the Fiscal Year 1901*, 502.

49. *Ibid.*

50. Telegram, J.H. White to Wyman, 10 January 1901, *Annual Report of the Supervising Surgeon-General of the Marine-Hospital Service of the United States for the Fiscal Year 1901*, 502; "Untitled." *The Chronicle*, 9 January 1901.

51. Telegram, J.H. White to Wyman, 10 January 1901, *Annual Report of the Supervising Surgeon-General of the Marine-Hospital Service of the United States for the Fiscal Year 1901*, 502.

52. *Ibid.*

53. *Ibid.*

54. Telegram, Kinyoun to Surgeon-General Wyman, 10 December 1901, *Annual Report of the Supervising Surgeon-General of the Marine-Hospital Service of the United States for the Fiscal Year 1901*, 503.

55. *Ibid.*

56. Telegram, Wyman to Kinyoun, 11 January 1901, *Annual Report of the Supervising Surgeon General of the Marine-*Hospital *Service of the United States for the Fiscal Year 1901*, 503.

57. Telegram, White to Surgeon Surgeon-General Wyman, 12 January 1901, *Annual Report of the Supervising Surgeon-General of the Marine-Hospital Service of the United States for the Fiscal Year 1901*, 503.

58. Telegram, White to Wyman, 12 January 1901, *Annual Report of the Supervising Surgeon-General of the Marine-Hospital Service of the United States for the Fiscal Year 1901*, 503.

59. *Ibid.*

60. Telegram, Walter Wyman to Surgeon White, 13 January 1901, *Annual Report of the Supervising Surgeon-General of the Marine-Hospital Service of the United States for the Fiscal Year 1901*, 503.

61. *Ibid.*

62. *Ibid.*

63. Letter, Mayor James A. Phelan to Dr. R.A. Forrest, 21 January 1901.

64. Letter, F.M. Cockrell to My Dear Dr. Kinyoun, 14 January 1901, 1–2.
65. *Ibid.*, 1.
66. *Ibid.*
67. *Ibid.*
68. *Ibid.*
69. *Ibid.*
70. *Ibid.*, 2.
71. Letter, J.J. Kinyoun to Senator F.M. Cockrell, 24 January 1901, 1–13.
72. *Ibid.*, 2.
73. *Ibid.*, 3.
74. *Ibid.*, 3–4.
75. *Ibid.*, 5.
76. *Ibid.*
77. *Ibid.*, 6.
78. *Ibid.*, 7.
79. *Ibid.*, 9.
80. *Ibid.*, 7.
81. *Ibid.*, 8.
82. *Ibid.*, 7–8.
83. *Ibid.*, 9.
84. *Ibid.*
85. *Ibid.*
86. *Ibid.*, 8–11.
87. *Ibid.*, 8.
88. *Ibid.*
89. *Ibid.*
90. *Ibid.*, 10.
91. *Ibid.*
92. *Ibid.*
93. *Ibid.*, 10–11.
94. *Ibid.*, 11–12.
95. *Ibid.*, 12.
96. "Kinyoun Is Under Fire." *The Chronicle*, 9 January 1901.
97. *Ibid.*
98. "The Message of Governor Gage." *The Bulletin*, 9 January 1901.
99. *Ibid.*
100. *Ibid.*
101. *Ibid.*
102. "State Senate Demands Dr. Kinyoun's Removal." *The Call*, 24 January 1901.
103. *Ibid.*
104. *Ibid.*
105. *Ibid.*
106. *Ibid.*
107. *Ibid.*
108. "The Removal of Kinyoun." *The Chronicle*, 25 January 1901.
109. *Ibid.*
110. *Ibid.*
111. *Ibid.*
112. *Ibid.*
113. "Dr. Kinyoun's Head Demanded-Paris Probers' Extravagance." *Los Angeles Times*, 27 February 1901.
114. "Another Case of Plague Found in San Francisco." *The Bee*, 12 January 1901.
115. *Ibid.*
116. *Ibid.*
117. *Ibid.*
118. "The Lesson of Kinyounism." *The Call*, 22 June 1900.
119. "Truth Is Mightier Even than California's Executive." *The Evening Bee*, 15 January 1901.
120. *Ibid.*
121. *Ibid.*
122. *Ibid.*
123. *Ibid.*
124. *Ibid.*
125. "Still Roaring About the Bubonic Plague." *The Honolulu Republican*, 19 January 1901.
126. *Ibid.*
127. *Ibid.*
128. "Bubonic Plague Conference." No publisher, but likely *The Bee*, 19 January 1901.
129. *Ibid.*
130. "The Plague Situation." *Occidental Medical Times*, 1901; "The Plague Question Again." *Pacific Medical Journal*, February 1901.
131. Telegram, White to Surgeon-General Wyman, 14 January 1901, *Annual Report of the Supervising Surgeon-General of the Marine-Hospital Service of the United States for the Fiscal Year 1901*, 503–504.
132. Telegram, White to Surgeon-General Wyman, 15 January 1901, *Annual Report of the Supervising Surgeon-General of the Marine-Hospital Service of the United States for the Fiscal Year 1901*, 504.
133. *Ibid.*
134. Telegram, Wyman to Surgeon White, 18 January 1901, *Annual Report of the Supervising Surgeon-General of the Marine-Hospital Service of the United States for the Fiscal Year 1901*, 504.
135. L.J. Gage, Secretary, "Letter of Appointment," 19 January 1901.
136. *Ibid.*
137. *Ibid.*
138. Letter of Instructions, Walter Wyman to Prof. Simon Flexner, 23 January 1901; Loreen George Lipson, M.D., *Plague in San Francisco 1900* (*Annals of Internal Medicine*, Volume 77, August 1972), 306–307.
139. Letter of Instructions, Walter Wyman to Prof. Simon Flexner, 23 January 1901.
140. *Ibid.*
141. *Ibid.*
142. Loreen George Lipson, M.D., *Plague in San Francisco 1900*, 306.
143. *Ibid.*
144. *Ibid.*
145. Telegram, Geo. C. Perkins to Hon. Henry T. Gage, Governor, 25 January 1901, *Annual Report of the Supervising Surgeon-General of the Marine-Hospital Service of the United States for the Fiscal Year 1901*, 507.
146. *Ibid.*
147. Telegram, Henry T. Gage, Governor to President, 29 January 1901, *Annual Report of the Supervising Surgeon-General of the Marine-Hospital Service of the United States for the Fiscal Year 1901*, 509.
148. Telegram, L.J. Gage, Secretary to Hon.

Henry T. Gage, Governor, 30 January 1901, *Annual Report of the Supervising Surgeon-General of the Marine-Hospital Service of the United States for the Fiscal Year 1901*, 509.

149. *Ibid.*

150. *Ibid.*

151. Telegram, Wyman to Surgeon White, 31 January 1901, *Annual Report of the Supervising Surgeon-General of the Marine-Hospital Service of the United States for the Fiscal Year 1901*, 510.

152. Telegram, White to Surgeon-General Wyman, 31 January 1901, *Annual Report of the Supervising Surgeon-General of the Marine-Hospital Service of the United States for the Fiscal Year 1901*, 510.

153. Loreen George Lipson, M.D., *Plague in San Francisco 1900* (Annals of Internal Medicine, Volume 77, August 1972), 307.

154. Telegram, Flexner to Surgeon-General Wyman, 29 January 1901, *Annual Report of the Supervising Surgeon-General of the Marine-Hospital Service of the United States for the Fiscal Year 1901*, 509.

155. "Report of the Commission Appointed by the Secretary of the Treasury for the Investigation of Plague in San Francisco, Under Instruction from the Surgeon-General, Marine-Hospital Service." (Washington, D.C.: Government Printing Office, 1901), 7–8.

156. *Ibid.*

157. *Ibid.*

158. *Ibid.*

159. *Ibid.*

160. *Ibid.*

161. *Ibid.*

162. *Ibid.*

163. *Ibid.*

164. *Ibid.*, 9–13.

165. *Ibid.*, 13–23.

166. *Ibid.*, 13–22.

167. *Ibid.*, 13.

168. *Ibid.*, 22.

Chapter XVI

1. "Governor Gage at His Old Tricks." *The Bee*, 31 January 1901.

2. *Ibid.*

3. "Untitled." *The Chronicle*, 9 January 1901.

4. *Ibid.*

5. "Still Roaring About the Bubonic Plague." *The Honolulu Republican*, 19 January 1901.

6. *Ibid.*

7. *Ibid.*

8. "Kinyoun Plague Not Understood." *The Bulletin*, 1 February 1901.

9. "Committee Sides with Governor." *The Call*, 12 February 1901.

10. *Ibid.*

11. "Bubonic" Bills Are Received Favorably."

12. *Ibid.*

13. "The Passage of the $100,000 Plague Bill." *The Evening Bee*, 19 February 1901.

14. "Where the Bubonic Cases Were Discovered." *The Evening Bee*, 15 February 1901.

15. *Ibid.*

16. *Ibid.*

17. *Ibid.*

18. "Federal Commission Has Practically Finished." *The Evening Bee*, 18 February 1901.

19. *Ibid.*

20. "Governor Gage Fears Investigation of the Plague." *The Evening Bee*, 28 February 1901.

21. *Ibid.*

22. *Ibid.*

23. *Ibid.* "Truth Is Mightier Even than California's Executive." *The Evening Bee*, 15 January 1901.

24. "Governor Gage Fears Investigation of the Plague." *The Evening Bee*, 28 February 1901.

25. Loreen George Lipson, M.D., *Plague in San Francisco 1900* (Annals of Internal Medicine, Volume 77, August 1972), 308.

26. Letter, Walter Wyman, Surgeon-General M.H.S.

27. *Ibid.*

28. *Ibid.*

29. *Ibid.*

30. Telegram, Wyman to Dr. J.H. White, Undated, but an attachment to Endnote 26.

31. Telegram, Fremont Older to (Governor Gage), 9 March 1901.

32. *Ibid.*

33. "San Francisco Has Bubonic Plahue [*sic*]." *Oroville Mercury*, 8 March 1901.

34. *Ibid.*

35. *Ibid.*

36. *Ibid.*

37. *Ibid.*

38. *Ibid.*

39. "Bubonic Plague." *Fresno Evening Democrat*, 12 March 1901.

40. *Ibid.*

41. *Ibid.*

42. *Ibid.*

43. *Ibid.*

44. *Ibid.*

45. *Ibid.*

46. Letter, Walter Wyman, Surgeon-General M.H.S. to Doctor (Dr. Joseph James Kinyoun), 15 March 1901. 1–2.

47. *Ibid.*, 1.

48. *Ibid.*

49. *Ibid.*, 1–2.

50. *Ibid.*, 2.

51. *Ibid.*

52. *Ibid.*

53. *Ibid.*

54. *Ibid.*

55. *Ibid.*

56. Letter, J.J. Kinyoun to Dr. Walter Wyman, 28 March 1901.

57. *Ibid.*

58. "Infamous Compact Sign by Wyman." *The Evening Bee*, 16 March 1901.

59. *Ibid.*

60. *Ibid.*

61. *Ibid.*

62. *Ibid.*
63. *Ibid.*
64. *Ibid.*
65. *Ibid.*
66. *Ibid.*
67. *Ibid.*
68. *Ibid.*
69. *Ibid.*
70. "Governor Gage Has Been Forced to Act." *The Saturday Bee*, 22 March 1901.
71. *Ibid.*
72. *Ibid.*
73. *Ibid.*
74. "Other States Demand Suppressed Plague Report." *The Bee*, 19 March 1901.
75. *Ibid.*
76. *Ibid.*
77. "The Surgeon-General and His Suppression of Plague News." *The Evening Bee*, 17 May 1901.
78. Letter, Lewellys F. Barker to Dr. Kenyon [*sic*], 30 March 1901.
79. *Ibid.*
80. Letter, Walter Wyman to Surgeon J.J. Kinyoun, 26 May 1901.
81. "Plague Report at Last Sees the Light of Day." *The Evening Bee*, 15 April 1901.
82. *Ibid.*, "The Surgeon-General and His Suppression of Plague News." *The Evening Bee*, 17 May 1901; "Plague Reports from Washington." *The Bee*, 30 July 1901.
83. "Plague Report at Last Sees the Light of Day." *The Evening Bee*, 15 April 1901.
84. *Ibid.*
85. Letter, Walter Wyman to Surgeon J.J. Kinyoun, 26 May 1901.
86. Letter, Milton Campbell Pres. to Dr. J.J. Kinyoun, 14 March 1901.
87. Letter, W.H. Francis to Dr. J.J. Kinyoun & Enclosures, 6 May 1901.
88. Letter, Milton Campbell Pres. to Dr. J.J. Kinyoun, 14 March 1901.
89. *Ibid.*
90. *Ibid.*
91. Letter, Surgeon (Kinyoun) to Supervising Surgeon-General (Wyman), 25 April 1901.
92. *Ibid.*
93. Letter, Milton Campbell Pres. to Dr. J.J. Kinyoun, 1 May 1901.
94. *Ibid.*
95. David M. Morens, M.D., Victoria A. Harden, Ph.D., Joseph K. Houts, Jr., Antony S. Fauci, M.D. "The Indispensable Forgotten Man." (U.S. Department of Health and Human Services, National Institutes of Health, National Institute of Allergy and Infectious Diseases, August 2012), 33–34.
96. Telegram, Wyman to Surgeon J.J. Kinyoun, 7 May 1901.
97. *Ibid.*
98. *Ibid.*
99. Letter, Walter Wyman, Surgeon-General M.H.S. to Surgeon J.J. Kinyoun, 28 June 1901.
100. J.J. Kinyoun, *Bubonic Times* (Occidental Medical Times: August 1901), 9 & 14.
101. *Ibid.*, 1.
102. Letter, Dr. Young to My Dear Dr. Kinyoun, 20 April 1901.
103. *Ibid.*
104. *Ibid.*
105. *Ibid.*
106. *Ibid.*
107. John M. Barry, *The Great Influenza* (United States of America: Penguin, 2005), 1–7.
108. Ralph Chester Williams, *The United States Public Health Service 1798–1950* (Washington, D.C.: Commissioned Officers Association of the United States Public Health Service, 1951), 166.
109. *Ibid.* 167.
110. Letter, Henry Hurr to J.J. Kinyoun, M.D., 10 May 1901.
111. Letter, Walter Wyman to Surgeon J.J. Kinyoun, 26 May 1901.
112. *Ibid.*
113. Letter, W.W. McFay to My Dear Dr. Kinyoun, 28 June 1901.
114. *Ibid.*
115. Letter, Walter Wyman, Surgeon-General, M.H.S. to Surgeon J.J. Kinyoun, 28 June 1901.
116. Letter, Walter Wyman, Surgeon-General, M.H.S. to Surgeon J.J. Kinyoun, 28 June 1901.
117. *Ibid.*
118. Letter, Joseph to My dear Elizabeth, 26 July 1901.
119. *Ibid.*
120. *Ibid.*
121. *Ibid.*
122. *Ibid.*
123. *Ibid.*
124. *Ibid.*
125. *Ibid.*
126. *Ibid.*
127. *Ibid.*
128. Letter, M. Shiraishi, General Manager. to Professor H. Hozomi, Director of College of Law, 17 July 1901.
129. Letter, M. Shiraishi, General Manager. to S. Asano, Esq., President, Toyo Kisen Kaisha, 17 July 1901.
130. Letter, Joseph to My dear Elizabeth, 26 July 1901.
131. Letter, Your Husband Joseph to Sweetheart, 18 August 1901.
132. *Ibid.*
133. *Ibid.*
134. *Ibid.*
135. *Ibid.*
136. *Ibid.*
137. *Ibid.*
138. *Ibid.*
139. *Ibid.*
140. *Ibid.*
141. *Ibid.*
142. *Ibid.*
143. Letter, M. Murata to Dr. Joseph J. Kinyoun, 22 August 1901.
144. Letter, Unsigned to My dear Elizabeth, 3 September 1901.

145. Letter, Prof. Dr. Kitasato to Doctor Kinyoun, 17 August 1901.
146. *Ibid.*
147. *Ibid.*
148. *Ibid.*
149. *Ibid.*
150. *Ibid.*
151. Letter, Unsigned (Kinyoun) to Dr. John W. Kerr, 23 December 1901.
152. Letter, J.J. Kinyoun to Father, 4 October 1901.
153. *Ibid.*
154. Letter, Unsigned (Kinyoun) to My Dear twins (No. 1), 27 December 1901.
155. *Ibid.*
156. *Ibid.*
157. *Ibid.*
158. *Ibid.*
159. *Ibid.*
160. *Ibid.*
161. *Ibid.*
162. *Ibid.*
163. *Ibid.*

Chapter XVII

1. Letter, Kinyoun to Supervising Surgeon General, Undated. & Letter, J.J. Kinyoun to President, 1 February 1902.
2. Letter, G.M. Sternberg to Hon. F.M. Cockrell, 20 January 1902.
3. *Ibid.*
4. Letter, (Dr. Henry R.) Carter to Dr. Kinyoun, 27 January 1902.
5. *Ibid.*
6. *Ibid.*
7. Letter, Walter Reed to Dr. Kinyoun, 20 June 1903; Letter, Walter Reed to Doctor (Kinyoun), 24 July 1902.
8. Letter, Walter Reed to Dr. Kinyoun, 20 June 1903, 3.
9. *Ibid.*
10. Letter, Walter Reed to Doctor (Kinyoun), 24 July 1902.
11. Letter, W.M. Shaw to Surgeon J.J. Kinyoun, 14 February 1902.
12. Bess Furman, *A Profile of the United States Public Health Service 1798–1948.* (Washington, D.C.: National Library of Medicine, 1973), 248–249.
13. Victor H. Hass, *When Bubonic Plague Came to Chinatown.* (Bethesda, MD: National Institutes of Health, 1959), 143.
14. *Ibid.*, 146.
15. *Ibid.*, 147.
16. Furman, *A Profile of the United States Public Health Service 1798–1948*, xi.
17. https://en.wikipedia.org/wiki/Eugene_Schmitz, 1.
18. https://en.wikipedia.org/wiki/Abe_Ruef.
19. Lipson, *Plague in San Francisco 1900*, 308.
20. John M. Williamson, *Annual Report of the President of the San Francisco Board of Health for Year Ending June 3, 1902* (Reprint from "*Occidental Medical Times,*" September 1902).
21. *Ibid.*, 1.
22. *Ibid.*, 1–2.
23. *Ibid.*, 2.
24. *Ibid.*, 3.
25. *Ibid.*
26. *Ibid.*
27. *Ibid.*, 4.
28. *Ibid.*, 5.
29. *Ibid.*
30. *Ibid.*, 5–6.
31. *Ibid.*, 6–7.
32. *Ibid.*, 7.
33. *Ibid.*, 7–9.
34. *Ibid.*, 9.
35. *Ibid.*, 8–9.
36. Abe Ruef, accessed 5 February 2018. https://en.wikipedia.org/wiki/Abe_Ruef, 1–2; Eugene Schmitz, accessed 5 February 2018. https://en.wikipedia.org/wiki/Eugene_Schmitz, 1–2.
37. Lipson, *Plague in San Francisco 1900*, 309.
38. Henry Gage, accessed 19 January 2014 and 12 July 2006. http://en.wikipedia.org/wiki/Henry_T._Gage, 4–5.
39. Lipson, *Plague in San Francisco 1900*, 309.
40. Invitation, American Public Health Association to Dr. J.J. Kinyoun, December 1902.
41. *The Prophylaxis of Plague: 1903; Dysentery, with Special Reference to its Bacillary Form: 1904; the Action of Glycerin on Bacteria in the Presence of Cell Exudates: 1905; the Prevention of the Spread of Infectious Disease: 1906; Dried Tetanus Antitoxin as a Dressing for Wound: 1906; Uncinariasis in Florida: Undated* and an article on Diphtheria.
42. Invitation, American Public Health Association to Dr. J.J. Kinyoun, December 1902.
43. Invitation, L.O. Howard American Association for the Advancement of Science to J.J. Kinyoun, 1 January 1903.
44. Wedding Invitation, Mr. Francis Marion Cockrell to Kinyoun, 14 February 1903. Breakfast Invitation, Mr. Francis Marion Cockrell to Dr. & Mrs. Kinyoun, 14 February 1903.
45. Telegram, Duller A. Lovell to Dr. J.J. Kinyoun, 27 7 (1903).
46. David M. Morens, M.D., Victoria A. Harden, Ph.D., Joseph Kinyoun Houts, Jr., Anthony S. Fauci, M.D., *The Indispensable Forgotten Man* (Washington, D.C.: U.S. Department of Health, Education, and Welfare, National Institutes of Health, National Institute of Allergy and Infectious Diseases, 2012), 38.
47. *Ibid.*
48. *Ibid.*
49. Letter, M.J. Rosenau to Dr. J.J. Kinyoun, 11 January 1904.
50. Morens, Harden, Houts, Jr., Fauci, M.D., *The Indispensable Forgotten Man*, 38–39.
51. *Ibid.*, 38–39.
52. Invitation, American Public Health Association to Dr. J.J. Kinyoun, December 1902; Invitation, L.O. Howard American Association for the

Advancement of Science to J.J. Kinyoun, 1 January 1903.

53. Invitation, International Congress of Arts and Science Universal Exhibition, St. Louis to Mr. J.J. Kinyoun, 19–25 September 1904.

54. 78. Morens, Harden, Houts, Jr., Fauci, *The Indispensable Forgotten Man*, 38; Furman, *A Profile of the United States Public Health Service 1798–1948*, 268.

55. *Ibid.*

56. Invitation, Semi-centennial of the Founding of the Pathological Society of Philadelphia, 10–11 May 1907.

57. Irving Robbin and Samuel Nisenson, *Giants of Medicine* (New York: Grosset & Dunlap, 1962), 61.

58. Letter, Charles W. Needham to Doctor, 17 October 1907; Letter, (Kinyoun) to Dr. Chas. W. Needham, 21 October 1907.

59. Appointment William Ziudall, Secretary, Commissioners of the District of Columbia: Joseph J. Kinyoun Bacteriologists District of Columbia, 17 June 1907.

60. *Ibid.*

61. 93. Invitation, the President and Mrs. McKinley to P.A. Surgeon Joseph J. Kinyoun and Mrs. Kinyoun, 11 February 1898.

62. The President and Mrs. Wilson to Assistant Surgeon and Mrs. Kinyoun, 3 March 1916.

63. White House Invitations to Mrs. Joseph J. Kinyoun.

64. Invitation, the Cosmo Club to Mr. J.J. Kinyoun, March 1909.

65. Morens, Harden, Houts, Jr., Fauci, *The Indispensable Forgotten Man*, 38.

66. Interview Alice Kinyoun Houts to Joseph Kinyoun Houts, Jr. 16 June 1974.

67. Letter, Walter Wyman to State and Municipal Health Officers, Transportation Companies, and others whom it may concern, 7 September 1911.

68. Appointment Cumo H. Rudolph, President, Board of Commissioners of the District of Columbia to J.J. Kinyoun M.D., 28th February 1913.

69. American Medical Association Fellowship Certificate Rupert Blue M.D., President to Joseph J. Kinyoun, Undated.

70. Letter, Bacteriologists (Dr. Joseph J. Kinyoun) to the Commissioners of the District of Columbia, 22 March 1918.

71. *Ibid.*

72. Letter, W.C. Woodard M.D. to Dr. Joseph J. Kinyoun, Bacteriologist, 25 March 1918.

73. Letter, Bacteriologists (Dr. Joseph J. Kinyoun) to the Health Officer, 25 March 1918.

74. Letter, W.C.W. Health Officer, District of Columbia to Surgeon General, United States Army, 2 April 1918.

75. Letter, Major. M.O.R.C., Joseph J. Kinyoun to the Adjutant General U.S.A., 28 March 1918.

76. Letter, Joseph McDaniels, Navy Department to Assistant Surgeon Joseph J. Kinyoun, M.R.C., U.S.N.

77. *Ibid.*

78. Special Order, 80 Peyton C. March, Major General, Acting Chief of Staff to Maj. Joseph J. Kinyoun, 5 Aril 1918.

79. Prescription to Joseph J. Kinyoun, M.D. 2 July 1918.

80. Letter, Joseph J. Kinyoun to Elizabeth, 15 August 1918.

81. Morens, Harden, Houts, Jr., Fauci, *The Indispensable Forgotten Man*, 45.

82. Telegram, Harris to State Board of Raleigh NC, 4 December 1918.

83. Morens, Harden, Houts, Jr., Fauci, *The Indispensable Forgotten Man*, 45.

84. Kinyoun Genealogical Chart, Section B.

85. Interview Alice Kinyoun Houts to Joseph Kinyoun Houts, Jr. 16 June 1974.

86. *Ibid.*

87. Irving Robbin and Samuel Nisenson, *Giants of Medicine* (New York: Grosset & Dunlap, 1962), Contents.

88. Furman, *A Profile of the United States Public Health Service 1798–1948*, 217.

89. Ralph Chester Williams, *The United States Public Health Service 1798–1950* (Washington, D.C.: Commissioned Officers Association of the United States Public Health Service, 1951), 180–183.

90. David M. Morens, NIAID, NIH, Presentation, *"Abutment"* (Bethesda, Maryland, 28 May 2009).

91. *Ibid.*

92. "Genesis of a National Treasure: The NIN." *Mayo Clinic Proceedings, Vol. 62, No. 2* (1987), 32.

93. Furman, *A Profile of the United States Public Health Service 1798–1948*, 374.

94. "Genesis of a National Treasure: The NIN." *Mayo Clinic Proceedings, Vol. 62, No. 2.* (1987), 34.

95. Morens, NIAID, NIH, Presentation, *"Abutment"* 2009.

Bibliography

Primary Sources

Articles

Centers for Disease Control and Prevention. "Prevention of Plague: Recommendations of the Advisory Committee on Immunization Practices." Mortality and Morbidity Weekly Report, 1996.

Forrest, R.A., M.D. "Echoes of the Plague Scare in San Francisco." San Francisco, California. 17 November 1900.

Hass, Victor H. "When Bubonic Plague Came to Chinatown." Bethesda, Maryland. National Institutes of Health. 1959.

Lipson, Loreen George, M.D. "Plague in San Francisco 1900." Baltimore, Maryland. Annals of Internal Medicine. 1972.

Vaughan, George T. "Report of the Division of Sanitary Reports and Statistics." Annual Report of the Supervising Surgeon-General of the Marine-Hospital Service of the United States for the Fiscal Year 1900. Washington. 1900.

Genealogical

Houts Genealogical Papers in the author's possession.

Kinyoun Genealogical Paper in the author's possession.

The Mears Genealogical Questionnaire. Alice Eccles Kinyoun Houts. Undated.

Government and Legal

Affidavit, B.J. Lloyd. July 1900. (Private No. 233) An Act to authorize Joseph J. Kinyoun, passed assistant surgeon [*sic*] of the Marine Hospital Service, to accept a medal from the President of the Republic of Venezuela. Approved 2 March 1899.

Bacteriological Examination of the Potomac River, L.J. Gage. Letter from the Secretary of the Treasury to 55th Congress, 2nd Session, Senate. Document No. 211, 26 March 1898.

Bureau Order, W. Wyman, SupervisingSurgeon-General, M.H.S., to P.A. Surgeon J.J. Kinyoun. 16 May 1898.

Gage, Secretary L.J. Interstate Quarantine Regulation to Prevent the Spread of Plague in the United States. Washington, D.C.: Department Circular No. 73, 1900. Marine Hospital Service. 22 May 1900.

Harrison, Benjamin. President of the United States of America appoints Joseph J. Kinyoun Passed Assistant Surgeon in the Marine-Hospital Service of the United States. Entered in Book No. 1, page 203. 21 November 1890.

Missouri Loyalty Oath, Office Provost Marshal Warrensburg, Mo N W Perry to Edg Castelle Captain 7th REG'T. MO. VOL., Provost Marshall, Certify U Foster Capt. 7th MSM. 5 May 1862.

"Report of the Commission Appointed by the Secretary of the Treasury for the Investigation of Plague in San Francisco, Under Instruction from the Surgeon-General, Marine-Hospital Service." Washington, D.C.: Government Printing Office, 1901.

"Report of the Special Health Commissioners Appointed by the Governor to Confer with the Federal Authorities at Washington Respecting the Alleged Existence of Bubonic Plague in California Also Report of State Board of Health." Sacramento: Superintendent State Printing, 1901.

United States Civil Service Commission hereby designates Joseph J. Kinyoun to be a member of the Board of Civil Service Examiners. Washington, D.C., 1898.

U.S. Marine-Hospital Service Station Orders, Etc., Form 52, P.A. Surgeon J.J. Kinyoun, to install exhibit of Service at Trans Mississippi and International Exhibit at Omaha, Neb., May 12, 1898. Washington, D.C.: National Library of Medicine, National Institutes of Health.

U.S. Marine-Hospital Service Station Orders, Etc., Form 52, P. A. Surgeon J.J. Kinyoun, to represent Service at meeting of American Medical Association at Denver, Colorado, June 7–10, 1898. Washington, D.C.: National Library of Medicine, National Institutes of Health. May 18, 1898.

Wong Wai vs. Williamson et al., 103 Fed 384. 1900.

Interviews

Houts, Joseph Kinyoun, Jr. Personal observation of my father, Joseph Kinyoun Houts, who regularly laced his mother's (Alice Kinyoun Houts) fruitcake with a healthy dose of brandy prior to bedtime, 1962–1973.

Houts, Alice Kinyoun. Interview by author. Kansas City, MO, 16 June 1974.
Morens, Dr. David M. Interview by author. St. Joseph, MO, 13 May 2010.

Journals

Armstrong, Dr. S.T., and Kinyoun, Dr. J.J. "Observations on the Cholera Bacillus as a Means of Positive Diagnosis." *New York Medical Journal*. 1887.
Barde, Robert. "Plague in San Francisco: An Essay Review." *Journal of the History of Medicine and Allied Sciences*. Oxford University Press. 2004.
Barde, Robert. "Prelude to the Plague: Health and Politics at America's Pacific Gateway, 1899." *Journal of the History of Medicine*. Oxford University Press. 2003.
Boston Medical and Surgical Journal. 1892.
Forrest, R.A., M.D. "Echoes of the Plague Scare in San Francisco." 1900.
"Genesis of a National Treasure: The NIN." *Mayo Clinic Proceedings*, Vol. 62, No. 2. 1987.
Houts, Mrs. Hale. "Yadkin Boys." *Journal of North Carolina Genealogy*. 1963.
Kinyoun, Dr. John Hendricks. "Medical Journal 66th North Carolina Infantry Regiment." 1864–1865; Notation: Alice Kinyoun Houts, Alice Kinyoun to Joseph Kinyoun Houts, Jr., Joseph Kinyoun. 5 January 1963.
Kinyoun, Dr. Joseph James. "Animal Immunity against Diphtheria." *Hygienische Resndeschau*. 1892.
Kinyoun, J.J., M.D. "Rabies—Its Prevention and Treatment." National Medical Library, National Institutes of Health. 1892.
Kinyoun, J.J., M.D. "Bubonic Plague." *Occidental Medical Times*. 1901.
Kinyoun, J.J., Passed Assistant Surgeon. "Report on the Treatment of Diphtheria by Antitoxic Serum, and Notes on the Prevention of Diphtheria." Washington: Government Printing Office. 1894.
Kinyoun, J.J., Passed Assistant Surgeon. "Report on the Treatment of Diphtheria by Antitoxic Serum, and Notes on the Prevention of Diphtheria." 1894.
"Koch's Celebrated Lymph." *Atlantic Constitution*. National Library of Medicine, National Institutes of Health. 1891.
Link, Vernon B. "A History of Plague in the Unites States of America." Public Health Monograph. 1955.
"The Plague Question Again." *Pacific Medical Journal*. February 1901.
"The Plague Situation." *Occidental Medical Times*. 1901.

Lecture

Morens, David M., M.D., NIAID, NIH. "Abutment Joseph James Kinyoun, MD, PhD, America's First Microbiologists: Founder of the National Institutes of Health (and Almost-Founder of CDC & FDA?)." Presented to the colleagues in the National Institute of Allergy & Infectious Diseases, NIH. Bethesda, MD. 28 May 2009.
Morens, David M., M.D. "The Forgotten Indispensable Man: Joe Kinyoun & the Birth of NIH." Presentation: History of Medicine Seminar, National Institute of Allergy & Infectious Disease, NIH. 26 September 2011.

Letters (I)

Under few exceptions and unless otherwise cited, countless letters, telegrams, invitations, departmental orders, military orders and miscellaneous papers are in the Kinyoun Family Papers. This source is comprised of letters to and from Dr. Joseph J. Kinyoun and to and from other innumerable parties. All of these letters are documented in the Chapter Notes and accordingly reference is made to this source.

Kinyoun, Dr. Jos. J. (Abutment Code Name JJK) to Bailhache, Doctor. 9 August 1900.
Letter (Email), Bradley-Sanders, Colleen, Archivist, to Houts, Joseph K., Jr. New York: Ehrman Medical Library. 24 June 2009.

Letters (II)

The following letters were provided to the author courtesy Eva Ahren, Washington, D.C.: National Library of Medicine, National Institutes of Health, 2011:

Chas. P. Francis to Dr. Walter Wyman, Surgeon General [*sic*], 30 September 1898
H.C. Francis, to Dr. Walter Wyman, Supervising Surgeon General, 30 July 1898.
H.C. Francis, Chairman, to Dr. Walter Wyman, Supervising Surgeon General, 1 August 1898.
H.C. Francis, Chairman, to Walter Wyman, Supervising Surgeon General, M.H.S., 2 August 1898.
H.C. Francis, Chairman to Dr. Walter Wyman, Supervising Surgeon General, 12 September 1898.
Kensington Engine Works, Ltd., Francis, Bros., to Depot Quartermaster, 3 August 1898.
W.H. Francis, Secretary & Treasurer, to Dr. J.J. Kinyoun, P.A. Surgeon, 30 September 1898.
W.H. Francis, Secretary & Treasurer, to Dr. J.J. Kinyoun, P.A. Surgeon, 30 September 1898, 1–2.
W.H. Francis, Secretary & Treasurer, to Dr. J.J. Kinyoun, 30 September 1898, 1–2.
W. H. Francis, Secretary & Treasurer, to Walter Wyman, Supervising Surgeon General, 3 August 1898.
W.H. Francis, Secretary & Treasurer, to Dr. Walter Wyman, Supervising Surgeon General, 3 August 1898, 1–2.
W.H. Francis, Secretary & Treasurer, to Dr. Walter Wyman, Supervising Surgeon General, 4 August 1898.
W.H. Francis, Secretary & Treasurer, to Dr. Walter Wyman, Supervising Surgeon General, 4 August 1898.
W.H. Francis, Secretary & Treasurer, to Dr. Walter Wyman, Supervising Surgeon General, 18 August 1898.
W. H. Francis, Secretary & Treasurer, to Dr. Walter

Wyman, Supervising Surgeon General, 1 September 1898.
W.H. Francis, Secretary & Treasurer, to Dr. Walter Wyman, Supervising Surgeon General, 7 September 1898.
W.H. Francis, Secretary & Treasurer, to Dr. Walter Wyman, Supervising Surgeon General, 29 October 1898.
W.H. Francis, Secretary & Treasurer, to Dr. Walter Wyman, Supervising Surgeon General, 1 September 1898.
W.H. Francis, Secretary & Treasurer, to Dr. Walter Wyman, Supervising Surgeon General, 29 October 1898.
W. H. Francis, Secretary & Treasurer, to Walter Wyman, Supervising Surgeon General, 3 August 1898.

National Institutes of Health Publications

"Abstract of Sanitary Reports." 1892–1895.
"Correspondence." 1897.
"Domestic Correspondence." 1893.
"Memorandum." 1893.
"Miscellany." 1893, 1895–1897.
Morens, David M., M.D; Harden, Victoria A., PhD; Houts, Joseph K., Jr.; Fauci, Anthony S., M.D. "The Indispensable Forgotten Man." U.S. Department of Health, Education, and Welfare, National Institutes of Health, National Institute of Allergy and Infectious Diseases, 2012.
"Quarantine Station." Washington, D.C.: National Library of Medicine, National Institutes of Health, 1895.

Newspapers

The Argus. 1894.
The Atlantic Constitution. 1891.
The Baltimore Sun. 1888 and 1889.
[Did the paper go missing here?] Centerview, Missouri, 1903.
Chicago Daily Tribune. 1894.
The Daily Gazette. 1894.
The Daily Light. San Antonio. 1888.
The Daily Northwestern. 1894.
Daily Republican. 1894.
Daily State Press. 1894.
Evening Gazette. Cedar Rapids. 1888.
Fort Wayne News. 1894.
Journal Democrat. 1903.
Logan Sport Reporter. 1894.
The New York Times. 1894–1895.
Philadelphia Record. 1895.
St. Louis Post-Dispatch. 1887, 1889 and 1894.
Washington News. 1895.
The Washington Post. 1894–1896.
Waterloo Daily Reporter. 1898.
Weekly Wisconsin Cousin. 1894.

Plague Papers

The Bee. 1899–1905.
The Bulletin. 1899–1902.
The Evening Bee. 1899–1905.
Fresno Evening Democrat. 1901.
The Honolulu Republican. 1901.
Los Angeles Times. 1901.
Oroville Mercury. 1901.
The San Francisco Call. 1899–1902.
The San Francisco Chronicle. 1899–1902.
The San Francisco Examiner. 1899–1902.
The Saturday Bee. 1899–1905.

Telegrams

Under few exceptions and unless otherwise cited, countless telegrams are in the Kinyoun Family Papers and in the Annual Reports of the Marine Hospital-Service 1889–1902. This source is comprised of numerous telegrams to and from Dr. Joseph J. Kinyoun and to and from other innumerable parties. All of these letters and telegrams are documented in the Chapter Notes and accordingly reference is made to this source.

Secondary Sources

Annual Reports

MARINE HOSPITAL-SERVICE ANNUAL REPORTS:
"Annual Report of the Supervising Surgeon-General of the Marine-Hospital Service of the United States for the Fiscal Year 1889." Washington: Government Printing Office, 1889.
"Annual Report of the Supervising Surgeon-General of the Marine-Hospital Service of the United States for the Fiscal Year 1890." Washington: Government Printing Office, 1890.
"Annual Report of the Supervising Surgeon-General of the Marine-Hospital Service of the United States for the Fiscal Year 1891." Washington: Government Printing Office, 1891.
"Annual Report of the Supervising Surgeon-General of the Marine-Hospital Service of the United States for the Fiscal Year 1893, Volume II." Washington: Government Printing Office, 1895.
"Annual Report of the Supervising Surgeon-General of the Marine-Hospital Service of the United States for the Fiscal Year 1894." Washington: Government Printing Office, 1895.
"Annual Report of the Supervising Surgeon-General of the Marine-Hospital Service of the United States for the Fiscal Year 1895." Washington: Government Printing Office, 1896.
"Annual Report of the Supervising Surgeon-General of the Marine-Hospital Service of the United States for the Fiscal Year 1896." Washington: Government Printing Office, 1896.
"Annual Report of the Supervising Surgeon-General of the Marine-Hospital Service of the United

States for the Fiscal Year 1897." Washington: Government Printing Office, 1899.
"Annual Report of the Supervising Surgeon-General of the Marine-Hospital Service of the United States for the Fiscal Year 1900." Washington: Government Printing Office, 1900.
"Annual Report of the Supervising Surgeon-General of the Marine-Hospital Service of the United States for the Fiscal Year 1899." Washington: Government Printing Office, 1901.
"Annual Report of the Supervising Surgeon-General of the Marine-Hospital Service of the United States for the Fiscal Year 1901." Washington: Government Printing Office, 1901.
"Centennial Year Annual Report of the Supervising Surgeon-General of the Marine-Hospital Service of the United States for the Fiscal Year 1898." Washington: Government Printing Office, 1899.
Operations of the United States Marine-Hospital Service. National Library of Medicine, 1892.
"Operations of the United States Marine-Hospital Service 1901." Annual Report of the Marine-Hospital Service for the Fiscal Year 1901.
"Operations of the United States Public Health and Marine-Hospital Service 1902." Annual Report of the Marine-Hospital Service for the Fiscal Year 1902.

Other

Williamson, John M. "Annual Report of the President of the San Francisco Board."
"Of Health for Year Ending June 3, 1902." Reprint from *Occidental Medical Times*. September 1902.

Marine Hospital-Service Official List:

"Official List of Medical Officers and Acting Assistant Surgeons of the United States Marine-Hospital Service, with their Stations." Treasury Department. 1881.
"Official List of Medical Officers of the U.S. Marine-Hospital Service, Including Acting Assistant Surgeons and Hospital Stewards: Also, Lists of U.S. Marine Hospital and Quarantine Stations." Washington: Government Printing Office. 1885.
"Official List of Medical Officers of the U.S. Marine-Hospital Service Including Acting Assistant Surgeons and Hospital Stewards: Also, Lists of U.S. Marine Hospitals and Quarantine Stations." Washington: Government Printing Office. 1 January 1887.
"Official List of Medical Officers of the U.S. Marine-Hospital Service, Including Acting Assistant Surgeons and Hospital Stewards: Also, Lists of U.S. Marine Hospitals and Quarantine Stations." Washington: Government Printing Office. 1 January 1889.
"Official List of Medical Officers of the U.S. Marine-Hospital Service, Including Acting Assistant Surgeons and Hospital Stewards: Also, Lists of U.S. Marine Hospitals and Quarantine Stations." Washington: Government Printing Office. 1 January 1890.
"Official List of Medical Officers, Acting Assistant Surgeons, and Hospital Stewards of the U.S. Marine-Hospital Service: Also, List of U.S. Marine Hospitals and Quarantine Stations." Washington: Government Printing Office. 1 January 1895.

Kinyoun Publications

Kinyoun, J. J. "The Action of Glycerin on Bacteria in the Presence of Cell Exudates." 1905.
Kinyoun, J. J. "Diphtheria." Date Unknown.
Kinyoun, J. J. "Dried Tetanus Antitoxin as a Dressing for Wound." 1906.
Kinyoun, J. J. "Dysentery, with Special Reference to its Bacillary Form." 1904.
Kinyoun, J. J. "The Prevention of the Spread of Infectious Disease." 1906.
Kinyoun, J. J. "The Prophylaxis of Plague." 1903.
Kinyoun, J. J. "Uncinariasis in Florida." Undated.

Books

Adams, George Worthington. *Doctors in Blue*. Baton Rouge: Louisiana State University Press, 1980.
The American Heritage Dictionary, Fourth Edition. New York: Random House, 2007.
Barry, John M. *The Great Influenza*. New York: Penguin Books, 2005.
Boatner, Mark M., III. *The Civil War Dictionary*. New York: Random House, 1991.
Brownlee, Richard S. *Gray Ghosts of the Confederacy*. Baton Rouge: Louisiana State University Press, 1958.
Cane, Philip, and Nisenson, Samuel. *Giants of* Science. New York: Grosset & Dunlap, 1959.
Cartwright, Frederick F. *Disease and History*. New York: Thomas Y. Crowell, 1972.
Casstevens, Frances H. *The Civil War and Yadkin County, North Carolina*. Jefferson, NC: McFarland, 1997.
Castel, Albert. *William Clarke Quantrill: His Life and Times*. New York: Frederick Fell, 1962.
Cattell, J. McKeen. *American Men of Science*. New York: The Science Press, 1906.
Chase, Marilyn. *The Barbary Plague*. New York: Random House, 2004.
Clark, Walter. *Histories of the Several Regiments and Battalions from North Carolina in the Great War 1861–1865*. Published by the State, Raleigh, 1901.
Cunningham, H. H. *Doctors in Gray*. Baton Rouge: Louisiana State University Press, 1993.
Dabney, Jean Carter, and Houx, Ann Bennett. *Book of Houx Stories*. Warrensburg, MO, 1995.
The Daily News' History of Buchanan County and St. Joseph, MO. St. Joseph, MO: St. Joseph Publishing Company, 1898.
Furman, Bess. *A Profile of the United States Public Health Service 1786–1948*. Washington, D.C.: National Library of Medicine, 1973.

Garrett, Laurie. *The Coming Plague*. New York: Penguin Books, 1994.
Heaton, Charles, M.D. *History of the Bellevue Hospital Medical College*. New York: Ehrman Medical Library, 1941.
Heidler, David S., and Heidler, Jeanne T. *Encyclopedia of the American Civil War*. New York: W.W. Norton, 2000.
Hoff, Brent, and Smith III, Carter. *Mapping Epidemics, a Historical Atlas of Disease*. New York: Grolier, 2000.
The Holy Bible. Toronto: Thomas Nelson & Sons, 1952.
Houts, Joseph K., Jr. *A Darkness Ablaze*. St. Joseph, MO: Platte Purchaser Publishers, 2005.
Houts, Joseph K., Jr. *Quantrill's Thieves*. Kansas City, MO: Truman Publishing, 2002.
Jackson, W. *Rufus Missouri Democracy Volume I & III*. Chicago: S.J. Clarke, 1935.
LeFebvre, Georges. *Napoleon from Tilsit to Waterloo 1897–1815*. New York: Columbia University Press, 1969.
Lewis, Charlton T. *Elementary Latin Dictionary*. Oxford: Oxford University Press, 1966.
Logan, Sheridan A. *Old Saint Jo Gateway to the West, 1799–1932*. St. Joseph, MO: John Sublett Logan Foundation, 1979.
Long, E.B., and Long, Barbara. *The Civil War Day by Day: An Almanac 1861–1865*. New York: Da Capo Press, 1971.
McNeil, William H. *Plagues and Peoples*. New York: Anchor Books, 1976.
Miller, Judith; Engleberg, Stephen; and Broad, William. *Germs*. New York: Touchstone, 2002.
Mullet, Charles F. *The Bubonic Plague and England*. Lexington: University of Kentucky Press, 1956.
New York World. *The World Almanac and Encyclopedia*. New York: The Press Publishing Company, 1901.
Nohl, Johannes. *The Black Death*. Yardley, PA: Westholme Publishing, 2006.
Parrish, William E. *A History of Missouri, Volume III 1860 to 1875*. Columbia: University of Missouri Press, 1873.
Parson, Robert P. *Trail to Light*. Indianapolis: Bobbs-Merrill, 1943.
Pearson, James H. *The Sick Man's Companion, or Family Guide to Health*. Madisonville, KY: 1836.
Riedman, Sarah R. *Shots Without Guns*. Chicago: Rand McNally, 1960.
Ritchie, John W. *Primer of Sanitation*. Yonkers-on-Hudson, NY: World Book, 1910.
Robin, Irving, and Nisenson. *Giants of Medicine*. New York: Grosset & Dunlap, 1962.
Rosen, George. *A History of Public Health*. New York: MD Publications, 1958.
Rosen, William. *Justinian's Flea*. New York: Penguin Books, 2007.
Ruthledge, William E., Jr., and Welborn, Max O. *An Illustrated History of Yadkin County 1850–1965*. Yadkinville, NC, 1965.
Schroeder-Lein, Glenna R. *Confederate Hospitals on the Move*. Columbia: University of South Carolina Press, 1996.
Scott, Susan, and Duncan, Christopher J. *Return of the Black Death*. West Sussex: John Wiley & Sons, 2005.
Shoemaker, Floyd Calvin, LL.D. *Missouri and Missourians*. Chicago: The Lewis Publishing Company, 1943.
Todd, Frank Morton. *Eradicating Plague from San Francisco, Report of the Citizen's Health Committee* and an Account of its Work. San Francisco: C. A. Murdock, 1909.
Ward, Geoffrey C., and Burns, Ken. *The War: An Intimate History 1941–1945*. New York: Random House, 2007.
Ward, Geoffrey C.; Burns, Ric; and Burns, Ken. *The Civil War*. New York: Alfred A. Knopf, 1997.
Warner, Ezra J. *Generals in Gray*. Baton Rouge: Louisiana State University Press, 1987.
Watson, Irving A. *Physicians and Surgeons of America*. Concord, NH: Republican Press Association, 1893.
Webster's Collegiate Dictionary, Fifth Edition. Springfield, MA: G. & M. Merriam, 1947.
Who's Who in America. Chicago: A.N. Marquis, 1910–1911.
Williams, Ralph Chester. *The United States Public Health Service 1798–1950*. Washington, D.C.: Commissioned Officers Association of the United States Public Health Service, 1950.
Wright, Isaac. *Wright's Family Medicine or System of Domestic Practice*. Madisonville, TN: Henderson, Johnson & Co., 1833.

Web Pages

"Abe Ruef." Accessed 5 February 2018. https://en.wikipedia.org/wiki/Abe_Ruef.
"Angel Island (California)." Accessed 27 December 2013. http://en.wikipedia.org/wiki/Angel_Island_(California).
"Benjamin Tillman." Accessed 30 March 2013. http://en.wikipedia.org/wiki/Benjamin_Tillman.
"Bubonic Plague, Infection/Transportation." Accessed 11 July 2006. http://en.wikipedia.org/wiki/Bubonic_plague.
"Bubonic Plague, Types." Accessed 11 July 2006. http://en.wikipedia.org/wiki/Bubonic_plague.
"CDC, Clinical Features." Accessed 16 July 2006. www.cdc/ncidod/dvbib/plague/facts.htm.
"CDC, Diagnosis." Accessed 16 July 2006. www.cdc.ncidod/dvbid/plague/diagnosis.htm.
"CDC, Information on Plague." Accessed 16 July 2006. ww.cdc.gov/ncidod/dvbid/plague/info.htm.
"CDC, Natural History." Accessed 5 August 2008. www.cdc.gov/ncidod/dvbid/plague/history.htm.
"CDC, Questions and Answers About Plague." Accessed 16 July 2006. www.cdc.gov/ncidod/dvbid/plague/qa.htm.
"Clemson University." Accessed 30 March 2013. http://en.wikipedia.org/wiki/Clemson_University.
"Discovery Channel, Tracking the attack of the plague." Accessed 12 July 2006. www.exn.ca/Stories/2000/09/12/52.asp.

"Ellis Island History—A Brief Look." National Park Service, U.S. Department of the Interior. Accessed 13 December 2011. www.nps.gov/elis/contacts.htm.

"Eugene Schmitz." Accessed 5 June 2018. https://en.wikipedia.org/wiki/Eugene_Schmitz.

"Formaldehyde and Cancer Risk." Accessed 18 November 2012. www.cancer.gov/cancertopics/factsheet/Risk/formaldehde.

"George Miller Sternberg." Accessed 10 March 2012. http://wikipedia.org/wiki/George_Sternberg.

"Henry Gage." Accessed 19 January 2014 and 12 July 2006. http://en.wikipedia.org/wiki/Henry_T._Gage.

"Hemotoxin." Accessed 23 August 2010. http://en.wikipedia.org/wiki/Hemotoxin.

"Hershey's History." Accessed 29 December 2011. www.thehersheycompany.com/about-hershey/our-story/hersheys-history.aspx.

"John Sherman." Accessed 30 November 2012. http://en.wikipedia.org/wiki/Senator_John_Sherman.

"Leprosy." Accessed 5 December 2012. http://www.niaid.nih.gov/topics/leprosy/Understanding/Pages/today.aspx.

"Maurice Raynaud." Accessed 10 March 2012. http://en.wikipedia.org/wiki/Maurice_Raynaud.

"Neurotoxin." Accessed 23 August 2010. http://en.wikipedia.org/wiki/Neurotoxin.

"Order of the Liberator." Accessed 6 May 2012. http://en.wikipedia.org/wiki/Order_of_the_Librator.

"Public Health Program." National Park Service, U.S. Department of the Interior. Accessed 16 July 2006. www.nps.gov/public_health/inter/info/factsheets/fs_plague.htm.

"San Francisco Plague of 1900." http://en.wikipedia.org/wiki/San_Francisco_plague_of_1900.

"Spanish-American War." Accessed 30 March 2013. http://en.wikipedia.org/wiki/Spanish-american_war.

"Surgeon General of the United States Army." Accessed 4 July 2012. http://en.wikipedia.org/wiki/Surgeon_General_of_the_United_States_Army.

"Syringe." Accessed 18 November 2012. http://en.wikipedia.org/wiki/Syringes.

"Theodore Roosevelt." Accessed 3 May 2013. http://en.wikipedia.org/wiki/theodore_Roosevelt.

"Thomas Edison." Accessed 26 February 2012. en.wikipedia.org/wiki/Thomas_Edison.

"Track gauge." Accessed 8 December 2012. http://en.wikipedia.org/wiki/Track_gauge.

"Unification of Germany." Accessed 6 November 2012. http://en.wikipedia.org/wiki/Unification_of_Germany.

"United States Public Health Services." Accessed 16 June 2018. https://www.usps.gov/aboutsus/history.aspx.

"United States Revenue Cutter Service." Accessed 1 June 2014. http://en.wikipedia.org/wiki/Revenue_Cutter_Service.

"United States presidential election, 1896." Accessed 1 June 2012. http://en.wikipedia.org/wiki/United_States_presidential_election,_1896.

"Waldemar Haffkine." Accessed 30 March 2013. http://en.wikipedia.org/wiki/Waldemar_Haffkine.

"The White House, Grover Cleveland." Accessed 25 February 2012. www.whitehouse.gov/about/presidents/grovercleveland22.

"William Rufus Schaffer." Accessed 6 July 2014. http://en.wikipedia.org/wiki/William_Rufus_Shafter.

"Yellow journalism." Accessed 5 July 2014. http://en.wikipedia.org/wiki/Yellow_journalism.

Index

www.ingramcontent.com/pod-product-compliance
Ingram Content Group UK Ltd.
Pitfield, Milton Keynes, MK11 3LW, UK
UKHW050539150426
5217IPUK00026B/2003

9 781476 682907